Mental Health and Deafness

Edited by
Peter Hindley and Nick Kitson
South West London and St George's Mental Health NHS Trust

W

WHURR PUBLISHERS
LONDON AND PHILADELPHIA

First published 2000 by
Whurr Publishers Ltd
19b Compton Terrace
London N1 2UN
England and
325 Chestnut Street
Philadelphia PA19106
USA

Reprinted 2000

British Library Cataloguing-in-Publication
A catalogue record for this book is available from the British Library.

ISBN 1 897635 39 7

Printed and bound in Great Britain by Athenæum Press Ltd, Gateshead, Tyne & Wear.

Contents

Contributors

Sally Austen, Chartered Clinical Psychologist, National Deaf Services, South West London and St. George's Mental Health NHS Trust, London, UK.

Jeremy Bird, Consultant Psychiatrist and Honorary Senior Lecturer, Department of Psychiatry (Learning Disabilities), Merton & Sutton Community NHS Trust and St George's Hospital Medical School, London, UK.

Lynn Blennerhassett, Assistant Professor, Department of Psychology, Gallaudet University, Washington DC, USA.

David E Bond, Chartered Educational Psychologist, Audiologist and Principal, Royal School for Deaf Children, Margate, UK.

Patrick Brookhouser, Director and Otolaryngologist, Boys Town National Research Hospital, Omaha, USA.

Ken Checinski, Senior Lecturer and Honorary Consultant Psychiatrist, Department of Addictive Behaviour, St George's Hospital Medical School, London, UK.

Jane Douglas, Psychodynamic Counsellor, National Deaf Services, South West London and St George's Mental Health NHS Trust, London, UK.

Carol Erting, Cultural Anthropologist and Professor of Education, Gallaudet Research Institute, Gallaudet University, Washington DC, USA.

Janet Fernando, Head of Psychodynamic Psychotherapy, National Deaf Services, South West London and St. George's Mental Health NHS Trust, London, UK.

Katia Gilhome Herbst, Independent Consultant Researcher, London, UK.

Mark Greenberg, Professor of Human Development and Family Studies, Penn State University, USA.

Laurence Higgens, Dance and Movement Therapist, Course Organizer, Laban Centre, London, UK.

Peter Hindley, Consultant and Senior Lecturer in Child and Adolescent Psychiatry, National Deaf Services, South West London and St George's Mental Health NHS Trust and St George's Hospital Medical School, London, UK.

Val Huet, Art Therapist, London, UK.

Nick Kitson, Consultant Psychiatrist and Honorary Senior Lecturer, National Deaf Services, South West London and St. George's Mental Health NHS Trust and St George's Hospital Medical School, London, UK.

Herbert Klein, Service Support Manager, National Deaf Services, South West London and St George's Mental Health NHS Trust, London, UK.

Valerie Leach, Social Worker, National Deaf Services, South West London and St George's Mental Health NHS Trust, London, UK.

Kathryn P Meadow-Orlans, Professor Emerita at Gallaudet University, Washington DC, where she was Senior Research Scientist in the Center for Studies in Education and Human Development.

Sue O'Rourke, Principal Clinical Psychologist, John Denmark Unit, Queen Elizabeth Hospital, Birmingham, UK.

Michael Scanlan, Consulting Psychiatrist, Center for Abused Children with Disabilities, Boys Town National Research Hospital, Omaha, USA.

Patricia Sullivan, Director and Paediatric Psychologist, Center for Abused Children with Disabilities, Boys Town National Research Hospital, Omaha, USA.

Alice Thacker, Senior Research Fellow and Lecturer, Department of the Psychiatry of Disability, St George's Hospital Medical School, London, UK.

Joan Turner, Interpreter, National Deaf Services, South West London and St George's Mental Health NHS Trust, London, UK.

Barbara Warner, Family Therapy Supervisor, National Deaf Services, South West London and St George's Mental Health NHS Trust, London, UK.

Chris Williams, Consultant Clinical Psychologist, Exeter, UK.

Sarah Wilson, previously Head Occupational Therapist, National Deaf Services, South West London and St George's Mental Health NHS Trust, London, UK.

Sybil Yeates, Honorary Consultant Paediatric Audiologist (retd), Guy's Hospital, London and researcher in deafness and learning difficulties.

Preface

This book is intended to be an introductory text to mental health and Deaf people for two main groups of people: those familiar with Deaf people but not with mental health and those familiar with mental health but not with Deaf people. Each chapter, wherever possible, provides a general introduction to the area and a more detailed treatment with respect to Deaf people.

The authors use two main descriptors when talking about deaf people (see Chapter 1 for a more detailed treatment). Deaf people (with an upper case 'D') are people who use the sign language of their native Deaf community and identify with that community; deaf people (with a lower case 'd') are deaf but do not use sign language or identify with the Deaf community of their native country. The boundaries of these definitions can be porous but the authors have tried to use these conventions as far as possible.

In some areas published literature is relatively scarce and authors have had to rely on their own clinical experience to a greater extent. However, we have tried to provide a comprehensive coverage of published studies to enable more detailed study for those who are interested. Fictitious names have been used in these studies.

We should like to thank all the contributing authors. The quality of their work has been an inspiration to both of us.

Peter Hindley and Nick Kitson

Acknowledgements

This book would not have been possible without the insights provided to us by our patients and our colleagues, Deaf and hearing. We should like to thank them first and foremost. Mike Martin had the original idea for the book, and so we are especially grateful to him. We should also like to thank Michelle Hickey, Jean Drewett, Romaine West, Karen Kitson and Sandy McLaren for secretarial support. Mark Hindley kindly provided legal advice on child and family law, for which many thanks. Finally, we should like to thank our families for their patience, tolerance and support during a protracted birth!

Section A: Assessment

Chapter 1
Deaf People in Society

KAY MEADOW-ORLANS AND CAROL ERTING

Introduction

This chapter is designed to provide an introduction to deafness for professionals who have not had intensive long-term contact with people who are deaf. The first section provides a demographic landscape of incidence, prevalence, socio-economic and marital status, followed by sketches of the Deaf community and Deaf culture. Membership in the Deaf community assumes a visual approach to life, common experiences of disadvantage or oppression, and fluency in a natural sign language. However, identification with the Deaf community is not automatic and an effort is made to elaborate the wide range of experiences, attitudes, and situations found in this small and special population. Although they may not be full members of the Deaf community, hearing children of Deaf parents have a special place in that community and often serve as sign interpreters for those who are Deaf. After describing these groups and elements of Deaf culture, a brief discussion is provided of issues surrounding access to the larger community by means of technological devices and legal processes.

Terminology and definitions related to deafness shift constantly. As the Deaf community became more cohesive and self-conscious, Deaf people and their hearing advocates have become more sensitive to negative terminology and more insistent upon the use of language and descriptors which they have chosen themselves. In an effort to honour this perspective, the convention of capitalizing 'Deaf' has been adopted when referring to people who consider themselves members of the subgroup which shares a sign language and a culture. The lower case 'deaf' is used in reference to:

- The absence of or reduction in response to sound in the audiological sense.
- People who are deaf but do not consider themselves to be members of the signing Deaf community.

- People who are deaf but for whom we have no information about self-identification.

The terms 'impairment', 'disability', and 'handicap' have been used in accordance with the definitions proposed by the World Health Organization (WHO, 1980). Thus:

> In the context of health experience . . . an impairment is any loss or abnormality of psychological, physiological, or anatomical structure or function. A disability is any restriction or lack (resulting from an impairment) of ability to perform in the manner or within the range considered normal for a human being. A handicap is a disadvantage for a given individual, resulting from an impairment or a disability, that limits or prevents the fulfillment of a role that is normal (depending on age, sex and social and cultural factors) for that individual.

This example was provided by the WHO committee:

> ' . . . A patient with hypertension (disease) is affected by cerebral haemorrhage (impairment) which leads to right-sided hemiplegia causing walking, writing and speech difficulties (disabilities). If the patient does not recover sufficiently to resume work or to be able to live an independent life, his disadvantage is considered a handicap'. (WHO, 1986, p. 4)

There are certain problems in applying these definitions to deafness, which should become more clear as the chapter progresses. Some members of the Deaf community would deny that deafness is an 'impairment', or is not 'normal'. They may insist that it is a handicap only when society fails to provide full access to available resources, and might also point out that people who are deaf from birth have not experienced a hearing 'loss'. Those who are born deaf to Deaf parents may be less 'impaired' or 'disabled' than those who are born to hearing parents. Those deafened in adulthood may be more 'handicapped' than others born deaf (Meadow-Orlans, 1985; Ashley, 1992). Practitioners need to be aware of the possible range of responses to these terms as they are applied to people who are deaf.*

*A pamphlet providing guidelines for reporting and writing about people with disabilities has the following paragraph in reference to deafness: 'Deafness' refers to a profound degree of hearing loss that prevents understanding speech through the ear. Hearing-impaired is the generic term preferred by some individuals to indicate any degree of hearing loss . . . It includes both hard of hearing and deaf. Hard of hearing refers to a mild to moderate hearing loss that may or may not be corrected with amplification. Use 'woman who is deaf', 'boy who is hard of hearing', or 'people who are hearing-impaired' (Research and Training Center on Independent Living, 1990). In other words, it is seen as pejorative to write 'deaf woman', 'hard of hearing boy', or 'hearing-impaired people'. This convention has been adopted by all journals published by the Council for Exceptional Children. The guidelines were endorsed by 41 organizations, including the National Association of the Deaf, despite the fact that members of the Deaf community may consider the term 'Deaf' to be a badge of pride rather than a hostile label. These ideas reflect the maelstrom of current social change and some of the conflicts awaiting those who venture into the helping professions, offering services to Deaf people and their families.

Demographics of the Deaf population

One of the most common disabilities, the absence or loss of hearing has an estimated overall prevalence rate in the USA of about 70 per 1000 people. In the UK, it is estimated that almost 20% of the population has hearing losses > 25 decibels (dB)*, although that proportion increases to almost 75% for individuals aged over 70 years (Kyle, Jones and Wood 1985). In 1988, the Department of Health and Social Security (DHSS) in London reported almost 20 million people in the UK with a hearing loss > 20 dB (DHSS, 1988); more than two million with a hearing loss > 40 dB, more than 200 000 with a hearing loss > 60 dB (Woll, 1995).

Deafness, defined broadly as the inability to hear speech without a hearing aid, is relatively rare, with a rate of about eight per 1000. Deafness occurring before the age of 3 years has an estimated rate of one per 1000 (Schein, 1987). More recent studies estimate the prevalence of profound early onset deafness in children to be about $^{1}/_{2700}$ per birth cohort (Davis *et al.*, 1995). As adults, these children are most likely to consider themselves members of the Deaf community.

Most studies of sensory or physical disabilities show higher prevalence rates among men than women, and among lower rather than upper socio-economic groups (Dubose, 1979; Gliedman and Roth, 1980). In fact, there is a strong relationship between disability and poverty: three-fifths of disabled adults live at the poverty level; more than half are outside the labour force; the disability rate among African Americans is double that of other racial groups (Bowe, 1980). (See also Kyle and Pullen, 1980.)

At least 50% of congenital deafness is genetic (Israel *et al.*, 1992), but more than 90% of deaf individuals have hearing parents. Those who are deaf from an early age tend to marry deaf partners, at the estimated ratio of 9:1 (Schein and Delk, 1974). Nine of 10 children born to two deaf parents have normal hearing (Schein, 1987).

In developing or Third World countries, prevalence rates can be much higher and deaf adults, deprived of all but the most rudimentary educational opportunities, are usually found at the bottom of the socio-economic ladder, living in appalling conditions. In Nigeria, for example, education for deaf people began only 25 years ago:

> deaf children were regarded as accursed and [their] parents . . . were tagged as sinful individuals, penalised by the gods for their evil deeds (Alake, 1988, p. 1957).

---

*Severity of impairment is expressed in terms of decibel (dB) loss or hearing threshold level. To about 25 dB, the hearing loss is probably insignificant. A mild hearing loss (25–40 dB) means the individual has difficulty hearing whispers or faint speech; a moderate loss (41–55 dB) causes difficulties with normal speech. A moderately severe loss (56–70 dB) is serious enough for a child to have difficulties acquiring spoken language. A severe hearing loss (71–90 dB) creates difficulties in understanding even strongly amplified speech, and a profound loss (> 90 dB) means that maximally amplified speech is not understood (Dubose, 1979, p. 366).

In Ethiopia, there are 'possibly 400 000 hearing-impaired children' in a population of 42 million, but only one school that serves about 200 children (Nolan and Tucker, 1988, p. 2041).

Socio-economic status and employment

In their comprehensive review of the socio-economic status of deaf persons in the USA, Christiansen and Barnartt (1987) demonstrate that the educational levels of deaf people have improved considerably in the past 50 years, but not as much as those of hearing individuals; unemployment rates are higher for deaf than for hearing men, and 'at the very least . . . the incomes of deaf workers have decreased compared to hearing workers since the Depression years' (p. 176). Throughout this century in the USA, deaf people have been employed primarily in blue collar jobs requiring skilled, semi-skilled, or unskilled manual labour (Christiansen, 1994).

Kyle (1988) found from interviews with deaf young adults in England and Wales that 73% of respondents in a representative sample were employed seven years after leaving school. However, compared with young hearing adults, they were somewhat more likely to be unemployed, and 82% of those who had jobs thought it unlikely that they would ever be promoted. (See also Jones and Pullen, 1990).

The socio-economic status of the deaf population in a particular country or region has a snowball effect. In Nigeria, for example, one official estimated that only about 1500 of 30 000 deaf adults have regular jobs, because 'people still have their prejudices' (Iwuanyanwu, 1988, p. 2021). In Nepal 'The fate of disabled persons is no better than that of animals'; ironically, deaf people are relatively fortunate, since they can be expected to do heavy labour 'such as portering, ploughing, plumbing' (Maskey, 1988, p. 2028).

Demography of family life

It is of some interest that the earliest systematic State-wide census of family and mental health characteristics of deaf persons in a large geographic area was conducted under the auspices of a psychiatric institute in New York State. That survey of literate profoundly deaf people showed that 86% of women aged 45 or older were or had been married, compared with 89% of the general population; 70% of the married women were mothers, compared with 79% in the general population. About 5% of women born deaf (and 9% of those deafened adventitiously) were married to hearing men. In families where both spouses were deaf, 30% had at least one deaf child (Rainer, Altshuler and Kallmann, 1969).*

Diversity within the deaf population

Diversity within the deaf population is often overlooked. Developed countries have experienced a great influx of immigrants in the past decade, and the deaf population reflects the increasing heterogeneity of the general population. The former Inner London Education Authority (ILEA), abolished in 1989, served about 1400 hearing-impaired students, of whom only 52% were from English, Scots, Welsh or Irish backgrounds (Robson, 1988). In Manchester, in 1988, almost one-third of hearing-impaired students came from homes where a language other than English was spoken (Turner, 1988).

In the 1991–1992 Annual Survey of Hearing Impaired Children and Youth, conducted by Gallaudet University, fully one-third of 47 000 participating children were members of minority groups. The proportion of deaf Hispanic children was 15% in that year, compared with 11% in 1984–1985, not surprising since the Hispanic population of the USA grew by 53% during the 1980s (Schildroth and Hotto, 1993). It has been suggested that minority status often serves as a surrogate measure of socio-economic status. That relationship may help to explain differences in academic achievement reported for deaf children from various ethnic groups. On standard tests for reading comprehension in 1989–1990, white deaf students' scores were at grade level 5.4; Black students were at grade level 3.6; Hispanic students were at grade level 2.7 (Holt, 1993). The deaf minority students' poor school performance is mirrored in the world of work. One study found that these students 'had only 45% the likelihood of success as the non-minority' deaf students (Allen, 1994).

About 30% of deaf children enrolled in special education classes have disabling conditions with educational significance (Wolff and Harkins, 1986). Deaf children who have cognitive or physical disabilities are also at

---

*This survey provided the rationale for the first programme of mental health services for deaf people, and is the model for many programmes today. Efforts of other psychiatrists or psychoanalysts, however, have not always had the same positive effect. Indeed, they demonstrate the dangers of work done without a basic understanding of the Deaf experience and the Deaf community. Some psychoanalytic case-studies emphasize the negative aspects of the lives of hearing patients whose parents are deaf. Authors such as Arlow (1976), Bene (1977), Halbreich (1979), Dent (1982), and Wagenheim (1985) appear to be unfamiliar with the literature on deafness, and demonstrate a negative bias. All use 'deaf-mute' or 'deaf and dumb' to describe the parents of their patients, evidence that they are unfamiliar with current practice. (These terms have not been acceptable for at least 50 years.) A group of psychiatrists working at the Lexington School for the Deaf (without the benefit of sign language knowledge or interpreters) concluded that emotional problems observed in children with Deaf parents reflected disturbed mother-infant relationships, and that the mother's 'characterology' contributed to her infant's unstable sense of self and other (Galenson et al., 1979).

a disadvantage in academic achievement, scoring almost two grades below other deaf students (Holt, 1993).

Characteristics of the Deaf community and culture

Adults who are deaf from an early age share a bond created by their experiences as individuals who know and interact with the world primarily through vision and as members of a group that is frequently misunderstood and oppressed. These common experiences are manifest in the content of what has been labelled Deaf culture, the Deaf world, or the Deaf way of life (Padden and Humphries, 1988; Wilcox, 1989; Andersson, 1990; Erting et al., 1994;). The bond between deaf individuals is evident in the socializing and support found in local clubs and national and international organizations of Deaf people throughout the world. In most countries, there is a national association of deaf people as well as local Deaf clubs where Deaf people can socialize, participate in a variety of activities (especially sports), and acquire information important for survival and success, all in a supportive environment where communication is easily accessible (see Croneberg, 1965; Higgins, 1980; Stewart, 1991; Andersson, 1994; Hall, 1994; Romeo and Renery, 1994; Vasishta and Sethna, 1994). The World Federation of the Deaf, the World Recreation Association of the Deaf, and the Comité International des Sports des Sourds are three organizations that bring Deaf people together internationally. Local, national and international groups communicate with their members about issues of importance to deaf people through regular publications, meetings and congresses.

During the past two decades, Deaf people have become more aware of their own heritage and have developed pride in their lives and achievements. They have begun to recognize the importance of studying and preserving their history, language and culture. Although schools for deaf children and Deaf clubs and organizations have kept historical records for their own purposes, only recently have scholars recognized the legitimacy of the field of Deaf history (Gannon, 1981; Van Cleve and Crouch, 1989; Jackson, 1990; Fischer and Lane, 1993; Van Cleve, 1993; Erting et al., 1994). The first of several international conferences on sign language research was held in 1979 (Ahlgren and Bergman, 1980); by 1989, The Deaf Way attracted more than 6000 people to an international conference and festival on the language, culture, history and arts of Deaf people (Erting et al., 1994). The following year, the First International Deaf History Conference was held at Gallaudet University, followed by a second conference in Hamburg, Germany in 1994. In response to this burgeoning, several universities have instituted Deaf Studies departments or programmes, including the University of Bristol and the University of Durham in the UK; Gallaudet University, Boston University and California State University at Northridge (USA).

Visual lives: accent on the positive

Members of the Deaf community often emphasize the role or presence of vision in their lives rather than the lack or absence of hearing (Bahan, 1989; Bienvenu, 1994; Ladd, 1994a). Their information about the world and their primary language for face-to-face interaction, sign language, comes through vision rather than audition. Padden and Humphries (1988) refer to this visual orientation as providing a different centre for Deaf people, one organized around seeing rather than hearing. Although hearing people may emphasize the sense that Deaf people lack, labelling them as handicapped, disabled, or impaired, Deaf people stress their capabilities and their positive qualities as visual human beings. In the words of I King Jordan, the first Deaf President of Gallaudet University, 'Deaf people can do anything' (Jordan, 1994).

The unique role of vision and sign language in the lives of Deaf people is reflected in the importance afforded storytelling, jokes, folklore, and the visual performing arts in Deaf community life. Rutherford (1993) describes American Deaf folklore as central to the culture and identity of Deaf Americans. Through storytelling, jokes, puns and riddles in American Sign Language, Deaf people maintain their cultural traditions, educating the newer members of the community, finding comfort and relief from the inequities and injustices suffered at the hands of the hearing majority, and entertaining each other (Bienvenu, 1994; Bouchauveau, 1994a). Deaf folklore with sign language at its centre embodies 'the concerns, values, aesthetics and ethics of Deaf culture' (Hall, 1994, p. 526), and teaches Deaf people, often through humour, 'how to resist obstacles in the environment; how to take risks that may be beneficial to their intellectual, cultural, and psychological growth; and how to develop their imaginations and creativity' (Coleman and Jankowski, 1994, p. 57). (Additional sources for British materials can be found in Gregory and Hartley, 1991; Ladd, 1994b; Miles, 1991; Woll, 1995.)

Amateur theatre, mime and dance groups supported by local clubs are found in Deaf communities worldwide (Garretson, 1994). Professional companies, such as the American National Theatre of the Deaf (NTD), the French International Visual Theatre and the Australian Theatre of the Deaf, create and perform theatrical works in sign language for both deaf and hearing audiences (Baldwin, 1993; Aquiline, 1994; Bangs, 1994; Bouchauveau, 1994b). NTD was founded in 1965 in Hartford, Connecticut, 'under the leadership of a successful Broadway scenic designer, David Hays, and an experienced deaf actor and mime, Bernard Bragg . . .' (Schuchman, 1988, p. 14). Schuchman (1988) and others credit the NTD with provoking much positive public interest in sign language and improving the public image of deaf people. Eastman (1994) suggests that the arts can build bridges between hearing and deaf people. Deaf artists, however, point out that they still suffer discrimination in the entertainment industry and the Deaf community continues to be concerned about the issues of access as well as negative stereotyping by the media (Alker, 1994; Frelich et al., 1994; Silver, 1994).

Oppression of minority status

Deaf community members share not only a visual orientation to the world but also experiences deriving from their status as a misunderstood and oppressed minority (Meadow, 1972; Higgins, 1980; Kannapell, 1989; Coleman and Jankowski, 1994; Erting, 1994; Ladd, 1994a). They emphasize that the negative attitudes of the majority are more handicapping to deaf people than the physical inability to hear. These attitudes, arising from lack of information or from indifference, result in the exclusion of deaf people from full participation in the majority culture and the denial of access to educational options, a full range of employment opportunities, and other social benefits. The result has been widespread discrimination against deaf people as well as the suppression of their language and culture (Andersson, 1992; Dunn, 1992; Denmark, 1994; Dhalee, 1994; Paliza Farfan, 1994; Sawuka, 1994). Usually isolated in hearing families, historically, Deaf people have looked to one another for support, community and full access to communication through sign language.

As an adult, a Deaf individual is likely to marry a partner who is also Deaf; their children, deaf or hearing, usually communicate with them in sign language. As parents, their main functional difficulties lie in monitoring their children's safety or behaviour by means of the auditory channel and in their inability to teach and monitor spoken language (Meadow-Orlans, 1995). Deaf parents often utilize sound-sensitive baby monitors with flashing lights, mirrors and other visual adaptations to overcome these challenges. Similarly, Deaf parents usually find ways to ensure that their hearing children have the opportunity to interact with hearing people (such as day-care providers and relatives) thereby learning spoken language.

Sign language as communication mode and cultural symbol

Sign language (American, British, French or other) is more than a linguistic system and a means of intra-group, face-to-face communication, it is a central feature of Deaf culture (Meadow, 1972; Kyle and Woll, 1985; Padden and Humphries, 1988; Johnson and Erting, 1989; Kannapell, 1989; Bouchauveau, 1994b). A sign language in the visual-gestural modality, it is the most important and visible of all of the cultural symbols of the Deaf community. Sign languages were not recognized by scholars as linguistic systems independent of spoken languages until the 1960s (Stokoe, 1960). Only in the last two decades has research begun to accumulate on sign languages around the world. Contrary to popular belief, sign language is neither universal nor a code for a spoken language. For example, British Sign Language and American Sign Language are mutually unintelligible, even though they may share certain grammatical features related to the use of movement and space or to the universal properties of language, despite the fact that spoken English is the majority language in both the UK and the USA. Fingerspelling, a means for representing letters of the alphabet on the hands and spelling words 'in the air', is performed with two hands in the UK, whereas American fingerspelling uses only one hand.

In 1965, Stokoe and colleagues (Stokoe, Casterline and Croneberg) published the first dictionary of American Sign Language (ASL), in which ASL is described as a language with a basic structure built from handshapes, locations, and movements — a structure analogous to the phonological structure of spoken language. Since then numerous linguistic studies and dictionaries of natural sign languages have been published throughout the world (for example, Klima and Bellugi, 1979; Kyle and Woll, 1983, 1985; Brennan, Colville and Lawson, 1984; Moody, Vouc'h and Girod, 1986; Suwanarat and Reilly, 1986; Johnston, 1989; Brien, 1992; Fischer and Siple, 1990). Socio-linguistic studies of sign languages have documented the same kind of variation found in spoken languages around the world, demonstrating that sign language dialects in any particular country may vary by region, and by characteristics such as gender, class, age and ethnicity (Woodward, 1976; Deuchar, 1981; Lucas, 1989; Woll, Allsop and Spence, 1994).

Although there is no single universally comprehended sign language, negative attitudes leading to its suppression or devaluation have been almost universal. This was especially true after the Congress of Milan in 1880 led to a ban on the use of sign language in the education of deaf children in Europe. (This was also true for the most part in the USA and other parts of the world.) Signing was reintroduced into the educational system in the USA in the mid-1960s when an educational philosophy called Total Communication was developed (Denton, 1972). Rather than promoting the use of natural sign languages, such as ASL and BSL, educators adopted sign systems for the purpose of representing the spoken language manually — often with little or no advice from Deaf adults. These systems usually borrow lexical items from the natural sign language of the community, place them in the syntactical order of English, and add invented signs to represent certain English morphemes (Gustason, Pfetzing and Zawolkow, 1972; Bornstein, 1973; Wilbur, 1979).(For British references, see Evans, 1991; Peter and Barnes, 1982; Woll, 1995.)

These contrived systems are not to be confused with contact signing, also called Pidgin Sign English (PSE) (Woodward, 1973; Reilly and McIntire, 1980) or fluent English signing (Johnson and Erting, 1989), a form of signing that has developed naturally out of everyday contact between Deaf and hearing signers (Woll and Larson, 1990; Lucas and Valli, 1992). Members in the Deaf community generally reject invented sign systems as a means of communication, preferring to use ASL or contact signing, depending on the communicative situation (Padden and Humphries, 1988; Erting, 1994).

Membership in the Deaf community: born deaf

While some degree of hearing loss appears to be a necessary condition for membership in the Deaf community, hearing loss alone does not guarantee membership. Membership is an *achieved*, not an *ascribed* status (Higgins, 1987). Individuals must identify with the community and behave as a member by acting in accordance with its norms if they are to be considered members by others. In general, profoundly deaf individuals, deaf from birth or an early age, who use the sign language of their community and participate in its social life, identify themselves and are identified by others as Deaf community members. However, individuals who are audiologically hard of hearing but prefer to use sign language and associate with the Deaf community are also considered members. On the other hand, profoundly deaf persons who do not use sign language but prefer spoken communication and therefore do not socialize with Deaf signers, are not considered members. It is unlikely that individuals with normal hearing are ever seen as full members of the Deaf community, but hearing children of deaf parents, who are fluent in sign language and continue to interact with the group, have a special status.

Unlike other cultural and linguistic minorities, only a small proportion of Deaf people (those born to Deaf parents), acquire sign language and cultural knowledge in the way other native languages and cultures are acquired, that is, from their parents. Most Deaf people do not become members of the Deaf community through their own family culture. Transmission of the language and culture from one generation to the next occurs primarily through the Deaf peer group, usually on entry to school or the world of work. Most deaf children (>90%) are born to two hearing parents who know little or nothing about the Deaf community and sign language and who did not expect to be the parents of a deaf child. Thus, most Deaf people share the experience of being different from their parents and siblings. Initially, and perhaps for several years, hearing parents have a difficult time accepting their deaf child, and experience emotions that include anger, guilt and depression. These feelings are accompanied by the frustration of trying to communicate with a child who cannot hear or speak. Some hearing parents decide to learn to sign, others do not, but the primary path to membership in the Deaf community is the Deaf peer group and perhaps Deaf adults in educational settings.

Born hearing to deaf parents

The personal accounts of the children of deaf adults (CODAs) usually reflect positive family experiences: they did not as children, nor do they as adults, consider their parents 'handicapped' (Hoffmeister, 1985). Some recount the burden of interpreting for their parents (Mallory, Schein and Zingle, 1992) and the necessity of protecting parents from cruel strangers or insens-itive family members (including hearing grandparents), but they express strong affection and close emotional ties (Royster, 1981; Walker, 1986; Sidransky, 1990). Some of these personal reflections suggest that the authors' spoken language was delayed when they started school, but that contact with hearing teachers, relatives or neighbours helped them to match their classmates' speech within a short time. These recollections are supported by available research, as summarized by Schiff-Myers (1993).

Time and place become important determiners of the experience of the hearing child of Deaf parents. Sidransky (1990) and Walker (1986) grew up in a metropolitan area with a large and active Deaf community whose members attended one of several nearby residential or day schools. Walker (1986) is younger, her parents more like contemporary Deaf adults in their acceptance of and pride in being Deaf, whereas Sidransky's (1990) mother never ceased wishing that she could hear. Royster's (1981) parents were employed by a State residential school, the centre for a large community of Deaf professionals and skilled craft workers. These experiences are different from those described by Schuchman (1988), who grew up with Deaf parents in a small community near Indianapolis where both a car and a telephone were luxuries. The warm extended family knew only rudimentary signs and depended on him, the hearing son, to communicate complicated information to his Deaf parents. The flavour of the lives of Deaf parents and hearing children in the early 1990s is beautifully portrayed by Greenberg (1970). A recent book (Preston, 1994) contains a wealth of fascinating information about this group, summarizing interviews with 150 hearing adults who grew up with Deaf parents. Another useful source is a set of filmed interviews, edited and captioned for use by both hearing and Deaf groups (Davie, 1992).

Schools as socializing institutions

Public residential schools for deaf children, established in most American States, have been considered a primary institution for the socialization of deaf children to Deaf culture (Erting, 1987; Meadow-Orlans, 1987). The American School for the Deaf, founded in 1817, was the first of 25 residential schools in existence by 1867. During that period, public education for all deaf children was conducted in residential settings (Moores, 1992). Initially, the schools were built in urban areas, but increasingly they were placed in rural or small town settings.

This geographic isolation contributed to one (hearing) observer's conclusion that these students live in isolation:

> 'the children's lifeworld is structured against a narrower range of stimuli and their selves evolve along a more restricted path than that of children not located in a total institution' (Evans, 1987, p. 160).

A different perspective is expressed by most of those Deaf people who are themselves graduates of a residential school. (For a British view, see Taylor and Bishop, 1991 and Woll, 1995.) Often, school provided their first opportunity to meet another deaf person, either child or adult. This was the place where they were first introduced to sign language, and where they were given their name signs (Meadow, 1977; Supalla, 1992; Hedberg, 1994).

Despite the strong support from Deaf adults for residential schools, the trend in deaf education in the USA has been in the direction of greater 'integration' or 'mainstreaming' for several decades. In the 1920s, residential schools were identified almost exclusively with the enrolment of profoundly deaf students and instruction in the manual mode, whereas non-residential education was identified with less severely deaf students who were taught exclusively in the oral mode.

Today, the picture is greatly changed. In 1991–1992, 54% of deaf students participating in Gallaudet's Annual Survey were attending school in classrooms with hearing students (Schildroth and Hotto, 1993). Although the trend began earlier, it was accelerated by the passage of Public Law 94–142, called 'the mainstreaming law'. Debates about the nature of the 'least restrictive environment' and the 'total inclusion' of deaf students in hearing classrooms are combined with discussions about the relative educational merits of American Sign Language and Signed English and provoke some of the most bitter debates in deaf education (Johnson, Liddell and Erting, 1989; Higgins, 1990; Johnson and Liddell, 1990; Siegel, 1991; Stewart, 1990).

Communication barriers between hearing and deaf children are difficult to overcome and are the most frequent cause of problems of social interaction and acceptance faced by deaf children in integrated classrooms. These problems have been documented by many researchers (such as Devoney, Guralnick and Rubin, 1974; Vandell and George, 1981; Vandell, et al., 1982; Ramsey, 1994). Indeed, integration of deaf and hearing children may lead to increased rejection and reduced interaction, effects that are the opposite of those intended (Arnold and Tremblay, 1979; Antia, 1982; Vandell et al., 1982; Stinson and Lang, 1994). Some educators propose that such school experiences can be detrimental to the mental health and self-concept of deaf children (Reich, Hambleton and Houldin, 1977). In addition, there are misconceptions about the feasibility of education through an interpreter at the elementary and secondary levels (Schildroth and Hotto, 1994). Even if the shortage of qualified educational interpreters were not a serious problem, there are significant constraints on the kinds of classroom activities that are fully accessible to deaf students through interpreters. In the USA, classroom interpreters are available at least for some deaf students in integrated classes, but this is not the case in the UK, where none are provided (Woll, 1995).

Despite these negative findings, some qualitative reports describe positive interactions between young deaf and hearing children in settings where the hearing children were learning sign language (Giangreco and

Giangreco, 1980; Roman, Tucker and Wirht, 1987; Esposito and Koorland, 1989; Kluwin and Gonsher, 1994). Contact over longer periods of time and throughout the school day can also increase positive interactions (Lederberg, Ryan and Robbins, 1986; Lee and Antia, 1992). Positive outcomes are more likely if the numbers of deaf children equal or exceed those of hearing children, if Deaf as well as hearing teachers are represented in the classroom and, most importantly, if the classroom environment is totally accessible to children who learn primarily through vision (Higgins, 1990; Solit, 1990; Spencer, Koester and Meadow-Orlans, 1994). It is becoming increasingly clear that for deaf children who rely upon sign language as their primary means of communication, an accessible and least restrictive environment is most likely to be achieved when all teachers, staff and students are fluent signers.

Issues of access

The status of deaf persons in society results from a complex mesh of social, cultural, educational and political factors. When progress is made on one front, it often triggers advances in other areas. In the USA, several laws enacted for persons with disabilities have been applied to and have benefited deaf persons. Section 504 of the Civil Rights Act of 1964, enacted in 1973, extended protection against discrimination to persons with disabilities (Bowe, 1980). The 'Americans with Disabilities Act', adopted in July 1990, extended that legislation, with guarantees for access to employment and public accommodations (DeJong and Batavia, 1990). These include assistance for deaf people, such as the provision in public institutions of interpreters for those who sign, and audio loops for those who use hearing aids. The British Disability Discrimination Act 1998 offers similar rights to Deaf people but its powers are facilitatory and not mandatory.

New technological advances and innovations have also led to improvements in the lives of deaf people, enabling them to become more independent. These devices are related to telephone communication, broadcast media, face-to-face communication, and environmental awareness (Harkins, 1991). Telecommunications devices for the deaf (TDD) make communication by telephone possible, if both caller and receiver possess a TDD. Telephone relay services allow calls to be placed through a third party who serves as an interpreter, speaking for the deaf person and typing for the hearing person (called 'Typetalk' in the UK). Sign language interpretation and the captioning of television programmes and videotapes have made popular culture and public information programming newly available to this population (Collins, 1994; Woll, Allsop and Spence, 1994). These advances, and others related to fax, computer, the Internet and video/telephone technology serve to improve deaf people's access to the larger society.

As the number of sign language interpreters increases and federally funded institutions (including hospitals) are required to make their services accessible to people with disabilities, their horizons will be extended even further. Cost as well as lack of information about assistive technology are two major barriers to access to new technology, but these should not be insurmountable in the future.

Postscript

Contact with members of the deaf community can help mental health professionals to understand and appreciate the experiences that have contributed to their Deaf clients' strengths and weaknesses, their problems and their potentials for growth and recovery. Deaf people are valuable resources for information about what it means to be Deaf and for the expertise in sign language and visual communication that comes with a lifetime of experience.

Acknowledgements

We are grateful to Bencie Woll at the City University, London, for reviewing this chapter and suggesting additional information and British references. Peter Hindley also provided helpful suggestions.

References

Ahlgren I, Bergman B (eds) (1980) Papers from the First International Symposium on Sign Language Research. Leksand, Sweden: The Swedish National Association of the Deaf.

Alake SF (1988) Primary education for deaf children in Nigeria. In Taylor IG (ed) The Education of the Deaf: Current Perspectives, Vol. 4. Beckenham: Croom Helm, pp 1957–1963.

Alker D (1994) Misconceptions of Deaf culture in the media and the arts. In Erting CJ, Johnson RC, Smith DL, Snider BD (eds) The Deaf Way; Perspectives from the International Conference on Deaf Culture. Washington, DC: Gallaudet University Press, pp 722–725.

Allen TE (1994) School and demographic predictors of transition success: a longitudinal assessment. In Hotto SA, Schildroth AN (eds) Young Deaf Adults and the Transition from High School to Postsecondary Careers. Gallaudet Research Institute Occasional Paper 94–1. Washington, DC: Gallaudet University, pp 61–70.

Andersson YJ (1990) The deaf world as a linguistic minority. In Prillwitz S, Vollhaber T (eds) Sign Language Research and Application. Hamburg, Germany: SIGNUM Press, pp 155–161.

Andersson YJ (1992) Sociological reflections on diversity within the deaf population. In Garretson MD (ed) Viewpoints on Deafness, a Deaf American Monograph, Vol. 42. Silver Spring, MD: National Association of the Deaf, pp 7–12.

Andersson YJ (1994) The Stockholm deaf club: a case study. In Erting CJ, Johnson RC, Smith DL, Snider BD (eds) The Deaf Way, Perspectives from the International Conference on Deaf Culture. Washington, DC: Gallaudet University Press, pp 516–521.

Antia S (1982) Social interaction of partially mainstreamed hearing-impaired children. American Annals of the Deaf 127: 18–25.

Aquiline C (1994) Theater of the Deaf in Australia. In Erting CJ, Johnson RC, Smith DL, Snider BD (eds) The Deaf Way: Perspectives from the International Conference on Deaf Culture. Washington, DC: Gallaudet University Press, pp 746–750.

Arlow J (1976) Communication and character: a clinical study of a man raised by deaf-mute parents. The Psychoanalytic Study of the Child 31: 139–163.

Arnold D, Tremblay A (1979) Interaction of deaf and hearing preschool children. Journal of Communication Disorders 12, 245–251.

Ashley J (1992) Acts of Defiance. London: Reinhardt/Viking.

Bahan B (1989) Notes from a 'seeing' person. In Wilcox S (ed) American Deaf Culture. An Anthology. Burtonsville, MD: Linstok Press, pp 17–20.

Baldwin S (1993) Pictures in the Air: The story of the National Theatre of the Deaf. Washington, DC: Gallaudet University Press.

Bangs D (1994) What is a Deaf performing arts experience? In Erting CJ, Johnson RC, Smith DL, Snider BE (eds) The Deaf Way: Perspectives from the International Conference on Deaf Culture. Washington, DC: Gallaudet University Press, pp 751–761.

Bene A (1977) The influence of deaf and dumb parents on a child's development. The Psychoanalytic Study of the Child 32: 175–194.

Bienvenu MJ (1994) Reflections of Deaf culture in Deaf humor. In Erting CJ, Johnson RC, Smith DL, Snider BD (eds) The Deaf Way: Perspectives from the International Conference on Deaf Culture. Washington, DC: Gallaudet University Press, pp 16–23.

Bornstein H (1973) A description of some current sign systems designed to represent English. American Annals of the Deaf 118: 454–463.

Bouchauveau G (1994a) Deaf humor and culture. In Erting CJ, Johnson RC, Smith DL, Snider BD (eds) The Deaf Way: Perspectives from the International Conference on Deaf Culture. Washington, DC: Gallaudet University, pp 24–30.

Bouchauveau G (1994b) Access to culture in France. In The French-American Foundation (eds) Parallel Views: Education and Access for Deaf People in France and the United States. Washington, DC: Gallaudet University Press, pp 215–222.

Bowe F (1980) Rehabilitating America. Toward Independence for Disabled and Elderly People. New York: Harper & Row.

Brennan M, Colville MD, Lawson LK (1984) Words in Hand: A Structural Analysis of the Signs of British Sign Language (second edition). Edinburgh, Scotland: Moray House College of Education.

Brien D (ed) (1992) Dictionary of British Sign Language. London: Faber & Faber.

Christiansen JB (1994) Deaf people and the world of work: a case study of deaf printers in Washington, DC. In Erting CJ, Johnson RC, Smith DL, Snider BD (eds) The Deaf Way: Perspectives from the International Conference on Deaf Culture. Washington, DC: Gallaudet University Press, pp 826–828.

Christiansen JB, Barnartt SN (1987) The silent minority: the socioeconomic status of Deaf people. In Higgins PC, Nash JE (eds) Understanding Deafness Socially. Springfield, IL: Charles C Thomas, pp 171–196.

Coleman L, Jankowski K (1994) Empowering Deaf people through folklore and story-telling. In Erting CJ, Johnson RC, Smith DL, Snider BD (eds) The Deaf Way: Perspectives from the International Conference on Deaf Culture. Washington, DC: Gallaudet University Press, pp 55–60.

Collins J (1994) Deaf people's civil rights to information. In Erting CJ, Johnson RC, Smith DL, Snider BD (eds) The Deaf Way: Perspectives from the International Conference on Deaf Culture. Washington, DC: Gallaudet University Press, pp 826–828.

Croneberg CG (1965 revised 1976) The linguistic community. In Stokoe WC, Casterline DC, Croneberg CG. A Dictionary of American Sign Language on Linguistic Principles. Silver Spring, MD: Linstok, pp 297–311.

Davie C (Writer and Producer) (1992) Passport Without a Country [Film]. Queensland, Australia: Queensland University of Technology Educational Television Facility.

Davis A, Wood S, Healy R, Webb H, Rowe S (1995) Risk factors for hearing disorder: Epidemiologic evidence of change over time in the UK. Journal of the American Academy of Audiology 6: 365–370.

DeJong G, Batavia AI (1990) The Americans with Disabilities Act and the current state of US disability policy. Journal of Disability Policy Studies 1: 65–75.

Denmark C (1994) Training Deaf people as British Sign Language tutors. In Erting CJ, Johnson RC, Smith DL, Snider BD (eds) The Deaf Way: Perspectives from the International Conference on Deaf Culture. Washington, DC: Gallaudet University Press, pp 425–431.

Dent K (1982) Two daughters of a deaf mute mother: implications for ego and cognitive development. Journal of the American Academy of Psychoanalysis 10: 427–441.

Denton D (1972) A rationale for total communication. In O'Rourke TJ (ed) Psycholinguistics and Total Communication: The State of the Art. Washington, DC: American Annals of the Deaf, pp 53–61.

Department of Health and Social Security (1988) Say It Again. London: DHSS.

Deuchar M (1981) Variation in British Sign Language. In Woll B, Kyle J, Deuchar M (eds) Perspectives on British Sign Language and Deafness. London: Croom Helm, pp 109–119.

Devoney C, Guralnick M, Rubin H (1974) Integrating handicapped and non-handicapped preschool children: effects on social play. Childhood Education 50: 360–364.

Dhalee SP (1994) Discrimination against deaf people in Bangladesh. In Erting CJ, Johnson RC, Smith DL, Snider BD (eds) The Deaf Way: Perspectives from the International Conference on Deaf Culture. Washington, DC: Gallaudet University Press, pp 788–790.

Dubose RF (1979) Working with sensorially impaired children, Part II: Hearing impairments. In Garwood SG (ed) Educating Young Handicapped Children. A Developmental Approach. Germantown, MD: Aspen Systems Corp., pp 361–398.

Dunn LM (1992) Intellectual oppression of the Black Deaf child. In Garretson MD (ed) Viewpoints on Deafness. A Deaf American Monograph. Volume 42. Silver Spring, MD: National Association of the Deaf, pp 53–58.

Eastman G (1994) Cultural arts accessibility. In The French-American Foundation (eds) Parallel Views: Education and Access for Deaf People in France and the United States. Washington, DC: Gallaudet University Press, pp 208–214.

Erting CJ (1987) Cultural conflict in a school for deaf children. In Higgins PC, Nash JE (eds) Understanding Deafness Socially. Springfield, IL: Charles C Thomas, pp 129–150.

Erting CJ (1994) Deafness, Communication, Social Identity: Ethnography in a Preschool for Deaf Children. Linstok Press Dissertation Series. Burtonsville, MD: Linstok Press.

Erting CJ, Johnson RC, Smith DL, Snider BD (eds) (1994) The Deaf Way: Perspectives from the International Conference on Deaf Culture. Washington, DC: Gallaudet University Press.

Esposito B, Koorland M (1989) Play behavior of hearing impaired children: integrated and segregated settings. Exceptional Children, 55: 412–419.

Evans AD (1987) Institutionally developed identities. An ethnographic account of reality construction in a residential school for the deaf. Sociological Studies of Child Development 2: 161–184.

Evans L (1991) Total communication. In Gregory S, Hartley GM (eds) Constructing Deafness. London: Pinter Publishers (in association with the Open University), pp 131–136.

Fischer R, Lane H (1993) Looking Back: A Reader on the History of Deaf Communities and their Sign Languages. Hamburg, Germany: SIGNUM Press.

Fischer SD, Siple P (eds) (1990) Theoretical Issues in Sign Language Research: Volume 1: Linguistics. Chicago, IL: University of Chicago Press.

Frelich P, Matlin M, Seago H, Waterstreet E, Bove L, Fjeld J, Terrylene C (1994) Hollywood through Deaf eyes: a panel discussion. In Erting CJ, Johnson RC, Smith DL, Snider BD (eds) The Deaf Way: Perspectives from the International Conference on Deaf Culture. Washington, DC: Gallaudet University Press, pp 736–745.

Galenson E, Miller R, Kaplan E, Rothstein A (1979) Assessment of development in the deaf child. Journal of the American Academy of Child Psychiatray 18: 128–142.

Gannon JR (1981) Deaf Heritage: A Narrative History of Deaf America. Silver Spring, MD: National Association of the Deaf.

Garretson MD (1994) Foreword. In Erting CJ, Johnson RC, Smith DL, Snider BD (eds) The Deaf Way: Perspectives from the International Conference on Deaf Culture. Washington, DC: Gallaudet University Press, pp xvii–xix.

Giangreco C, Giangreco M (1980) Reverse mainstreaming, a different approach. American Annals of the Deaf 125: 491–494.

Gliedman J, Roth W (1980) The Unexpected Minority. Handicapped in America. New York and London: Harcourt Brace Jovanovich.

Greenberg J (1970) In This Sign. New York: Holt, Rinehart & Winston.

Gregory S, Hartley GM (eds) (1991) Constructing Deafness. London: Pinter Publishers (in association with the Open University).

Gustason G, Pfetzing D, Zawolkow E (1972) Signing Exact English. Rossmoor, CA: Modern Signs Press.

Halbreich U (1979) Influence of deaf-mute parents on the character of their offspring. Acta Psychiatrica Scandinavia 5: 729–738.

Hall SA (1994) Silent club: an ethnographic study of folklore among the deaf. In Erting CJ, Johnson RC, Smith DL, Snider BD (eds) The Deaf Way: Perspectives from the International Conference on Deaf Culture. Washington, DC: Gallaudet University Press, pp 522–527.

Harkins JE (1991) Visual Devices for Deaf and Hard of Hearing People: State-of-the-Art. GRI Monograph Series (Monograph Series A, No. 3) Washington, DC: Gallaudet Research Institute.

Hedberg T (1994) Name signs in Swedish Sign Language: their formation and use. In Erting CJ, Johnson RC, Smith DL, Snider BD (eds) The Deaf Way: Perspectives from the International Conference on Deaf Culture. Washington, DC: Gallaudet University Press, pp 416–424.

Higgins PC (1980) Outsiders in a Hearing World. Beverly Hills, CA: Sage.

Higgins PC (1987) The Deaf Community. In Higgins PC, Nash JE (eds) Understanding Deafness Socially. Springfield, IL: Charles C Thomas, pp 151–170.

Higgins PC (1990) The Challenge of Educating Together, Deaf and Hearing Youth. Making Mainstreaming Work. Springfield, IL: Charles C Thomas.

Hoffmeister RJ (1985) Families with deaf parents: a functional perspective. In Thurman SK (ed) Children of Handicapped Parents, Research and Clinical Perspectives. Orlando, FL: Academic Press, pp 111–130.

Holt JA (1993) Stanford Achievement Test — 8th edition: reading comprehension subgroup results. American Annals of the Deaf 138: 172–175.

Israel J, Cunningham M, Thumann H, Arnos KS (1992) Genetic counseling for deaf adults: Communication/language and cultural considerations. Journal of Genetic Counseling 1: 135–153.

Iwuanyanwu EO (1988) Employment of Deaf persons in Imo state of Nigeria. In Taylor IG (ed) The Education of the Deaf. Current Perspectives, Vol. 4. Beckenham, Kent: Croom Helm, pp 2020–2024.

Jackson PW (1990) Britain's Deaf Heritage. Edinburgh: Pentland Press.

Johnson R, Erting C (1989) Ethnicity and socialization in a classroom for deaf children. In Lucas C (ed) The Sociolinguistics of the Deaf Community. New York: Academic Press, pp 41–83.

Johnson R, Liddell S (1990) The value of ASL in the education of deaf children. In Garretson MD (ed) Eyes, Hands, Voices. A Deaf American Monograph 40: 58–64.

Johnson R, Liddell S, Erting C (1989) Unlocking the Curriculum: Principles for Achieving Access in Deaf Education. Gallaudet Research Institute Working Paper 89–3, Washington, DC: Gallaudet Research Institute.

Johnston T (1989) AUSLAN Dictionary: A Dictionary of the Sign Language of the Australian Deaf Community. Petersham, NSW: Deafness Resources, Australia Ltd.

Jones L, Pullen G (1990) Inside We Are All Equal: A Social Policy Survey of Deaf People in the European Community. London: European Community Regional Secretariat of the World Federation of the Deaf.

Jordan IK (1994) The Deaf Way: Touchstone 1989! In Erting CJ, Johnson RC, Smith DL, Snider BD (eds) The Deaf Way: Perspectives from the International Conference on Deaf Culture. Washington, DC: Gallaudet University Press, pp xxxiii–xxxv.

Kannapell B (1989) Inside the Deaf Community. In Wilcox S (ed) American Deaf culture, An Anthology. Burtonsville, MD: Linstok Press, pp 21–28.

Klima E, Bellugi U (1979) The Signs of Language. Cambridge, MA: Harvard University Press.

Kluwin T, Gonsher M (1994) Social Integration of Hearing Impaired and Hearing Children in a Team taught Kindergarten. Paper presented at the annual meeting of American Educational Research Association. New Orleans, LA: April.

Kyle JG (1988) Deaf children beyond school: prospects and progress. In Taylor IG (ed) The Education of the Deaf. Current Perspectives, Vol. 4. Beckenham: Croom Helm, pp 2260–2265.

Kyle JG, Jones LG, Wood PL (1985) Adjustment to acquired hearing loss: a working model. In Orlans H (ed) Adjustment to Adult Hearing Loss. San Diego: CA: College-Hill Press, pp 119–138.

Kyle JG, Pullen G (1980) Young Deaf People in Employment. Report to MRC. University of Bristol: School of Education.

Kyle JG, Woll B (1985) Sign Language. The Study of Deaf People and Their Language. New York: Cambridge University Press.

Kyle JG, Woll B (eds) (1983) Language in Sign: An International Perspective on sign Language. London: Croom Helm.

Ladd P (1994a) Deaf culture: finding it and nurturing it. In Erting CJ, Johnson RC, Smith DL, Snider BD (eds) The Deaf Way: Perspectives from the International Conference on Deaf Culture. Washington, DC: Gallaudet University Press, pp 5–15.

Ladd P (1994b) Review of 'The Deaf comedians cabaret.' Newsletter (January). University of Bristol.

Lederberg A, Ryan H, Robbins B (1986) Peer interaction in young deaf children: the effect of partner status and familiarity. Developmental Psychology 22: 691–700.

Lee C, Antia S (1992) A sociological approach to the social integration of hearing-impaired and normally hearing students. Volta Review 95: 425–434.

Lucas C (ed) (1989) the Sociolinguistics of the Deaf Community. New York: Academic Press.

Lucas C, Valli C (1992) Language Contact in the American Deaf Community. New York: Academic Press.

Mallory BL, Schein JD, Zingle HW (1992) Hearing offspring as visual language mediators in deaf-parented families. Sign Language Studies 76: 193–213.

Maskey SR (1988) Fate of a disabled person in Nepalese society. In Taylor IG (ed) The Education of the Deaf. Current Perspectives, Vol. 4. Beckenham: Croom Helm, pp 2028–2030.

Meadow KP (1972) Sociolinguistics, sign language, and the deaf sub-culture. In O'Rourke TJ (ed) Psycholinguistics and Total Communication: The State of the Art. Washington, DC: American Annals of the Deaf, pp 19–33.

Meadow KP (1977) Name signs as identity symbols in the deaf community. Sign Language Studies 16: 237–246.

Meadow-Orlans KP (1985) Social and psychological effects of hearing loss in adulthood: a literature review. In Orlans H (ed) Adjustment to Adult Hearing Loss. San Diego, CA: College-Hill Press, pp 35–58.

Meadow-Orlans KP (1987) Understanding deafness: socialization of children and youth. In Higgins PC, Nash JE (eds) Understanding Deafness Socially. Springfield, IL: Charles C Thomas, pp 29–58.

Meadow-Orlans KP (1995) Parenting with a sensory or physical disability. In Bornstein MH (ed) The Handbook of Parenting, Vol. IV: Applied and Practical Considerations. Hillsdale, NJ: Lawrence Erlbaum, pp 57–84.

Miles D (1991) A Sign Poem: Art Gallery. Milton Keynes: The Open University.

Moody B, Vouc'h A, Girod M (1986) La Langue des Signes. Paris: Ellipses.

Moores DF (1992) An historical perspective on school placement. In Kluwin TN, Moores DF, Gaustad MG (eds) Toward Effective Public School Programs for Deaf Students. Context, Process, and Outcomes. New York, NY: Teachers College Press, pp 7–29.

Nolan M, Tucker IG (1988) A pilot project on hearing impairment in Ethiopia. In Taylor IG (ed) The Education of the Deaf. Current Perspectives, Vol. 4. Beckenham: Croom Helm, pp 2041–2042.

Padden C, Humphries T (1988) Deaf in America: Voices from a Culture. Cambridge, MA: Harvard University Press.

Paliza Farfan A (1994) The problem of the Peruvian deaf person. In Erting CJ, Johnson RC, Smith DL, Snider BD (eds) The Deaf Way: Perspectives from the International Conference on Deaf Culture. Washington, DC: Gallaudet University Press, pp 804–810.

Peter M, Barnes R (1982) Signs, Symbols and Schools. Chester: National Council for Special Education.

Preston P (1994) Mother Father Deaf, Living Between Sound and Silence. Cambridge, MA: Harvard University Press.

Rainer JD, Altshuler KZ, Kallmann F (eds) (1969) Family and Mental Health Problems in a Deaf Population, second edition. Springfield, IL: Charles C Thomas.

Ramsey C (1994) The price of dreams: who will pay it? In Johnson RC, Cohen OP (eds). Implications and Complications for Deaf Students of the Full Inclusion Movement. Gallaudet Research Institute Occasional Paper 94–2. Washington, DC: Gallaudet Research Institute, pp 41–54.

Reich C, Hambleton D, Houldin B (1977) The integration of hearing impaired children in regular classrooms. American Annals of the Deaf 122: 534–543.

Reilly JS, McIntire M (1980) American Sign Language and Pidgin Sign English: What's the difference? Sign Language Studies 27: 151–192.

Research and Training Center on Independent Living (1990) Guidelines for Reporting and Writing about People with Disabilities (third edition), Lawrence KS: Bureau of Child Research, University of Kansas.

Robson PI (1988) Multi-ethnic issues in the education of the hearing-impaired population of an inner-city area. In Taylor IG (ed) The Education of the Deaf. Current Perspectives, Vol. 4. Beckenham: Croom Helm, 2070–2075.

Roman A, Tucker P, Wirht P (1987) Enjoying each other's company: our model mainstream classroom, Perspectives 58: 8–10.

Romeo O, Renery LJ (1994) The role of 'silent sports' in Italian Deaf culture. In Erting CJ, Johnson RC, Smith DL, Snider BD (eds) The Deaf Way: Perspectives from the International Conference on Deaf Culture. Washington, DC: Gallaudet University Press, pp 538–541.

Royster MA (1981) Deaf parents: a personal perspective. The Deaf American 34: 19–22.

Rutherford SD (1993) A Study of American Deaf Folklore. Linstok Dissertation Series. Burtonsville, MD: Linstok Press.

Sawuka AA (1994) The oppression of deaf people as cultural minorities in developing countries. In Erting CJ, Johnson RC, Smith DL, Snider BD (eds) The Deaf Way: Perspectives from the International Conference on Deaf Culture. Washington, DC: Gallaudet University Press, pp 794–799.

Schein JD (1987) The demography of deafness. In Higgins PC, Nash JE (eds) Understanding Deafness Socially. Springfield, IL: Charles C Thomas, pp 1–27.

Schein JD, Delk MT (1974) The Deaf Population of the United States. Silver Spring, MD: National Association of the Deaf.

Schiff-Myers N (1993) Hearing children of deaf parents. In Bishop D, Mogford K (eds) Language Development in Exceptional Circumstances. Hove: Lawrence Erlbaum Associates, pp 47–61.

Schildroth AN, Hotto SA (1993) Annual survey of hearing-impaired children and youth: 1991–92 school year. American Annals of the Deaf 138: 163–171.

Schildroth AN, Hotto SA (1994) Deaf students and full inclusion: who wants to be excluded? In Johnson RC, Cohen OP (eds) Implications and Complications for Deaf Students of the Full Inclusion Movement. Gallaudet Research Institute Occasional Paper 94–2. Washington, DC: Gallaudet Research Institute, pp 7–30.

Schuchman JS (1988) Holly Speaks: Deafness and the Film Entertainment Industry. Urbana, IL: University of Illinois Press.

Sidransky R (1990) In Silence: Growing Up in a Deaf World. New York: St Martin's.

Siegel L (1991) The least restrictive environment. In Garretson MD (ed) Perspectives in Deafness, A Deaf American Monograph, Vol. 41: 135–140.

Silver A (1994) How does Hollywood see us, and how do we see Hollywood? In Erting CJ, Johnson RC, Smith DL, Snider BD (eds) The Deaf Way: Perspectives from the International Conference on Deaf Culture. Washington, DC: Gallaudet University Press, pp 731–735.

Solit G (1990) Deaf and hearing children together: a cooperative approach to child care. Perspectives 8: 2–6.

Spencer PE, Koester LS, Meadow-Orlans KP (1994) Communicative interactions of deaf and hearing children in a day care center: an exploratory study. American Annals of the Deaf 139: 512–518.

Stewart DA (1991) Deaf Sport. The Impact of Sports within the Deaf Community. Washington, DC: Gallaudet University Press.

Stewart L (1990) Sign language: some thoughts of a Deaf American. In Garretson MD

(ed) Eyes, Hands, Voices. A Deaf American Monograph, Vol. 40: pp 117–124.
Stinson M, Lang H (1994) The potential impact on deaf students of the full inclusion movement. In Johnson RC, Cohen OP (eds) Implications and Complications for Deaf Students of the Full Inclusion Movement. Gallaudet Research Institute Occasional Paper 94–2. Washington, DC: Gallaudet Research Institute, pp 31–40.
Stokoe WC (1960) Sign language structure: An outline of the visual communication system of the American Deaf. Studies in Linguistics: Occasional papers 8. Buffalo, NY: University of Buffalo. (Reprinted 1976, 1993: Silver Spring, MD: Linstok).
Stokoe WC, Casterline DC, Croneberg CG (1965 revised 1976) A Dictionary of American Sign Language on Linguistic Principles. Silver Spring, MD: Linstok.
Supalla SJ (1992) The Book of Name Signs. San Diego, CA: Dawn Sign Press.
Suwanarat M, Reilly C (1986) The Thai Sign Language Dictionary. Bangkok, Thailand: The National Association of the Deaf in Thailand.
Taylor G, Bishop J (eds) (1991) Being Deaf: The Experience of Deafness. London: Pinter Publishers (in association with the Open University).
Turner SB (1988) Some problems of ethnic minority hearing impaired children and their families in the city of Manchester. In Taylor IG (ed) The Education of the Deaf. Current Perspectives, Vol. 4. Beckenham: Croom Helm, pp 2081–2086.
Van Cleve JV (ed) (1993) Deaf History Unveiled: Interpretations from the New Scholarship. Washington, DC: Gallaudet University Press.
Van Cleve JV, Crouch BA (1989) A Place of Their Own: Creating the Deaf Community in America. Washington, DC: Gallaudet University Press.
Vandell D, Anderson L, Ehrhardt G, Wilson K (1982) Integrating hearing and deaf preschoolers: an attempt to enhance hearing children's interactions with deaf peers. Child Development 53: 1354–1363.
Vandell D, George L (1981) Social interaction in hearing and deaf preschoolers: successes and failures in initiations. Child Development 52: 627–635.
Vasishta MM, Sethna M (1994) Clubs for Deaf people in India. In Erting CJ, Johnson RC, Smith DL, Snider BD (eds) The Deaf Way: Perspectives from the International Conference on Deaf Culture. Washington, DC: Gallaudet University Press, pp 532–534.
Wagenheim HS (1985) Aspects of the analysis of an adult son of deafmute parents. Journal of the American Psychoanalytic Association 33: 413–435.
Walker LA (1986) A Loss for Words: The Story of Deafness in a Family. New York: Harper & Row.
Wilbur RB (1979) American Sign Language and Sign Systems. Baltimore, MD: University Park Press.
Wilcox S (ed) (1989) American Deaf Culture: An Anthology. Silver Spring, MD: Linstok Press.
Wolff AB, Harkins JE (1986) Multihandicapped students. In Schildroth AN, Karchmer MA (eds) Deaf Children in America. San Diego, CA: College-Hill Press, pp 55–82.
Woll B (1995) Personal communication.
Woll B, Allsop L, Spence R (1994) Sign language varieties in British television: an historical perspective. In Erting CJ, Johnson RC, Smith DL, Snider BD (eds) The Deaf Way: Perspectives from the International Conference on Deaf Culture. Washington, DC: Gallaudet University, pp 373–378.
Woll B, Larson L (1990) British Sign Language. In Hayes E, McClure JD, Thomson DS (eds) Minority Languages Today. Edinburgh: Edinburgh University Press.
Woodward JC (1973) Some characteristics of Pidgin Sign English. Sign Language Studies 3: 39–46.
Woodward JC (1976) Black Southern signing. Language in Society 5: 211–218.

World Health Organization (1980) International Classification of Impairments, Disabilities, and Handicaps. Resolution WHA 29.35 of the Twenty-Ninth World Health Assembly, May, 1976. Geneva, Switzerland: WHO.
World Health Organization (1986, December). Disability concepts: A position paper prepared in connection with The United Nations' Decade of Disabled Persons (UNDDP) 1983–1992, Second draft. UN Regional Office for Europe, mimeo.

Chapter 2
Audiological Assessment of People with Special Difficulties

SYBIL YEATES

Testing subjects with special difficulties

Most children are apprehensive about a visit to hospital unless they have been carefully prepared beforehand. There are now books and leaflets which can help, especially those which are suitably illustrated for younger children. Most importantly, parents can explain, and general family conversations are important. The child then feels 'important' and this should be reinforced by hospital staff. However, it is immediately apparent that these methods may be useless for children with learning or emotional disabilities. Pictures may be meaningless and conversation not understood. How can the situation be ameliorated?

Diagnosis in very early infancy

This is the optimal time of diagnosis for any child with a hearing loss. For children with special difficulties it is particularly useful. However, different geographical areas have different methods of selecting infants to be tested in the neo-natal period. Optimally, all infants would be examined, but financial considerations often mean that an 'at risk' register determines those who are tested. The following factors place an infant on the at-risk register (Yeates, 1989; 1992).

Family history of hearing loss

This may be a clinically undifferentiated recessive or dominant loss or a syndrome of recessive or dominant type.

Conditions occurring during pregnancy

Maternal rubella was formerly the most common condition in this group, but the introduction of the measles, mumps and rubella (MMR) vaccine has dramatically reduced the number of infants with rubella syndrome and consequent problems with hearing, vision, learning difficulties and congenital heart defects. Those cases which are still being found tend to come from countries where mothers have been unable to obtain protection in earlier life by vaccination.

However, there are other infections which have to be considered. Cytomegalovirus (CMV) is a viral infection that produces negligible symptoms in the mother, similar to 'flu-like ones, but can severely damage the foetus. This may result in hearing problems and developmental delay leading to learning disability.

Toxoplasmosis, a fungal infection similar to CMV in that it produces few symptoms in the mother, can also profoundly affect the foetus, giving rise to visual, hearing and learning problems. Diagnosis of both CMV and toxoplasmosis infection can be made reliably only after birth.

Drugs given during pregnancy are now rarely a problem. Gentamicin and drugs of the streptomycin (antibiotic) group were formerly the chief culprits in producing a hearing loss in the child, but these are now rarely used in pregnancy, except in the occasional case where they might be considered life-saving.

Conditions at or around birth

These are connected with poor foetal brain oxygenation hypoxia or anoxia, at crucial times before, at or after birth. Examples include prematurity, severe toxaemia of pregnancy with possible eclamptic fits, prolapsed cord, placenta praevia, difficult presentations with inadequate treatment, post-partum haemorrhage and respiratory distress syndrome (also known as hyaline membrane disease) in the newborn.

Increased serum bilirubin levels (shown as jaundice in the newborn) may mean that pigment is laid down in the cochlea, in the basal ganglia and the auditory pathway in the brain. The main cause of this was formerly Rhesus (Rh) factor incompatibility. However, susceptible mothers are now given anti-D immunoglobulin in the immediate post-partum period after the first pregnancy. This has drastically reduced the number of cases where haemoglobin is broken down because of Rh incompatibility, leading to pigment being laid down in significantly dangerous areas. It must be mentioned, however, that some cases of AB–O incompatibility do still occur.

Conditions after birth

Meningitis, occurring either in the perinatal period or at any other time later in life, may lead to hearing loss, learning disability or both. The hearing loss is often severe or profound and it is important to diagnose it as soon as possible.

Primary chromosomal abnormalities

Any infant showing a primary chromosomal abnormality should have a hearing test as soon as the diagnosis is made, as many of these conditions include a hearing loss as one of their features. The most common chromosomal abnormality is Down's syndrome (Cunningham, 1982), in which both children and adults (Dalton and Cropper, 1984) are very often found to have a hearing loss. In childhood the problem is one of repeated attacks of chronic secretory otitis media (SOM), leading to conductive hearing loss. Although Down's syndrome children show varying degrees of limitation of speech and language development, there is no doubt that a hearing loss exacerbates the problem. Treatment is very important and cannot, as sometimes happened in the past, be ignored. Recurrent attacks of SOM must be treated surgically by insertion of grommets or Good's tubes. If there is a contraindication to surgery, such as the presence of a congenital heart lesion, then the use of a hearing aid must be considered seriously. Teachers of the deaf must be prepared to work hard to achieve regular hearing aid use, and the enthusiastic co-operation of parents is essential in this.

Other, much rarer, chromosomal abnormalities which may show hearing loss include Patau's syndrome (extra chromosome in pairs 13–15), Edwards' syndrome (trisomy of chromosomes 17–18) and cri-du-chat syndrome (deletion of the short arm of chromosomes 4–5). Down's syndrome shows a trisomy of chromosome 21 in 95% of cases. But there are two other rarer conditions, the translocation and mosaic types, in which the chromosomal material is arranged abnormally but which may not result in an extra chromosome at 21. It is not yet clear whether the two latter types are similarly prone to hearing problems, although it is known that where there is no extra chromosome at 21, individuals may be less severely affected (Heaton-Ward and Wiley, 1984; Holland, 1986).

Tests used in early infancy: the perinatal period

These tests are particularly useful as the three that are normally carried out can all be performed when the infant is sleeping. There is no question of apprehension and no need for any form of anaesthesia.

The test, which was first used in a few selected centres, was the Auditory Response Cradle (ARC). This apparatus seeks to measure the infant's head turn, startle reflex, body activity and changes in respiration, in response to a high-frequency sound at approximately 85 dB. The ARC is controlled by a microprocessor system and contains sensors to measure head turn, startle reflex, body activity and respiration.

The ARC is a quick and easy test which can be carried out by nursing staff. However, it does have two main drawbacks. Firstly, it does not appear to detect a hearing loss of <45 dB; also, it may not identify loss because of recruitment. This can mean that a severe hearing loss is missed. Secondly, it has been found that approximately 20% of infants with a perinatal hearing problem give a false positive result. Obviously this is very significant for those infants who subsequently show learning disability.

The ARC, therefore, should be used only as a screening tool, not to provide a reliable diagnosis. Further tests are needed to provide this.

The most modern tool is the oto-acoustic emission (OAE) test (Bray and Kemp, 1987). This technique depends on the fact that, in the normal ear, the cochlea itself produces sounds which can be detected by placing a tiny microphone in the external auditory canal. The microphone is housed in a probe, somewhat similar to that used in tympanometry, and the rubber-tipped end fits snugly into the infant's external auditory canal. There are two types of measurement: the first picks up spontaneous sounds made without any stimulation, whereas the second measures sound following stimulation by the application of broad-band clicks (Burr, Mulhera and Degg, 1996). Recent work shows that the number of emissions recorded is greater following stimulation by clicks. Work continues on this test — which would appear to be of considerable value — especially as it can be performed in the earliest days of life and is completely non-invasive.

If abnormal responses are obtained by use of either of the above then a third test should be undertaken. The brainstem evoked response (BSER) test is almost certainly the most reliable test available to date. It detects electrical changes in the lower part of the auditory pathway, as far as the inferior colliculus. An electrode is placed on the vertex and the sound stimulus is a sharp-onset click. As each electrical response is tiny it is necessary to use over 1000 clicks to produce a result that can be recorded by the use of an averaging computer. This means that the test takes 30–45 minutes — considerably longer than the two tests already described. However, BSER may be performed while the infant is sleeping and obviously the optimal time for doing so is in the earliest days of life when the child is most likely to have long periods of sleep.

These three tests are not only most easily performed in the neo-natal period, but they enable diagnosis to be made at the earliest possible (and best) time. Many of the problems encountered when testing older children and adults are avoided by testing in the early days of life.

Other tests used in the first year of life

The test performed at 8 months of age is the distraction or localization test (Yeates, 1986). By this age the baby with normal hearing and normal development is able to localize sounds of 35–40 dB SPL at the distance of three feet (one metre), and out of visual field. The sounds used are:

- That produced by rubbing a teaspoon very gently along the rim of a china cup. This sound is not frequency-specific and many people omit this test. However, it has some interest and can be used as an introduction. This particularly applies to children with developmental delay when responses may not be obtained to the other stimuli described below.

- The high-frequency sound, i.e. 8 kHz, produced by gently turning a Manchester rattle or by holding a Nuffield rattle like a pen and turning it as if stirring a cup of coffee.
- The high-frequency sound, i.e. 4 kHz, produced by the human voice when repeating a *'ss–ss–ss'* sound. Soft humming is another useful voice sound and, lastly, a conversational voice, not a whisper, but measured at 35–40 dB SPL and including the child's name.

The distraction test should be carried out by two people, generally health visitors or practice nurses, who have been carefully trained and who have attended revision courses to ensure that standards are maintained. It is most satisfactory if the pair continue to work together and monitor each other. The first person gains the baby's visual attention while the infant is sitting on the parent's lap. A small toy is used for this purpose and when attention is satisfactory, the visual distraction is removed. Simultaneously, the second tester, standing in the correct position behind the baby, produces the sound stimulus. Only a full turn of the baby's head in the correct direction is counted as a positive response.

Distraction tests are useful only if they are carried out accurately, and poor tests are dangerous in as much as they give false reassurance. The intensity of the sounds used must be measured with a sound level meter to ensure that they are presented at 35–40 dB. The tester must be sure to remain out of the child's visual field and must ensure that no other clues are given to the baby, for example the noise of shoes moving from one side to another or the smell of strong perfume, again moving from side to side. Localizing tests are used between the ages of 7 months and 2 years. However babies with developmental delay may be unable to localize sounds by this age. Therefore the tests can be used for older children and even for adults with learning disability. However, as the child gets older it becomes more and more difficult to achieve an accurate test. Children do not co-operate by sitting on the parental lap and watching the visual distraction (which probably holds little interest for them). Sometimes a skilled operator may change the visual distraction and allow the test partner enough time to produce the auditory distraction. But even then the child may find little of interest in the sound and may not be motivated to look for it. As children's mobility increases they wriggle off someone's lap or climb down from a small chair and find it more interesting to explore the room. It is sensible to remove all tempting objects from the room and certainly to put them out of reach of investigating fingers! A distraction test may even degenerate further — with the tester chasing the child, vainly attempting to see whether he will turn to *any* soft sound from behind. In no way can this be called a hearing assessment, and arrangements should be made for an objective test to be conducted on another occasion.

In summary, it may be seen that there are many obstacles that prevent distraction tests from producing a satisfactory measurement of hearing in both children and adults, with either learning disability or psychiatric disorders. Many people without audiological training or experience will use the wrong apparatus, for example the sound of a bell, the jingle of coins or keys, etc., or they will use the correct apparatus in the wrong way, such as tapping the side of a cup, which will produce a sound of 60–70 dB or more, or using an ordinary voice which varies between 30 and 60 dB. If a response is obtained, the subject's hearing is recorded as 'normal'. It should be remembered that the distraction test is only as good as the testers using it, and is useful only if all the criteria described are met. As this proves hard to achieve with many 'difficult' children, an honest report must acknowledge that an electrophysiological test is required.

Other subjective tests

It has already been intimated that hearing tests can be divided into those known as 'subjective', in which some degree of co-operation is required from the subject, or 'objective', in which a result is obtained without subject co-operation (Yeates, 1995). In many cases of learning disability the subject is unable to give the help required. In cases of psychiatric problems, for example autism, the problem is different. These subjects may have certain skills and it is the job of the examiner to utilize them, incorporating them in the way the test is introduced.

Tests involving spoken language

In a child without problems, distraction tests are followed by simple tests involving verbal comprehension. These may commence at the age of 18–24 months. However, children of this age who are 'difficult to test' rarely have sufficient verbal comprehension to use them. But, as language develops (or if it develops), language tests can be very useful. Adults with learning disability can use — and enjoy — such tests if their verbal comprehension is sufficient. The following tests may be used as comprehension develops.

Five-object test

By the time normal children reach 18–24 months of age they have acquired a small vocabulary of single words. By age two they can join two words together. The first words acquired are usually nouns and by the ages of 2;0–2;3 children can join a noun with a verb, i.e. noun–verb or verb–noun constructions. The first use of verbs is a very important milestone in the development of speech. The five-object test can be used when the subject has acquired a small noun vocabulary. The objects usually used are a cup, a spoon, a brush, a car and a doll or a model aeroplane. These normally evince a good deal of interest, even in older people. The use of toy objects is often criticized when they are presented to adults. However, it has been found (when used for a large subject sample) that individuals did not appear demeaned, but rather appeared to enjoy the test. It seems that the attitude of the examiner is the important factor.

The objects are placed on a table in front of the test subject, one at a time, and each is named in a clear conversational voice. Suitable comments about each object help to increase interest. Subjects are asked to identify each object in turn (to ensure comprehension) again using a strong, clear voice. The tester then explains that a 'soft' voice will then be used and subjects will be asked to indicate the objects in the same manner. The intensity of the examiner's voice is measured with a sound level meter. It should be noted that the test subject is not required to demonstrate expressive language, although a conversation may result spontaneously. As comprehension develops before expression this is a useful 'by-product'. Satisfactory hearing means that the subject hears a voice of 35–40 dB SPL at a distance of three feet (one metre).

McCormick test

If the subject is able to co-operate with the five-object test it is useful to try the McCormick test (McCormick, 1977, 1988) which requires a considerably larger vocabulary. The purpose of this test is to ascertain whether there is satisfactory discrimination of consonants, or high-frequency sounds. These are the sounds which give the intelligibility to speech, whereas low-frequency sounds (or vowels) give speech its energy, carrying power and emotional quality. An inability to distinguish the consonants in speech can lead to mistakes in intelligibility, often with dire consequences. 'Mishearing' words can lead to the wrong 'labels' being attached by subjects with a high-frequency hearing loss. Children may be called 'inattentive', 'disobedient', 'dreamy', 'naughty' or even 'maladjusted', whereas adults may be said to 'hear when they want to' and to lack concentration or to show challenging behaviour or even signs of senility. Thus it can be seen that tests which detect high-frequency hearing loss are extremely useful and that the diagnosis of this condition is very important (Downs and Balkany, 1977; Yeates, 1992).

The McCormick test uses seven pairs of objects, each pair having a common vowel but differing consonants in their names:

- Cup and duck.
- Plate and plane.
- House and cow.

- Lamb and man.
- Key and tree.
- Shoe and spoon.
- Horse and fork.

The test is administered in the same way as the simpler five-object test. The items are placed randomly in front of the subject, and named in a clear, conversational voice. The subject is then asked to identify each object to ensure verbal comprehension. Next, the subject is told that the examiner is going to use a 'soft' voice and the subject must listen very carefully as he did in the five-object test. In each case the examiner covers his mouth to exclude any possibility of lip-reading. Again, the intensity of voice is measured with a sound level meter.

After the subject has completed the five-object test successfully praise and encouragement must be unstinting. This certainly leads to maximum effort when attempting the harder McCormick test. If this too is successful, or it is obvious that the subject has made a real effort we should, again, be generous with praise so that the next test is attempted happily. Each test is a little harder than the preceding one and success at each stage means that the subject is motivated to attempt each in turn. Experience has shown that the best results are obtained by commencing with the easiest test, producing encouragement, and then proceeding in an orderly manner until it is obvious that the subject has reached the level at which he is no longer able to co-operate. It must be remembered that everyone enjoys praise, and interest in the tests is more likely to be sustained when succeeding.

It has already been mentioned that criticism of the use of toy objects when testing adults has been voiced by some people working with older subjects. Although probably a criticism of the way in which the test is presented, nevertheless, a test designed specifically for use by adults would be a useful addition to the test battery. A test now undergoing validation has been suggested by Moorey (1996). The principle behind this test is the same as that of the McCormick test, but the pairs of objects used are more 'adult'. The South London Object Test (SLOT) (Moorey, 1996) uses six pairs of words with matched vowels and differing consonants:

- Key and cheese.
- Ball and fork.
- Bread and pen.
- Soap and comb.
- Jam and bag.
- Cake and tape.

Replica foodstuffs are available, are very life-like and provoke much interest. Some subjects even attempt to sample the cake or the cheese!

The SLOT (Moorey, 1996) is used in exactly the same way as the tests already described.

There are other tests, such as the Kendall Toy Test (Kendall, 1957) and Mary Sheridan's Picture Tests (Sheridan, 1973) which are not described here, but which use the same principle of consonant differentiation.

Of course, there are many children and adults who never reach the development required for language tests of even the simplest type. However, it is sensible to spend time encouraging the comprehension of words that are used when testing hearing. Concentrated work by a speech therapist, working as a member of the team, in the development of a child with learning disability or autism can produce highly useful results. Children or adults with psychiatric problems may vary from day to day in their ability to co-operate with language tests. In such cases it appears best to wait for the time when co-operation is forthcoming, and not to provoke ill will by persevering with a situation that may only lead to shouting or throwing the apparatus. Calming the situation by producing a favoured toy and talking about this, and then leaving the scene when peace has been restored, appears to give the best chance of having a second attempt on another occasion. Although this may appear to be rewarding bad behaviour, it is also a method of commencing a friendly relationship with the subject. If this can be established the subject may eventually be willing to please the examiner by co-operating.

There may be those who ask why a lot of time is spent establishing co-operation when an objective hearing test under anaesthesia could be substituted, with a quicker result. Although the objective test, such as BSER, can provide a result it gives nothing else. A language test gives an idea of how the subject is functioning in his or her environment and helps those who are designing programmes of help for individuals.

Conditioning tests

The next set of tests are based on 'conditioning' or, more accurately, are simple modelling techniques (Yeates, 1980). They do not require the use of speech and some subjects who have not developed any spoken language can be taught to use them. Conditioning tests are also useful for people whose first language is not English. Subjects are taught to respond to a sound with a simple motor action. The first sound that is normally used is the word *'Go'*, said in a very loud voice. It is immaterial whether the word is meaningful as it is simply a good low-frequency sound to which the subject is taught to respond. A useful response is the dropping of a brick into a box or a bowl. The examiner and a partner demonstrate the action several times, attempting to arouse the interest of the subject until he or she takes a brick and joins the 'game'. It is often necessary to place a brick into the subject's hand and help him or her to respond at the correct time. This action is then repeated many times, still using a loud voice, and finally removing the examiner's hand to see whether the principle of the 'game' has been grasped. If there is no success the parents or care staff are asked to practise the 'game' with the subject every day until it can be ascertained whether there will eventually be success. Short, frequent practice sessions are recommended to maintain the interest of the subject. The motor response can also be changed to maintain interest. Some children enjoy dropping a brick on to the floor when they hear the word *'Go'*. Some examiners use 'peg men' in a boat, a peg man being placed in a hole in response to the sound. (However, this apparatus requires manipulative ability which is possibly beyond the developmental stage of the subject, who may also be hindered by a physical disability such as cerebral palsy.) It is up to the examiner to devise a motor response which will maintain the subject's interest and be within his or her capabilities.

When the examiner is satisfied that the principle of the 'game' has been understood, the intensity of the voice can gradually be lessened until there is no response from the subject; this intensity is measured with a sound level meter. This gives a reasonable estimate of low-frequency hearing. High-frequency hearing may be estimated by substituting the sound *'ss–ss–ss'* for the word *'Go'*. It has already been mentioned that the sound *'ss–ss–ss'* is a high-frequency sibilant sound of approximately 4 kHz. If the subject has sufficient comprehension the high-frequency sound can be made into a game where the sound imitates that of a snake. But, with both low- and high-frequency sounds success can be achieved by helping the subject to copy the examiners, by frequent repetition and practice sessions with a speech therapist or care staff, or both.

Free field audiometer and warble tone audiometer

Once the above has been achieved, pure tones can be substituted for voice sounds, i.e. the test gets a little harder but the results become more accurate. The free field audiometer produces sounds between 5 dB and 80 dB, at frequencies between 125 Hz and 4 kHz. Use of this technique depends on the proper understanding of the 'conditioning' or 'modelling' with the use of voice described above. The subject is required to make the same motor responses as have been used previously when a pure tone is heard. This action is demonstrated several times by the examiner and partner and it will be seen that repeated demonstration at all the frequencies and at the loudest intensity can be achieved without the use of speech. Sometimes a subject who has appeared to understand the principle of the test when the voice is used cannot make the transition to pure tones. In these cases the use of an objective test should be considered. The free field audiometer gives a very useful result but it must be remembered that the device measures only binaural hearing.

The warble tone audiometer is useful because the sounds it produces are more interesting for the subject. Each sound is a narrow band, centred on a specific frequency, giving the effect of a 'warble'. Audiologically this is also more accurate than pure tones used without headphones, when the phenomenon known as 'standing waves' may distort the intensity of the sound used. The frequencies and intensities available are the same as those produced by the free field audiometer. The warble tone audiometer has been found to produce sounds that are interesting to babies and thus it can also be added to the list of stimuli used in distraction tests.

When a subject has been able to give reliable results with a free field or warble tone audiometer it is only a small step to the use of the pure tone audiometer and the production of an audiogram showing the subject's hearing in right and left ears separately.

The pure tone audiometer

If taken step by step, a surprising number of people are able to use the pure tone audiometer. This instrument measures the hearing in the right and left ears separately, measuring the intensity from –10 dB to 120 dB at frequencies from 125 Hz to 8 kHz. In a sample of 500 adults with learning disabilities (Yeates, 1995) an audiogram was completed by 280 people (56%).

The measurement of a 'minus quantity' may be queried. Measurement of intensity is the measurement of the pressure of a sound. Initially, a group of healthy young adults was taken and sounds at each frequency between 125 Hz and 8 kHz were played to them (Jerger, 1973; McCormick, 1988). The subjects were asked to indicate when each sound was no longer heard and the pressure of the sound was measured at this point. The average pressures at which this happened for the group were calculated and this pressure was then named 0 dB for each frequency. The smallest pressure detected by the human ear is at 1 kHz. Thus, anyone hearing a sound at –5 dB or –10 dB is able to decipher a sound softer than the average subject.

The main problem when proceeding from the use of a free field or warble tone audiometer to a pure tone audiometer is that the latter requires the use of headphones so that sounds can be played into each ear separately. Surprisingly, children (and adults) with learning disability or psychiatric problems resent the use of headphones. Watching others using a 'walkman' and then trying it themselves may be useful preparation for pure tone audiometry. Curiosity about the obvious pleasure given by the 'walkman' is very helpful in overcoming the apprehension felt about wearing headphones. Even watching a friend using headphones can be a useful precursor to trying them out. Once the subject has overcome his apprehension it is sensible to start with a sound at 1 kHz and approximately 60 dB. If previous tests have indicated a more severe hearing loss, then a louder sound should be chosen initially. It is sensible to use the same motor reaction that has been used when testing with voice and pure tone or warble tones. This is now very familiar to the subject and will seem a confirmation of what has been done before. In many cases it is helpful to assist the subject in the response to the first sounds by putting the examiner's hand over that of the subject, holding the brick (or similar), waiting until the sound is produced and then helping him or her drop it into the bowl. It may be necessary to do this several times, altering the frequency of the sound. When the subject has demonstrated that he or she has understood what is wanted, help from the examiner is stopped and the intensity of the sound at 1 kHz is reduced in 10 dB steps. When there is no further response the intensity is raised in 5 dB increments until the point is reached at which the subject responds again. This requires considerable concentration from the subject and it may be sensible to stop the test after obtaining an accurate response at one frequency in both ears. Other frequencies may be tested at subsequent sessions and it is always very important to give a lot of praise and encouragement for what has been achieved.

If the programme already described is followed, it is surprising how often the subject will be willing to respond to sounds at 500 Hz, 1, 2 and 4 kHz, in both ears, in one session. Examiners must be prepared to meet a wide range of abilities, deal with many different behaviours and adapt their test material accordingly. They must be sufficiently flexible to alter the day or time of the test in order to obtain optimal results from someone whose behaviour is erratic.

Visual reinforcement

There are some subjects whose response is greatly enhanced if the initial sounds are reinforced by an interesting visual clue (Bamford, 1988). However, when the response to sound plus visual reinforcer has been well established the visual element is removed and it can be seen whether the subject will respond to sound alone.

This type of apparatus (right- and left-hand speakers with a light above) can eventually ascertain whether the subject turns to sounds at 250 and 500 Hz, 1, 2 and 4 kHz. The light above the speakers can be made more interesting by being enclosed in a toy such as a small animal or a doll.

The use of visual reinforcement can, of course, only be used in tertiary centres where the apparatus is available. It is useful for testing children with problems and may be used for those subjects whose development is still at the localizing stage. It may also be used for those who are beginning to understand the conditioning process but who require a little more help in the initial stages. The optimal sound stimulus is that made by a warble tone audiometer, but younger children or those whose development is still at a very early stage may respond better to narrow-band noise.

Objective tests for children and adults

Many examiners may attempt the subjective tests without a great deal of effort in helping the subject to succeed. They may feel that it is easier and perhaps more accurate to ask for an objective hearing test. However, examiners may forget that by spending more time with the subject they are learning more about his or her strengths and weaknesses. By doing so the examiner may find ways in which to encourage the subject, and ways which will encourage him or her to succeed in a simple subjective hearing test. In a research project carried out on 500 people with learning disability in Lewisham and north Southwark (Yeates, 1995) it was found that time taken in this way was certainly not wasted. It does, however, mean that subjects need to have a special service provided for their needs and that they cannot be referred to a large, busy ENT clinic, where they may be placed in a sound-proofed cubicle and expected to respond to pure tones. Obviously the learning-disabled person is frightened and will behave correspondingly. The whole episode is a disaster and will yield no results.

If the examiner has proceeded through the subjective tests as suggested and the subject cannot understand what is required, and his or her behaviour is such that results cannot possibly be called meaningful then an electrophysiological test should be attempted (Tucker and Nolan, 1986). There are four such tests:

- Post-aural myogenic response (PAM) or crossed acoustic response (CAR).
- Electrocochleography (ECoG).
- Cortical evoked response (CER).
- Brainstem evoked response audiometry (BSER).

These tests do not require any co-operation from the subject, but at least two of them require anaesthesia. This is a problem when subjects are adults as they are the only people who can legally give consent for this.

Post-aural myogenic response

In humans, the post-aural muscle is vestigial, but in many animals it is well developed and useful. It is connected with the 'fight or flight' mechanism used by many animals. This means that there is a well-developed electrical response in the muscle when a sound is heard.

In the post-aural myogenic response (PAM) test electrodes are placed behind the ears and the sounds used are sharp-onset clicks. In humans the response requires over 100 clicks so that an averaging computer can record a result. The test takes approximately 10 minutes and is totally non-invasive. Unfortunately, if muscle tone is poor the result is not accurate and it cannot be relied upon in some people with learning disability. So although PAM has advantages, the test is sometimes unreliable and should only be used in cases where other, more reliable tests cannot be used.

Electrocochleogram

In the electrocochleogram (ECoG) it is necessary to place a needle electrode through the tympanic membrane and position it against the promontory of the cochlea, under anaesthesia. The sound stimuli used are, again, sharp-onset clicks and the electrical responses come from the cochlea and the adjacent part of the auditory nerve. An averaging computer is used to record the result. This is an accurate test.

Brainstem evoked response audiometry (BSER)

This is probably the objective test of choice, but it generally requires anaesthesia. The electrode is placed on the vertex and electrical changes are picked up from the lowest part of the auditory pathway, reaching as far as the inferior colliculus. But over 1000 clicks are required to obtain a response that can be recorded by use of the averaging computer. This means that the subject must remain still for 30–45 minutes, something that is by no means easy, even for someone who has no other problems. When the subject has a learning disability or psychiatric problems it may be almost impossible, and anaesthesia is necessary.

Cortical evoked response

The responses of this test are derived from the cortex and the stimuli are pure tones of long duration. It is the only electrophysiological test in which pure tones can be used. However, the responses may be obscured by EEG alpha rhythm and this limits its use.

Impedance testing (admittance audiometry)

This technique falls in between a subjective and an objective test. It requires the subject to allow a probe to be placed in the external auditory canal so that an air-tight seal is obtained. Obviously, people who are touch-defensive will not allow this and the test cannot be carried out. But no other co-operation is required.

The probe contains three tubes. The first contains a low-frequency sound generator. The second contains a pump and the third contains a tiny microphone. If the middle ear is filled with fluid, as in 'glue ear' or SOM, the sound cannot pass through the tympanic membrane and is reflected back to the microphone. If the middle ear is healthy and air-filled, the sound passes normally through the middle ear and on towards the inner ear. If the Eustachian tube is blocked by catarrhal material this produces a negative pressure in the middle ear. The sound passes through optimally when the pump has corrected this. A graph is produced showing which condition is present in the middle ear, i.e. a normal middle ear, filled with air, via the Eustachian tube; a middle ear filled with thick 'glue'-like material or a middle ear connected to a Eustachian tube which is blocked by the same type of material. As children with Down's syndrome are very liable to get chronic SOM, this test is very useful for them and when approached with sensitivity they will often allow the probe to be placed in each ear in turn. A demonstration of how the probe is inserted will diminish apprehension.

Use of anaesthesia in objective hearing tests

It will be seen that sedation, light anaesthesia or both may be needed for several of the objective hearing tests described. Consent for anaesthesia is then required. With children, the consent form may be signed by a parent after a careful explanation of the test and why it is needed. It is worth taking time over this explanation and making sure that the parents understand what is happening. Whilst doing this, time should be made to discuss what the child is missing if he or she has a hearing loss, and what can be done to help if a loss is discovered. If the parents have a very negative attitude which cannot be changed by long and thoughtful discussion it is probably best to leave them to consider and return at a later date. Some parents may be very frightened of an anaesthetic and it is best not to be over-persuasive but to leave them to talk to others in the family.

For adults who are unable to give meaningful consent to anaesthesia the problem is worse. In the research project mentioned previously (Yeates, 1995) a Mental Health Commissioner was consulted, who took legal advice. The result was still somewhat unclear, but the main object was to consider 'the best interest of the patient'. It was suggested that a meeting should be arranged between the parents (if still in contact with the subject) and all the professionals working with the subject. At this meeting the test should be described carefully and if those present agreed that the test was in the best interest of the subject and that help could be given if a hearing loss was confirmed then the consent form for anaesthesia could be signed by the senior professional attending the meeting. This would normally be the doctor concerned or the specialist speech therapist treating the subject. It should be mentioned that some anaesthetists are unhappy about dealing with subjects who are frightened and who behave in a very difficult manner. To ameliorate this situation it is often sensible to sedate the subject so that he or she is sleeping lightly before reaching the anaesthetist. Of course, if the subject is capable of understanding a simple explanation of the procedure every effort should be made to give this. Unfortunately, this is rarely the case as anyone capable of such understanding will almost certainly have been able to complete a subjective hearing test.

General comments on tests

Before attempting any test, the examiner should take time to see the subject and to make contact with him or her as far as possible. With some subjects it is possible to hold a (limited) conversation. This means that the examiner is not a complete stranger when the first test is undertaken. The subject should always be accompanied by someone he or she knows and trusts; this is beneficial for both subject and examiner as the companion should be able to provide a useful history. If the subject is not known and the companion is not a regular member of the care staff the situation is useless for the examiner who seeks a history. Nothing is more irritating than someone who says they are 'agency staff', know nothing of the subject and are merely a means of transport.

Setting up a special service

If all the special needs for testing difficult subjects are considered, it will be seen that the optimal method is to establish a special service for people with learning disability or psychological problems (Yeates and Moorey, 1996). More and more districts are setting aside finance for this (Wilson and Hare, 1990). The motivating force for doing this has come largely from speech therapists (Yeates, 1991). They realize that their work is impossible if the hearing level of their patients is unknown. This led on to the formation of special teams working to gather information on hearing. Often the teams were led by speech therapists. Other important members of the team were parents, audiologists (or consultants in audiological medicine, wherever possible), psychologists and support staff (when subjects were in some form of residential care). Support staff or parents are very important members of the team, especially when a hearing loss is being treated. They are the individuals who help and persevere with the use of hearing or other environmental aids. If they are not convinced of the enormous benefits that can be achieved, the cause is often completely lost and hearing aids end up in drawers or cupboards.

The special service should, optimally, be peripatetic as this can overcome many of the problems involved in hearing testing we have seen. Both adults and children seen in their own homes are less apprehensive and are obviously with people they know. There is no long waiting period in an outpatient department and they are not frightened by the normal clinic paraphernalia. Also, it is not possible to devote the time required for subjective hearing tests in a busy ENT clinic.

A sympathetic ENT surgeon is an important member of the team, but if all the subjective hearing tests have been performed prior to an ENT appointment this obviously provides much information before the ENT examination. Liaison with reception staff at the clinic will often mean that a first appointment can be arranged in order to cut down the waiting period, when unacceptable behaviour, often exacerbated by apprehension, may occur.

In summary, anyone attempting to work with 'difficult' subjects, whether children or adults, must be patient and prepared to find good points which can be developed and then used in the testing sessions. They must be prepared to work hard to develop a relationship that can be enjoyed by the subject. This may be very time consuming, but is ultimately satisfactory. Lastly, they should be working as part of a team, with mutual help and understanding, and believe that they can achieve success and the rehabilitation of people with a hearing loss.

References

Bamford J (1988) Visual reinforcement audiometry. In McCormick B (ed) Practical Aspects of Audiology: Paediatric Audiology 0–5 Years. London: Whurr Publishers. pp 117–134.

Bray P, Kemp D (1987) An advanced cochlear echo technique suitable for infant screening. British Journal of Audiology 21: 191–204.

Burr SA, Mulhera M, Degg C (1996) Characterization of Click-synchronized spontaneous Oto-acoustic Emissions in Humans. Paper presented at the Annual Meeting of the British Society of Audiology. Cambridge, 22–23 September.

Cunningham C (1982) Down's Syndrome: An Introduction for Parents. London: Souvenir Press.

Dalton AJ, Cropper DR (1984) Incidence of memory deterioration in ageing persons with Down's syndrome. In Berg JM (ed) Perspectives and Progress in Mental Retardation. Baltimore, MD: University Park Press.

Downs M, Balkany T (1977) Audiological and Otological Findings in Down's Syndrome. Paper presented at the American Speech and Hearing Convention, Chicago.

Heaton-Ward WA, Wiley Y (1984) Mental Handicap. Bristol: Wright.

Holland A (1986) Genetic aspects of visual and auditory impairment in mentally handicapped people. In Ellis D (ed) Sensory Impairments in Mentally Handicapped People. London: Croom Helm, pp 149–165.

Jerger N (1973) The theory of signed detectability and the measurement of hearing. In Modern Developments in Audiology. London: Academic Press, pp 437–466.

Kendall DC (1957) Mental development of young children. In Ewing AWG (ed) Educational Guidance and the Deaf Child. Manchester: Manchester University Press.

McCormick B (1977) The Toy Discrimination Test: an aid for screening the hearing of children above the mental age of two years. Public Health 91: 67–69.

McCormick B (1988) Screening for Hearing Impairment in Young Children. London: Croom Helm.

Moorey M (1996) South Lewisham Object Test: From Specialist Audiology Services for Adults with Learning Disabilities. Booklet prepared for study day. London: Guy's Hospital, November.

Sheridan M (1973) Children's Developmental Progress from Birth to Five Years, the Stycar Sequences. Windsor: NFER-Nelson.

Tucker I, Nolan M (1986) Methods of objective assessment of auditory function in subjects with limited communication skills. In Ellis D (ed) Sensory Impairments in Mentally Handicapped People. London: Croom Helm, pp 218–237.

Wilson AN, Hare A (1990) Health care screening for people with mental handicap living in the community. British Medical Journal 301: 1379–1381.

Yeates S (1980) The Development of Hearing. Manchester: MTP Press.

Yeates S (1986) Medical and otological aspects of hearing impairment in mentally handicapped people. In D Ellis (ed) Sensory Impairments in Mentally Handicapped People. London: Croom Helm, pp 115–148.

Yeates S (1989) Hearing in people with mental handicaps: a review of 100 adults. Mental Handicap 17: 33–37.

Yeates S (1991) Hearing loss in adults with learning disabilities. British Medical Journal 303: 427–428.

Yeates S (1992) Have they got a hearing loss? Mental Handicap 20: 126–133.

Yeates S (1995) The incidence and importance of hearing loss in people with severe learning disability: the evolution of a service. British Journal of Learning Disabilities 23: 79–84.

Yeates S, Moorey M (1996) Specialist Audiology Services for Adults with Learning Disabilities: Development and Operation. Optimum Health Services National Study Day in co-operation with the British Society of Audiology.

Chapter 3
Child and Adolescent Psychiatry

PETER HINDLEY

Introduction

Most parents assume that their children will grow up and talk. Most clinicians assume that, age and other factors allowing, they will be able to talk to the children that they see and that these children will talk to their parents and brothers and sisters with ease. Profound early onset deafness challenges all these assumptions. As Meadow-Orlans and Erting have described in Chapter 1, most deaf children are born into hearing families with little or no previous experience of deafness. In most countries parents of deaf children are not encouraged to acquire sign language early in their children's lives, countries such as Sweden and Finland being exceptions to this rule (Sinkonnen, 1994; Heiling, 1995). Even in the USA, where most deaf children are now educated in Total Communication (TC) environments, the majority of their parents do not use sign (Jordan and Karchmer 1986). And so distortions in family communication and delays in the child's language development are the rule (Gregory, 1976; Gregory, Bishop and Sheldon 1995).

The consequent difficulties in communication have a profound influence on the development of the child and his or her family and on clinical practice and pose a question which is at the centre of our understanding of the mental health of deaf children and their families. Should difficulties in communication be considered the primary factor in the mental health problems of deaf children or just another risk factor to which deaf children happen to be exposed? In other words, should we think of deaf children as essentially ordinary children coping with extraordinary circumstances (see Chapter 14) rather than children at a higher risk of mental health problems?

It is clear that problems of communication are not the only difficulties that face deaf children and their families. Although 90% of deaf children are born into hearing families, it seems that a majority of deaf children will grow up to use sign language in some form (Gregory, Bishop and Sheldon

1995) and although not all deaf adults will feel themselves core members of the Deaf community, the majority will feel a strong identification with other deaf people — both sign language users and oral deaf people. In this respect deaf children growing up can be thought of as making a transition from the culture of their families to that of their peers. How they make this transition can have a powerful influence on deaf children's identity (Cole and Edelman, 1991) and mental health. Although communication between deaf children and their parents has a powerful impact on this process, the parents' thoughts and feelings about their child's deafness are of equal importance (Gregory et al., 1995), as are the child's relationships with his or her hearing and deaf peers.

Additionally, deaf children are exposed to risk factors which are indirectly related to their deafness. Although being deaf may not be considered as an impairment by many Deaf people (see Chapter 1) deaf children are at greater risk of additional impairments (see Chapter 5). As David Bond points out in Chapter 6, these can be impairments of learning or vision as well as central nervous system (CNS) disorders such as brain damage or epilepsy and other physical impairments, which are well recognized as risk factors for child psychiatric disorder in their own right. Deaf children are also more likely to experience emotional, physical and sexual abuse than hearing children (see Chapter 7).

This chapter tries to strike a fine balance between the cultural perspective and the medical perspective. At times it succeeds but at others it fails. However, trying to synthesize these apparently conflicting views lies at the heart of practising psychiatry with deaf children and their families.

This chapter provides a brief introduction to child and adolescent psychiatry and a guided reading list to set the context for those interested in the area. Consideration is given to some aspects of the social and psychological development of deaf children as a context in which to explore the mental health problems of deaf children and their families.Two recent publications provide detailed accounts of the research (Hindley, 1997) and clinical (Roberts and Hindley, 1999) aspects of this area.

Child and adolescent psychiatry

Child and adolescent psychiatry is a broad discipline. It draws on developmental psychology, systems theories, psychodynamic theories, neurophysiology, genetics and psychiatry to understand the wide range of emotional, behavioural and psychiatric disorders presenting during childhood and adolescence. Child and adolescent psychiatry differs from adult psychiatry in four important ways. Firstly, many problems presenting as child psychiatric disorders are most helpfully thought of as deviations from normal behaviour which cause distress to either the child or important people in his or her environment, such as parents or teachers. In this respect it is often more important to consider why a particular child is a focus of concern rather than whether its behaviour is abnormal. Secondly, other people in a child's life are more likely to voice concern about a particular child rather than the child itself, although older adolescents may seek help in their own right. Thirdly, child and adolescent psychiatry covers the major period of development; the difficulties that a toddler faces will differ massively from those that a late teenager faces. Finally, children's difficulties arise in the context of an interaction between the social system in which they live and the process of their development — their difficulties are dynamic and changing.

History

The concepts of childhood, development and psychopathology intertwined to create the environment in which child psychiatry as a speciality emerged in the early 20th century. Parry-Jones (1994) provides a comprehensive account of this process. In the UK the emergence of child psychiatry was initially closely associated with psychodynamic theory and practice. Anna Freud (1946) and Melanie Klein (1932) were major influences in the emergence of the Child Guidance Movement in Great Britain, and other countries, in the 1920s and 1930s. Child psychotherapy and psychodynamic theory continue to play an important part in the field, and Winnicott's work (1958) provided a vital link to paediatric practice, but their influence began to diminish with the publication of the first epidemiological studies of child psychiatric disorder (Rutter, Graham and Yule, 1970). As a consequence of Rutter's studies our understanding of the epidemiology and aetiology of child psychiatric disorders began to change, and more clearly defined diagnostic systems were introduced. At the same time understanding of the functioning of systems and a growing awareness of the importance of seeing children in the context of their social system — family, school, etc. — led to a growing influence for family therapy and systems theory (Minuchin 1974; and Warner, this Volume). In the 1980s studies of psychological development led to the emergence of stress-coping theories (Lazarus and Folkman, 1984 and Greenberg, this Volume) in which children's responses to highly stressful events and experiences (life-threatening illness, parental death or divorce, physical and sexual abuse) were seen as attempts by children to cope and thus in normative rather than pathological terms. Finally in the late 1980s and 1990s the influence of genetic predisposition on the emergence of disorders e.g. autism (Rutter, 1991) and obsessive compulsive disorder and Tourette's syndrome (Pauls, Reymond, Stevenson and Leckman, 1991) has become more apparent and theories linking neurophysiological (Goodman, 1994) and biochemical processes have been advanced. As a result, there has been a growing recognition of the influence of biological factors on the development of child psychiatric disorders.

Classification of child psychiatric disorder

Two international systems of classification exist — the *American Psychiatric Association Diagnostic and Statistical Manual* (DSM), the most recent edition being the fourth, DSM–IV (APA, 1994), and the tenth edition of the *World Health Organization International Classification of Diseases*, ICD–10 (WHO, 1992). Both systems use multi-axial systems of classification and allow clinicians to assess domains of disorder and functioning which are separate but related. ICD–10 describes four different axes: clinical disorders, mental retardation, physical health and psychosocial factors. DSM–IV uses five axes: clinical disorders; personality disorders and mental retardation; general medical conditions; psychosocial and environmental factors; and a global assessment of functioning

Both DSM–IV and ICD–10 allow practitioners to make multiple diagnoses, e.g. major depressive episode and attention deficit disorder, but ICD–10 encourages the clinician to give precedence to the diagnosis that is most relevant to the purpose of the assessment and to make other diagnoses subsidiary to the main diagnosis. Both systems include diagnoses that are specific to childhood, such as elimination disorders, and disorders which occur in both children and adults, such as depression or schizophrenia.

For children there are five areas of disorder: disturbances of behaviour, called Conduct Disorder, Hyperkinetic Disorder and Mixed Disorders of Emotion and Conduct in ICD–10 and Attention and Disruptive Behaviour Disorders in DSM–IV; disturbance of emotions or affective disorder; disturbances of relationship; disorders of development such as infantile autism; and major mental illnesses such as schizophrenia and bipolar affective disorder.

Assessment

Children cannot be seen in isolation; the assessment of a referred child involves assessing both the child and the environment in which he or she is developing. Information needs to be gathered from a variety of people important in the child's life. It is necessary to establish who has concerns about a particular child at an early point in the assessment process (if a teacher is the person most concerned, whilst parents are not, it is essential to ensure that these concerns have been shared and discussed before starting the assessment) and why they arise at this particular time. An assessment would usually involve discussions with the child and his or her family (Jenkins, 1994), discussions with the child alone (Angold, 1994), his or her parents or carers alone (Cox, 1994) and, if appropriate, the brothers and sisters. Information would be gathered from the child's school and other professionals involved with the child. In particularly complex cases, a child in local authority care or with complex educational needs, it can be helpful to convene a network meeting of all relevant professionals to facilitate full sharing of information, before an assessment or as the assessment proceeds.

In most circumstances it is most appropriate to start by interviewing the whole family together. This allows the clinician to get a picture of the problem and the family's understanding of the difficulty, to become familiar with the relationships within the family and the family's life-cycle stage. However, separate interviews with parents and children are essential to gain a complete picture. Equally, the assessment process allows the child and the family to assess the people offering them help and to decide whether or not this help is appropriate for them. In this sense, assessment involves finding out what parents and children want and trying to match this up to what the professionals believe they need; often these are not the same thing at the start of assessment.

Practically all interventions used in child and adolescent psychiatry involve the parents in some way or other, and often involve the whole family. In order to intervene effectively, the clinician must engage with the family. Engagement entails understanding the family's concerns, making them feel that the clinician understands, coming to a shared agreement about intervention, and obtaining the family's and/or the child's consent. Intervention without the parents' and/or child's consent is at best ineffective and at worst counterproductive.

However, in certain circumstances, the problems presented by the child or family may be so severe as to warrant treatment without either the child's or family's consent. In these circumstances the powers provided by either child care or mental health legislation may be used to intervene without consent (see Chapter 9).

In this model of assessment, information from a wide variety of sources is integrated or formulated to provide an explanation of the child's or family's difficulties and then to suggest a framework for intervention. Very often the formulation is in the form of a hypothesis, very similar to cognitive behavioural therapy (see Chapters 5 and 17) that can then be tested and modified as intervention proceeds. If the parents are seeking understanding and explanation, assessment alone can be sufficient. If intervention is appropriate, it should be tailored to the needs of the family and child as far as possible.

Aetiology

The causes of psychiatric problems in childhood can be described in two ways. Firstly, different mechanisms: what predisposed the child to develop a particular problem; what started or precipitated the problem; and what maintains the problem. Secondly, as different factors which fall into three broad groups: biological, e.g. a genetic predisposition to autism or the presence of brain damage; psychological, e.g. a lowered sense of self-esteem; and social, e.g. social deprivation or child sexual abuse. Many factors interact with each other and at different times. The following example gives a flavour of how these interactions work.

> Joanna was a 13-year-old deaf girl, the youngest in her family and the only deaf person. The confirmation of Joanna's deafness had come as a profound shock to her mother, causing much sadness, feelings that were still fresh 12 years later. These feelings led to Joanna's mother overprotecting her and always thinking of her as 'my little girl', but Joanna had always felt closer to her father than her mother. Joanna's parents had a stormy relationship. At 9 Joanna was sexually abused by a fellow pupil at school; she reported this to her head teacher but this was not disclosed to her parents. At 13 she started her first serious relationship with a boy and began to experiment sexually. At the same time her father left the family home. Within weeks Joanna became angry and defiant at school, falling out with peers and staff. She was excluded from school and on return home became progressively more angry and aggressive towards her mother.
>
> Joanna's early history of sexual abuse predisposed her to emotional difficulties when she entered her first relationships with boys, which coincided with her father leaving home. This led to an escalation in her problems, precipitating a crisis. Her mother's feelings of sadness and overprotection coupled with Joanna's close relationship with her father prevented her mother from supporting Joanna through the pain of her first serious relationship and maintained the problem that had first started in school. Joanna's parents felt unable to communicate with each other directly. One of the results of Joanna's problems was that her parents were forced to communicate with each other but through Joanna, so perpetuating her difficulties.

Intervention

Given the multifactorial nature of psychiatric disorders in children, it is appropriate to tailor interventions to the particular child and family and their difficulties. For Joanna this consisted of initial family work to encourage the parents to communicate directly rather than through Joanna. After this, Joanna was offered individual counselling to think through her feelings about her sexuality. Whilst Joanna's personal distress diminished, her relationship with her mother deteriorated and an alternative family placement was found at Joanna's request and with her mother's agreement. Thus, for Joanna interventions were at all levels: individual, family and social but also involved other agencies such as social services and education.

A wide range of interventions are used with children; these can again be grouped into biological, psychological and social:

- Biological: medication and dietary manipulation
- Psychological: psychotherapy (psychodynamic, cognitive behavioural, behavioural); family therapy; social skills training.

- Social: involving other agencies; social and financial support; respite care; fostering and adoption; legal interventions and child protection.
- Educational: assessment of needs; provision through extra support in mainstream classes and special educational provision.

Deaf child and adolescent psychiatry

Disease/disorder or language and culture?

Like other branches of medicine, child and adolescent psychiatry uses a variety of models to explain children's distress. One of these is the disease/disorder model. In this instance, assessment involves the making of diagnoses and the ascertainment of risk and protective factors that contribute to the child developing a disorder. It is in this respect that medical models of child psychiatry clash most clearly with the social/cultural model of deafness used in this book. In this model, the development of most deaf children is understood as a transition from the hearing culture of their parents, to the Deaf culture of their peers. Thus, many of the difficulties that they present are understood as attempts to cope with the extraordinary demands that this process places on them.

By describing the social and psychological development of deaf children it may be possible to clarify which aspects of emotional and behavioural disorder in deaf children can be best understood as attempts to cope with exceptional circumstances and which aspects can be best understood as psychiatric disorders.

The social and psychological development of deaf children

The social context of deaf children

In reviewing the social and psychological development of deaf children it is important to consider the social context into which these children are born and develop. In many societies deafness is regarded as a disability, and medical and educational efforts are directed at helping the deaf child to make maximum use of his or her residual hearing and promote the development of spoken language. Efforts are made to normalize the deaf child by integrating deaf children into schools for hearing children, either in units for hearing-impaired children or in fully integrated settings. In many countries parents of deaf children are actively discouraged from using sign language during the early years of their child's life, sign being introduced late in childhood when the child has 'failed' to develop spoken language. Although the situation is changing, it is still the exception rather than the rule that the hearing parents of deaf children are encouraged and enabled to develop sign language early in their child's life and that deaf children are taught in sign language, be it either in schools for deaf children or in mainstream establishments. Even in schools where sign language is used as an educational medium it is still rare for teachers to be themselves deaf and for teachers (deaf or hearing) to use native sign languages; more often than not some form of simultaneous communication (Signed Exact English, Signed French) or manually coded spoken language is used. Thus, deafness is presented as an unfortunate sad occurrence and deaf children as in need of help to try to become, as near as possible, hearing children.

By contrast, a social/cultural view of deafness would encourage the early development of native sign language, the promotion of deafness as a positive experience and the fostering of a sense of Deaf identity through the use of sign, interaction with Deaf peers and experience of Deaf culture. From this perspective a number of factors can be identified as potential risk factors:

- lack of an adequate early language environment
- continuing difficulties in communication with parents and siblings
- inappropriate language environments in school
- restrictions in access to appropriate peer groups
- negative/discriminatory attitudes towards Deaf people leading to a lowered sense of self-esteem.

It is going to be important to see how each of these factors, alone and in combination, affect social and psychological development. In turn, it may be possible to consider the extent to which emotional and behavioural disturbance is a manifestation of a child's and family's coping strategies and to what extent it can be considered a disorder. By considering the experience of deaf children born into deaf families we may be able to identify environmental factors which enable deaf children to develop to their full potential.

Deaf children of Deaf families

Some 5–10% of deaf children are born to Deaf parents (Rawlings and Jensema, 1977). For most Deaf parents, the birth of a deaf child does not come as a shock and is often a relief, tempered by knowledge of the difficulties that that child will face (Erting, 1987). A study using the Still Face paradigm* (Cohn and Tronick, 1983) showed that within the first six

* An artificially stressful situation for babies, in which mothers are asked to maintain an expressionless face, the 'Still Face', which mimics the affect of depressed mothers.

months of life deaf infants rely on visual information more than hearing control subjects and that Deaf mothers used more positive facial expression than hearing mothers of deaf infants (Meadow-Orlans et al., 1987). In addition, Deaf mothers ensure that their hands, faces and eye gaze are within the infant's visual field (Erting, Prezioso and O'Grady Hynes, 1989).

Using simultaneous videotaping of Deaf mothers and their deaf infants, Erting et al. (1989) have shown that the mothers slow and enlarge their signing and use repetition — changes which the authors compare to spoken 'Motherese'. These adaptations of signs seem intended to enable shared attention and joint referencing to occur. In turn, deaf infants develop manual babbling (Pettito and Marentette, 1991) which shares many linguistic features with spoken babbling.

These studies point to a fundamental difficulty for deaf children in establishing language, that is how to ensure that linguistic symbol and referent object can, as far as possible, be within the same visual field. How can a deaf child see what he or she is doing and see what the mother or father are talking about, whether they use sign or speech? This problem, the problem of 'divided attention' (Wood et al., 1986; Harris, 1992), is central to the language development of deaf children because there are a number of essential conditions that must be fulfilled for language to develop. In particular, the meaning of the adult's language must be clearly related to the child's activity, or salient to it, and be led by the child's activity that is contingent upon it.

Hearing children can divide their attention *between* visual and auditory fields; they can listen to what their parents are talking about whilst doing it. Deaf children must either divide their attention *within* their visual field or between touch and vision. Deaf parents use a variety of methods to manage the field of shared attention. Deaf parents use both touch and adaptations of sign language to overcome divided attention (Harris, 1992). These adaptations include moving signs within the signing space and signing on the child's body. These adaptations and Deaf mothers' sensitivity to their deaf infants' activities have an impact on their social interaction. Thus, after one year, Deaf mothers are more able than their hearing counterparts to establish and sustain meaningful interactions with their children (Gregory and Barlow, 1986).

It may be that for deaf children of Deaf parents the establishment of shared attention and joint referencing, and the mutuality that these imply, form the basis for the relatively normal pattern of development that follows. Thus, the developments of attachments (Meadow, Greenberg, Erting and Carmichael, 1981; Meadow, Greenberg and Erting, 1983), symbolic play (Spencer, Deyo and Grindstaff, 1990) and sign language (Caselli and Volterra, 1989) in deaf children of Deaf parents parallel those of hearing children of hearing parents. The exception to these findings is a study of attachment formation in deaf children of oral deaf parents, in which delayed and deviant patterns of attachment predominated (Galenson et al., 1979). Bonvillian and Folven (1993) have suggested that this may primarily be a reflection of the oral deaf mothers' negative self-perceptions, which in turn were a consequence of their oral education.

As Deaf children of Deaf parents pass through the school system their levels of attainment in all areas are on average superior to those of their deaf counterparts, when groups matched for non–verbal IQ are compared (Balow and Brill, 1972; Meadow, 1968b). In fact, the IQs of Deaf children of Deaf parents are on average eight points higher than those of their hearing peers (Braden, 1994, p.99). In adult life, Deaf people with Deaf parents are often community leaders.

Deaf children of hearing families

Early interaction and attachments

Many hearing parents of deaf children suspect that their infants are deaf before the diagnosis is made (Hall, 1989). In the past these suspicions have often been denied by professionals (Freeman, Hastings and Malkin 1975; Meadow, 1968a; Gregory, 1976) and the parents labelled as neurotic, contributing to delays in diagnosis. However, the delay between suspicion and diagnosis means that for some parents the confirmation of their fears yields an initial sense of relief. For others, the abrupt manner in which the news is broken leaves a long-lasting sense of distress and anger (Hindley, 1993; Gregory, 1976).

It has been suggested that the intensity of emotion surrounding diagnosis is akin to grief (Schlesinger and Meadow, 1972) and that if these feelings remain unresolved they can lead to a persistent sense of powerlessness in the parents (Schlesinger, 1988). By contrast, in a total population survey of deaf children (ages 5–16) in the Greater Vancouver area, most parents were thought to have accepted that their child was deaf and adjusted well to its needs (Freeman et al., 1975). However, Sue Gregory's longitudinal study (Gregory et al., 1995) suggests that a significant minority of parents either never accept their child's deafness or have great difficulty in doing so, with understandable effects on the child's views of him or herself.

In adjusting to their deaf child, some parents talk of the need to re-examine themselves and of re-discovering their deaf child and themselves as parents. The findings of Meadow-Orlans et al. (1987) suggest some of the direction that this re-discovery takes. Deaf infants of Deaf and hearing mothers made much greater use of the visual environment when stressed, but Deaf mothers were more successful in comforting their deaf infants. As hearing parents are given the opportunity to meet Deaf adults and find out more about Deaf culture they also talk of discovering a new world that was previously hidden from them.

As hearing people, we are highly attuned to auditory signals of distress or delight; hearing parents of hearing babies recognise their own infant's cry and the different types of crying — hunger, discomfort, pain, etc. — within days of their child's birth, and in turn use their voices to calm and comfort their babies. Could it be that hearing parents need particular help in identifying visual means of communicating and caring for their deaf babies?

A significant proportion of hearing mothers (and other hearing carers) of deaf children have been consistently described as overcontrolling and intrusive in their interactions with their deaf pre-school children (see Lederberg, 1993 for a comprehensive review). This style of interaction can be understood in a number of ways. Firstly, as a response to a child with delayed language, with the adult trying to create a more structured language environment in which the deaf child can acquire language (Lederberg, 1993 p. 105). Secondly, as a response to grief-like feelings provoked by the confirmation of deafness (Schlesinger, 1988) and finally as a response to the pragmatic problem of divided attention. This appears to be reflected in the finding that hearing mothers have much greater difficulty in gaining and sustaining their deaf children's attention in comparison with deaf mothers. However, some hearing mothers appear to adapt intuitively to their deaf children, making use of exaggerated facial expression and gestures to engage their deaf infants (Koester and Trim, 1991).

These features of deaf infants' relationships with their carers have led to suggestions that the deaf infants of hearing parents are more likely to develop an insecure attachment (Ainsworth et al., 1978) relationship (Gregory, 1976; Schlesinger and Meadow, 1972). However, there have been no empirical studies to confirm this. Greenberg and Marvin (1979) used Ainsworth and Bell's (1970) Strange Situation* to study separation-reunion behaviour between deaf preschoolers and their parents. They found that immature attachment was associated with parents who used oral communication alone, that is either without sign or gesture, this being particularly related to the mother's communication with the child before separation occurred.

In summary, it appears that in general hearing parents do have greater difficulty interacting with their deaf infants and young children for a variety of reasons, some practical and some emotional. Anecdotal evidence suggests that poor communication is associated with insecure attachment. The experience of Deaf mothers offers important guidance as to how to overcome these difficulties.

---

* An experimental situation in which 12–18 month-old infants' behaviour is video-taped. The mother/carer brings the child into the experimental room, leaves it and a stranger comes in whilst the mother is away. The mother then returns and the child's behaviour towards the mother is coded as secure, resistant, avoidant and disorganized. The last three are commonly grouped as *insecure*.

Early language development and the emergence of play

Even with early identification and audiological intervention, deaf children's spoken language development is significantly delayed (Gregory and Mogford, 1982; Marschark, 1993) and is often deviant. A longitudinal study of deaf children born in the 1970s in the UK, when oral education was the norm, showed that the majority grew up to use sign language in adulthood (Gregory et al., 1995). Although most deaf children in the USA are now educated in settings that use some form of sign, only a minority of parents report themselves as using signing at home (Jordan and Karchmer, 1986). How do deaf children of hearing parents acquire sign language?

Families that have chosen to use signing from the outset are faced with the task of acquiring a language whilst getting used to a new baby. A number of programmes offer families the opportunity of a Deaf language aide to come into parents' homes, both to advise about communication and help parents and siblings to learn to sign.

Supporters of purely oral education have suggested that sign interferes with the deaf child's acquisition of spoken language. There is no evidence to support this (Marschark, 1993 p. 109). Children raised in purely oral homes develop systematic gesture which some authors suggest shares features of native sign languages such as American Sign Language (ASL) (Goldin-Meadow and Mylander, 1984). Parents using Total Communication (TC) methods tend to use simplified language and miss out important information in their communication (Swisher, 1984). Their deaf children do use sign as their first language (Johnson et al., 1989) and the emergence of semantic relations in their sign parallels that of hearing children (Marschark, 1993 p.116).

As with parents, teachers can use overcontrolling strategies in their interactions with their pupils (Wood et al., 1986). Wood et al. found that children whose teachers were most controlling were least likely to initiate conversations and showed the poorest language use. However, they found that teachers could change their interaction with their pupils through the use of video feedback.

The development of play in deaf children appears to be influenced by language development. A study conducted in the 1970s with children who were predominantly orally educated showed that although deaf children's play emerged at the same chronological age as hearing children, it was less well elaborated. Additionally, their play contained elements that did not appear to be clearly related to each other (Gregory and Mogford, 1982). Studies of children educated in TC settings suggest that the level of sophistication of deaf children's play is related to their language ability (Spencer, Deyo and Grindstaff 1990).

In summary, it appears that although the sign language presented to deaf children of hearing parents is relatively simple, they do develop sign.

However, it appears that the style of interaction between child and parent or teacher is of equal importance. Deaf children who experience overcontrolling interactions develop less fluent language and are pragmatically less skilled. These factors should be borne in mind by both educators and professionals leading early intervention programmes.

Peer relationships

Given that most deaf children are now being educated in various mainstream environments, what effect does this have on their relationships with their peers and with adults in their environment? Many will be using a different language to that of their hearing peers, or will have spoken language which is significantly delayed. They are likely to stand out as different.

For many deaf children their first contacts outside the home will be with hearing children and adults. Hearing adults appear to have difficulties initiating and maintaining interactions with deaf preschoolers (Lederberg, 1984). Deaf preschoolers appear to be less socially skilled than their hard-of-hearing and hearing peers (Levy-Schiff and Hoffman, 1985) but it is not clear if the diminished social interaction seen between deaf and hearing children is a consequence of self-selection or peer rejection (Levy-Schiff and Hoffman, 1985; Arnold and Tremblay, 1979)

Kennedy's prospective sociometric study of deaf and hard-of-hearing children in integrated settings suggests that they are popular in their early school careers (Kennedy and Bruininks, 1974). However, as they progress their popularity wanes (Kennedy, Northcott, McCauley and Williams 1976), so that in their third year of school they are significantly less likely to be selected as friends. In adolescence, deaf and hard of hearing children make use of both hearing and deaf peer groups at school (Ladd, Munson and Miller, 1984; Markides, 1989). But this does not extend to friendships and activities out of school (Ladd et al., 1984). Markides' findings suggest that hearing children are extremely unlikely to choose a deaf peer as a friend.

Two factors have been proposed to account for these differences. Firstly, difficulties in communication and secondly, lack of knowledge about deafness. Brackett and Henniges (1976) found that deaf children with good oral skills showed no preference for deaf over hearing children. An intervention designed to increase hearing preschoolers' understanding of deafness led to a decrease in peer interaction (Vandell et al., 1982). It appears that where hearing children and deaf children do form friendships, it is as a result of familiarity developed at home rather than in school. Lederberg, Ryan and Robbins (1986) found that interaction between deaf children and hearing children from home was more similar to that between deaf–deaf dyads than interaction between deaf children and their hearing peers at school. However, this difference was not maintained when the hearing children with deaf friends at home met unfamiliar deaf children. Lederberg et al. suggest that these differences stem from differences in motivation, which in turn stem from the greater familiarity that develops in home-based friendships.

Schools for the deaf provide children with a larger peer group but there are no studies to tell us what use children make of it. Informally, deaf adults often refer to their peers at school as their real brothers and sisters, and Deaf authors cite the residential school as the arena in which children join Deaf society and culture (Higgins, 1987).

Incidental learning and social and psychological delay

Children acquire an understanding of the world in which they live through direct experience or by overseeing and overhearing the experience of others, in other words through incidental learning. The two factors described above, difficulties of communication and interaction within the family and with hearing peers, reduce deaf children's opportunities for incidental learning. What are the consequences for deaf children?

Cognitive development and social maturity: developmental delay or cultural difference

The cognitive development of deaf children has been the subject of much study, partly in the belief that studying deaf children will help us to understand the role that language plays in all children's cognitive and social development. Greenberg and Kusché (1987) summarize the literature in a comprehensive review of deaf children's social and psychological development. They caution that many of the studies that they reviewed were conducted before the extensive introduction of TC into the American educational system and that the groups of children were often not homogeneous. They summarize their findings in a number of areas.

With respect to cognitive development (Greenberg and Kusché, 1987 pp. 108-109) they suggest that deaf children show greater reliance on visual spatial perception and show strengths in holistic, simultaneous visual processing. By contrast, deaf children are weak in the areas of sequential and abstract processing. They highlight the wide range of cognitive skills (e.g. abstraction, memory, problem-solving) that are mediated by language and conclude that deaf children's opportunities to develop skills such as these are limited by language deprivation. They speculate that this may also result in different patterns of brain organization and functioning.

These delays in cognitive development have a significant impact on deaf children's academic achievement. Despite similar abilities when tested using non-verbal measures of intelligence (see Chapter 6), deaf children's reading ability and overall academic achievement is significantly below that of hearing children. This is so for complex problem-solving and reasoning (Greenberg and Kusché, 1987, p. 109).

Greenberg and Kusché (1987 p. 113) suggest that these delays in cognitive development, in combination with communication difficulties, affect deaf children's social development. They confirm earlier findings that deaf children tend to be more impulsive and egocentric than hearing children and that they show delays in social–cognitive abilities such as recognizing emotions and social problem-solving. In addition, they suggest that the self-esteem of deaf children is likely to be adversely affected.

However, they suggest that these delays are susceptible to amelioration. Citing findings from their early intervention study (Greenberg, Kusché and Calderon, 1984) and the PATHS project (see Chapter 12), they describe a range of interventions that benefit deaf children's social development. These include early parent counselling to help families adjust to their deaf child, the introduction of TC as early as possible and teaching social problem-solving skills within school settings. Greenberg (1996) has pointed out that two aspects of communication need to be borne in mind when implementing these interventions. Firstly, that deaf children of hearing parents have little experience of language as a means of communic-ating, and so regulating oneself. Hearing children experience adults talking to themselves from an early age, whilst they undertake difficult tasks or calm themselves down when emotionally aroused. Deaf children only see people talking to each other, unless hearing teachers and parents deliberately sign to themselves. Secondly, hearing people working with deaf children frequently adjust their language use down to the deaf child's level to ensure that they understand everything that is said to them, unlike hearing children with whom adults frequently use language that they have to struggle to understand. Greenberg (1996) cites a personal experience when he used 'sad' when he really meant 'disappointed' to describe an able deaf child's experience of trying but failing in a test situation. This linguistic overprotection constrains deaf children's social and emotional development.

Psychiatric disorders in deaf children

The epidemiology of psychiatric disorder in deaf children

There have been a number of studies of psychiatric disorder in deaf and hard-of-hearing children and adolescents (see Table 3.1). Four studies have used control groups (Rutter et al., 1970; Fundudis et al., 1979; Sinkkonen, 1994) or comparison groups (Schlesinger and Meadow. 1972). All of these studies, except the most recent, suggested that rates of disorder were higher in deaf children than in hearing children, with rates ranging from 15.4% to 60%, two to five times that seen in the comparison groups. In contrast, Sinkkonen (1994) studied all Finnish deaf and hard-of-hearing children, using a modified version of the Rutter B scale and a comparison group of hearing children. He found no significant increase in the rate of disorder in the deaf and hard-of-hearing children.

Three sets of mechanisms are likely to contribute to the differing findings. Firstly, there were differences in the methods of ascertainment, sizes and other characteristics of the populations studied. Secondly, different rating instruments were used (see Table 3.2) and prevalence rates were calculated in different ways. Thirdly, there have been significant changes in deaf children's education over the 30 years spanned by these studies.

The studies used two different methods to ascertain their populations of deaf children. Some studies used either whole populations of children (Rutter et al., 1970) or whole populations of deaf children (Freeman et al., 1975). The other studies used populations of deaf children attending school. It is likely that most profoundly deaf children will be known to

Table 3.1 Prevalence of psychiatric disorders in hearing-impaired children and adolescents and hearing control subjects

Study	Number of HI Children	Range of HI	Prevalence of disorder (%) HI Group	Control subjects
Rutter, Graham and Yule (1970)	13	moderate–profound	15.4	6.6
Schlesinger and Meadow (1972)	512	severe – profound	31.2	9.7
Freeman, Malkin and Hastings (1975)	120	severe–profound	22.0	–
Fundudis, Kolvin and Garside (1979)	54	moderate –profound	deaf: 54 H/H : 28	18
Aplin (1985)	61	profound	36.1	–
Aplin (1987)	42	mild – profound	16.6	–
Hindley, Hill, McGuigan and Kitson (1994)	81	moderate–profound	deaf: 41.3 H/H : 60	–
Sinkkonen (1994)*	294	funct. def.	deaf: 18.7 H/H : 25.3 HIMH: 42.4	15.8

HI =hearing impaired, deaf: severe to profound, early onset hearing impairment.
H/H (hard of hearing): moderate to profound acquired hearing impairment.
HIMH: hearing impaired (deaf and H/H) with additional handicaps
* Sinkkonen used a functional definition of deaf and hard of hearing

Table 3.2 Psychiatric rating scales in prevalence studies

Study	Teacher scale	Parent scale	Parent interview	Child interview
Sinkkonen (1994)	√			
Aplin (1985/87)	√			
Schlesinger and Meadow (1972)	√			
Fundudis et al. (1979)	√	√	√	
Freeman et al. (1975)*	√	√	√	
Hindley et al. (1993)	√	√	√	√

* Freeman et al. included an observation of the child but did not interview the child.

educational authorities, barring the handful of deaf children and adolescents who are out of school because of major behaviour problems, but this is less likely for children with mild–to–moderate hearing impairment, some of whom may be unknown to educational services.

The children in these studies varied in age. Some studies (Rutter et al., Schlesinger and Meadow, Freeman et al., Aplin and Sinkkonen) included all children from ages 5 to 16 years. Fundudis et al. studied children from ages 5 to 11 and Hindley et al. children and young people aged 11 to 16 years. Freeman et al.'s findings suggest that younger children are more susceptible to psychiatric disorder but this is not confirmed by Aplin's studies.

The children in these studies had varying degrees of hearing impairment. Some studies included only deaf children (Schlesinger and Meadow, 1972 and Freeman et al., 1975) whilst others included deaf children, and children with mild and/or moderate hearing impairments (Fundudis et al., 1979; Aplin, 1985/87; Hindley et al., 1994 and Sinkkonen, 1994). Hindley et al. and Aplin suggest that degree of hearing impairment alone is not a significant factor in the aetiology of psychiatric disorder. Fundudis et al. suggest that deaf children are at greater risk of developing psychiatric disorder than children with less severe hearing impairment, whilst Sinkkonen's findings suggest that hard-of-hearing children may be at greater risk. However, two factors, apart from communication, may indirectly account for these inconsistent findings. Firstly, differences in school setting (see below) and, secondly, differences in the rates of additional impairments which in themselves are a significant risk factor (see Chapter 6).

Finally, these various studies have taken place over almost 30 years and over this period of time educational practice has changed significantly. Sinkkonen's (1994) study shows the most striking change. He compared parents' communication with their children with a study carried out in 1978. In 1978 only 23% of hearing mothers and 9% of hearing fathers had any sign language skills and sign language was the main mode of communication in only 4% of families (Sinkkonen, 1994 p.95). In 1994 all mothers and 94% of fathers had sign language skills and sign language was used in every family in the 80% who returned their questionnaires.

A variety of rating instruments were used in these studies. All but one used scales developed in hearing populations and suitably adapted. However, speech-related items in some scales made them unreliable (Fundudis et al., 1979 and Prior, Glazner, Sanson and Debelle, 1988). Hindley et al. (1994) developed teacher and parent scales to screen for psychiatric disorder in deaf children but psychiatric ratings were based on interviews with parents and children, using a BSL interpreter with the deaf children. Studies using teacher or parent questionnaires found a preponderance of conduct disorders (Fundudis et al., 1979; Aplin, 1985) but when children were interviewed there was a preponderance of anxiety disorders. However, although Hindley et al. (1994) interviewed all children who had screened positive for psychiatric disorders they interviewed only a proportion of children screened negative and an adjusted prevalence rate was calculated using a pre-established false negative rate. In contrast, Freeman et al. (1975) interviewed all parents and so were able to calculate a true prevalence rate.

Risk factors

Degree of deafness alone does not appear to be an important risk factor in psychiatric disorder in deaf children. There has been considerable interest in the role of impaired communication in the genesis of psychiatric disorders. Some authors have asserted that lack of communication accounts for much of the disorder seen in deaf children (Lesser and Easer, 1972; Schlesinger and Meadow, 1972; Stokoe and Battison, 1975). This can be understood in relation to distortions of parent–child interaction and deprivation of social experiences (Feinstein, 1983). Rainer (1976) suggested that the absence of the anxiety-reducing effects of the mother's voice may also account for increased personality difficulties in deaf adolescents and adults. Sinkkonen's study (1994) shows the most convincing link between psychopathology and communication in two ways. Firstly, poor communication in the child was a significant risk factor for children with and without additional impairments. Secondly, changes in family communication appear to be associated with a decreasing rate of psychiatric disorder in the population of deaf children.

In Chapter 1 Meadow-Orlans and Erting have described the key role of deaf schools in the Deaf community. Difficulties in peer relationships in integrated settings suggest that school should be an important factor in the genesis of psychiatric disorder. However, attempts to study the effects of different school settings are difficult to interpret. School placement is dictated by a number of factors, some of which are likely to affect rates of psychiatric disorder (Fundudis et al., 1979). Thus children with additional impairments and children with behavioural problems are more likely to go to deaf schools.

To date, findings about the effects of school placement are inconsistent. Hindley et al. (1994) found lower rates of disorder amongst children attending a deaf school. In contrast both Fundudis et al. (1979) and Aplin (1985;1987) found increased rates of disorder amongst children attending deaf schools against those attending units for the hearing impaired or in integrated settings. However, neither of these studies involved interviews with the children. At interview the hard-of-hearing children in the study by Hindley et al. reported more unsatisfactory school experiences, had fewer friends and had poorer self–images. All these factors were significantly related to psychiatric disorder. Anecdotally, the hard-of-hearing children reported much higher rates of stigmatization and victimization. Recent studies of bullying in mainstream schools suggest that up to 70% of deaf children experience serious bullying (Smith and Sharp, 1994) but growing awareness of bullying has led people to realize that severe bullying can also occur in deaf schools (Lewis, 1995).

Just as in studies of hearing children, in deaf children IQ score is inversely related to risk of psychiatric disorder (Williams, 1970; Schlesinger and Meadow, 1972; Aplin, 1985). In a similar vein, certain aetiological groups seem to be at risk. The most extensively studied group are children with congenital rubella syndrome (Vernon, 1967; Chess, Korn and Fernandez, 1971; Chess and Fernandez, 1980; Desmond et al., 1978). In addition to increased rates of impulsivity and attention difficulties, the rate of autism seems to be higher, particularly amongst the deaf–blind group (Chess et al., 1971). Vernon (1967) suggests that there are increased rates of central language disorder in children with congenital rubella. However, although standardized instruments to assess sign language are now available (Woll and Herman 1996; Newport et al., 1996) the widely varying linguistic environments of deaf children make the assessment of language disorder extremely difficult.

In clinical practice family interaction seems to be a key feature. In a clinical sample of 130 deaf children, almost 50% were described as marginalized and scapegoats within their families (Hindley, 1994) and a further 25% had experienced either physical or sexual abuse (see Chapter 7). A typical example of these difficulties would be Sophie:

> Sophie was a 13-year-old deaf girl who was referred by her school because of extreme attention-seeking behaviour and poor peer relationships. Assessment revealed that she had experienced serious neglect during early childhood and from 8 years of age had been involved in sexual abuse initiated by her father. Once sexualized, her mother had encouraged Sophie to have sexual relationships with various men in the neighbourhood. Child protection proceedings led to Sophie's removal from her family. A period of individual psychotherapy led to an improvement in Sophie's self-esteem and peer relationships but she remained highly vulnerable to sexual exploitation.

Referral and assessment

Many deaf children with emotional and behavioural problems will not be referred to services for hearing children. Referrals to specialist services are more likely to come from agencies in the Deaf world than through GPs or other medical sources. In a study of all the children referred to a specialist service (the Deaf Child and Family Team, National Deaf Services) over 70% of referrals came from either social services for deaf people or schools and other educational services (Hindley, 1994).

Language usage is the single factor most likely to determine whether referral to specialist services for deaf children is needed. Almost 80% of children referred to the Deaf Child and Family Team (DCFT) used sign language – either British Sign Language (BSL) or Sign Supported English (SSE) – (Hindley, 1994) and amongst the other 20% we have become used to meeting deaf children referred from oral schools whose language choice is clearly sign – when they are given the choice. Because many families of deaf children have limited or no understanding of sign, an interpreter is routinely included in assessments (see Chapters 13 and 15).

In the DCFT interpreters play a dual role, interpreting for the child and family and for Deaf and hearing members of the team. This can create a dilemma for the interpreter – at which level should he interpret and to what extent should he interrupt the assessment if he feels the child is not understanding the interpretation. In addition, for many deaf children attendance at a mental health assessment may be their first experience of meeting an interpreter. The child will need direct explanation of how an interpreter works and the interpreter will need time to gain an idea of the linguistic level at which the child is operating. At times this arrangement can create clumsy and stilted assessments but close and regular work with a limited number of interpreters diminishes these problems.

A general child psychiatrist undertaking an assessment of a Deaf child, is strongly advised to work with an interpreter. Both clinician and interpreter will have to adapt, primarily because the clinician will find that the interpreter becomes their ears and eyes, especially when assessing non-verbal communication and interaction (Hoyt, Siegelman and Schlesinger, 1981; Hindley, 1993). The interpreter will need to consult with the clinician prior to and after the assessment and this may conflict with his professional and ethical position as a neutral facilitator of communication (Stansfield and Veltri, 1987). If the clinician has a limited knowledge of sign but undertakes the assessment alone he or she should do so with caution. Well intentioned attempts to engage the child may well colour the interaction. This can lead to the clinician missing important non–verbal cues and prevent the child from disclosing painful feelings and experiences (Hindley, Hill and Bond, 1993).

Oral/aural children may well manage without an interpreter, but some benefit from a speech reader/communicator. Given the experience of the

DCFT, it would make sense to engage an interpreter if seeing a child from an oral/aural school. Many younger children and multi-handicapped children may not have sufficient language to take part in an interview, and direct observations at home and in school will then be essential.

Residential schools are often where deaf children begin to develop their Deaf cultural identity. For children attending residential schools, close liaison with teaching and care staff is essential. However, many parents find it understandably disturbing to send their children away from home. Envy and jealous feelings can develop between parents and school staff. For some parents these feelings are compounded by the ease with which children and staff communicate. Equally, staff members may see themselves as more competent and caring than parents. The nature of these relationships adds to the importance of involving parents in any psychiatric consultation, except in exceptional circumstances. For Deaf parents, consideration needs to be given to their earlier experience of hearing professionals. Deaf parents may see such people as interfering and intrusive, attempting to dominate and control by providing counselling rather than information (Erting, 1987). A Deaf mental health worker can provide vital insights in all these areas.

Two aspects of mental state assessment can be particularly difficult with Deaf children. Inexperienced clinicians may find it difficult to distinguish written sign language from thought-disordered writing (Evans and Elliot, 1981; Kitson and Fry, 1990). Even the experienced can find it difficult to distinguish idiosyncratic sign from thought-disordered sign. Again, a Deaf colleague can be helpful. Assessment of mood and affect can also pose problems. How can one distinguish between narrative-related changes of affect and true affect? Developmental studies suggest that the shape of the mood contour can help to make the distinction (Snitzer Reilly et al., 1989). Abrupt changes in affect are associated with narrative-related mood, whereas true mood changes more smoothly (Kitson, 1991).

Finally, a central part of the assessment is an attempt by the clinician to understand how the deaf child and his or her family feel about the deafness. The presence of a deaf child can have a profound influence on the family but this will change as the family develops (Harvey, 1989). For the child, parental and societal attitudes will affect his or her self-image. He or she may see the deafness as unimportant, and may see him or herself as a proud member of the Deaf community, or as an impaired individual and his or her deafness as a source of shame (Hindley et al., 1993).

Diagnostic issues

Language and communication are central to any assessment of a child with psychiatric problems. What effect do differences in communication have on the presentation of disorders in deaf children? Overall, the pattern of problems seen by the DCFT appears similar to the pattern of problems seen in a general child psychiatry outpatient service (Hindley, 1994). Just over half of the children presented with either conduct disorders or mixed disorders of emotion and conduct and approximately 15 % presented with emotional disorders. The only exception was a significantly larger number of children with autism (10%) than one might expect. However, some problems seem to occur particularly frequently and other problems are difficult to assess, primarily because of communication differences.

Behaviour disorders associated with limited family communication

Limited communication between the deaf child and his or her family can lead to distortions of social and psychological development (see above) and particular patterns of behaviour. However, early intervention can alter these patterns:

> Tony was a 4-year-old boy referred because of severe behavioural problems at home and in school. He was being educated in an oral unit and his mother had limited signing skills. He had witnessed severe marital violence. Assessment revealed a warm, affectionate boy, whose mother displayed great affection but limited understanding as to how to communicate with him, and had difficulties in maintaining behavioural boundaries. Video feedback of her communication with Tony helped her realize that she frequently talked and signed without his visual attention and the use of the Parent Child Game (Forehand and McMahon, 1981) helped her alter her parenting style. Tony was transferred to a TC unit and his communication and behaviour improved significantly over six months.

By contrast, when these patterns become embedded they can take long periods of intensive treatment to change:

> Jim was a 12-year-old deaf boy. He was referred with a history of aggressive and defiant behaviour dating back to his early childhood, leading to permanent exclusion from school. He had been educated in an oral unit until age 7 when he had abruptly transferred to a residential TC school. His parents had limited or no signing skills and minor altercations rapidly escalated into physical violence. Jim's impulse control was extremely poor, as was his self-image and peer relationships. His treatment included inpatient, outpatient family therapy and psychotherapy. Over three years he was able to return to fulltime schooling. His relationships with his family are still strained and he blows up when under major stress but is now being considered for Further Education college.

Hyperkinetic disorder

Difficulties in attending and maintaining attention are a central feature of hyperkinetic disorder and attention deficit hyperactivity disorder (ADHD). Associated features include marked overactivity, restlessness and impulsivity. These difficulties are thought to reflect a combination of a CNS disorder which is often compounded by adults in the child's environment selectively attending to the difficult behaviour that children with hyperkinesis display. The cognitive processes that underpin children's ability to sustain attention are verbally mediated. Self-talk, in hearing children, emerges at 3–4 years of age and allows children to monitor themselves and begin to develop control over their behaviour. Given that many deaf children will have marked delays in language development, there appears to be a risk that hyperkinesis will be diagnosed when much of the child's behaviour might be better understood in the context of his or her abnormal language environment. Yet, many of the risk factors associated with deafness are also associated with hyperkinesis. In their study of students at a residential school for deaf children, Kelly et al. (1993) found that children with non-genetic causes of deafness were significantly more likely to score above the cut-off point on a hyperactivity scale (Conner's Parent Rating Scale) than children with genetic causes of deafness.

> Paul was a 6-year-old child referred because of markedly disruptive behaviour at home and in school. He had been permanently withdrawn within his mainstream school, spending all his time with one adult. Paul was eventually expelled. He had witnessed considerable marital violence and his sexualized play suggested that he had been exposed to inappropriate sexual experiences. At home his mother used little sign language and Paul's sign was limited to a total of 20 signs, despite being of normal intelligence. Paul transferred to a residential school for deaf children, his sign language began to develop rapidly and his behaviour slowly improved. He became less aggressive, related better to his peers but remained overactive and had great difficulty in attending for any longer than a few minutes, finding multiple sources of distraction within the classroom. The diagnosis of hyperactivity was made and he was treated with methylphenidate, leading to a significant reduction in overactivity and improved academic achievement, communication and peer relationships. He still showed intermittently destructive and defiant behaviour.

Depression and affective disorders

Depression and bipolar affective disease appear to present in similar ways but predisposing factors may be different and additional impairments can create difficulties in making a diagnosis.

> Mina had been deafened at 9 years of age when her moderate hearing loss deteriorated. She had transferred to a TC deaf school at age 11 and found sign helpful and enjoyed the company of Deaf peers. Her parents were high caste Hindus and greatly valued Mina's ability to use her voice and disliked Deaf cultural values. Mina was caught between two worlds and became severely depressed, with marked suicidal and self-denigratory thoughts. She was assessed as an emergency and treated with antidepressants, individual psychotherapy and family meetings. Although her family attitudes towards Mina's deafness did not alter, Mina recovered from her depression and was able to come to an accommodation by being Deaf with her peers and Hearing with her family.

Jerome, a 15-year-old boy, presented with periods of disturbed behaviour when he became overactive, easily distressed and preoccupied with his grandfather's death. His sleep was disturbed and his sign language production speeded up and became disordered. He had additional learning difficulties. In between these periods he was a cheerful and friendly young man. A diagnosis of rapid cycling bipolar affective disorder was made. He was treated initially with chlorpromazine but this led to a deterioration in his behaviour. Antidepressants were started but he remitted spontaneously. At his second episode he was treated with haloperidol and carbamazepine. Although haloperidol led to reduction in his overactivity, prolonged treatment with carbamazepine seemed to lead to a further deterioration. Finally he was commenced on lithium, leading to a sustained improvement.

Psychotic disorders

The assessment of functional psychoses (see Chapter 4) can be particularly difficult because of communication difficulties, but schizophrenia can present in a dramatic fashion:

Jasmine was an 11-year-old girl of Asian background who presented with marked anxiety, with a deterioration in academic achievement and social withdrawal. Her signed communication consisted of unconnected signs and examination of her written work revealed a progressive deterioration in her ability to link concepts, finally ending in written 'word salad'. She was able to sustain unusual postures for periods of hours and she showed marked social withdrawal. A diagnosis of early-onset schizophrenia was made and she responded well to pimozide.

Autism

Accurate assessments of children who are both deaf and autistic can be very difficult. Juré, Rapin and Tuchman (1991) describe a series of 46 children with both deafness and autism. For many, the diagnosis of either their deafness or their autism had been considerably delayed. There were seven autistic children whose deafness was not confirmed until they were 5 years old or more, and 16 deaf children whose autism was not diagnosed until they were 5 years old or more. Juré et al. found a high rate of hard and soft neurological signs in their group and a high rate of dysmorphic features. Our experience is that the developmental histories of deaf children with autism are similar to those of hearing autistic children, apart from their language development. Just as with hearing autistic children, social aloofness and disinterest, marked delays in the development of play and rituals and stereotypes set deaf autistic children apart from deaf children.

At face value it might seem that a deaf child with autism would face a greater challenge than a hearing child with autism in developing useful language. A child who avoids eye contact will surely have great difficulty in acquiring a visuospatial language. Our clinical experience does not support this. Deaf children with autism who are placed in environments that use sign language, are able to respond to the child's communicative intent, and manage inappropriate behaviour effectively, allow children to develop usable language. This can have a dramatic effect on their social skills:

> Geoff was a 6-year-old deaf child referred because of marked learning difficulties and challenging behaviour. He was physically aggressive and self-injuring. He showed no interest in other children in his class, was perseverative in his activities, preoccupied with flashing lights and twiddling small pieces of paper. He showed no imaginative play. Geoff's developmental history revealed gaze avoidance and social disinterest dating back to his first year. He appeared to have no functional language, apart from sign echolalia. Geoff transferred to a regional resource residential school for deaf children, initially joining the multi-handicapped class. Within six months he was signing two sign phrases, his social interaction had improved and he had changed classes, integrating with the mainstream classroom. His social interaction remained unusual and his signing could still be echolalic. He did not develop imaginative play.

Juré et al. (1991) point out that school placement for these children is often very difficult but they also found that deaf autistic children who were placed in signing environments with good behaviour management made significant improvements in their language and social functioning. Woll (1995) suggests that this is because eye gaze is used in a very clearly defined way in BSL and other signed languages and so removes the ambiguity of social eye gaze that autistic children find so confusing.

Intervention

Each child and family will need an intervention tailored to suit their unique set of circumstances. However, in most countries specialist services for deaf children cover large geographical areas, apart from Holland where a well co-ordinated range of outpatient services exist in a number of regions, served by an inpatient unit (Hoetink et al., 1994; van Gent and Hilberink, 1994). At the DCFT assessment and advice is offered to local services for approximately 25% of the children seen (Hindley, 1994). Consultation to schools (Hindley 1994) and other agencies is also offered, partly to provide early intervention and partly as means of serving a larger number of children.

Other chapters in this book will touch on cognitive behavioural therapy, psychotherapy and family therapy. As with deaf adults, linguistic competence, cultural awareness and a willingness to use visual means of communication and visual metaphors are vital in using psychological treatments with deaf children. These skills all come more easily to Deaf professionals.

> A teenage deaf girl with a very disturbed family background approached the Deaf tutor in her school. She had all sorts of terrible feelings about herself and didn't get on with her peers. She had been offered counselling but couldn't understand why. The Deaf tutor drew a picture of the girl, pointed at it and asked her where she came from. The girl looked puzzled and was at a loss to answer the tutor's question. The tutor drew another picture of a tree without roots; she pointed to it and asked the girl where the tree came from. Again the girl looked puzzled. The tutor drew in the roots and then showed the girl that her roots lay in her past. The girl suddenly understood what the tutor was explaining to her.
>
> (My thanks to Wendy Daunt for telling me this story)

Members of the DCFT conducting individual psychotherapy frequently turn to role play and re-enactment as means of engaging deaf children. Feinstein and Lytle (1987) show how differing communication abilities within a children's psychotherapy group can affect the group process.

Inpatient facilities

There is a distinct paucity of inpatient services for deaf children. The inpatient unit in Holland (Hoetink et al., 1994) uses a highly structured programme based on social skills training, with additional support from a child psychotherapist and family therapists. As yet they have no Deaf staff.

Burnes, Seabolt and Vreeland (1992) outline a residential programme for Deaf children with emotional and behavioural problems built around a cultural model of Deafness. At least half the staff are Deaf and ASL is the language of the community. The programme is highly structured using a combination of therapeutic approaches – particularly group, behaviour management, social skills and family therapy. The co-ordinated educational approach emphasizes ASL and English literacy skills through ASL.

In the main, deaf children and adolescents are admitted to inpatient units for hearing children and attempts are made to support them. McCune (1988) describes two such admissions and the additional support that was required. This included teaching sign language to staff and children, and deaf awareness training from local social services for deaf people. However, none of the staff had any previous experience of deaf children. Our experience is similar but we have been able to augment the staff groups with nursing staff who work in an adult unit for Deaf people and so have sign language skills and are Deaf aware. However, this has only given the deaf children limited access to the therapeutic milieu.

Mental health aspects of cochlear implants

Cochlear implants are electronic assistive hearing devices which process sound and deliver an electronically amplified signal directly to the acoustic nerve, unlike acoustic hearing aids which amplify sound to the ear. They have been demonstrated to be effective in helping postlingually deafened adults and children to hear speech but their effectiveness in prelingually deaf and perilingually deafened children and adults is unclear. Their use with deaf children is particularly controversial and has provoked fierce criticism from Deaf communities across the world. Mental health professionals have been involved in cochlear implant programmes in three ways:

- in highlighting the ethical dilemmas that surround their use (Power and Hyde, 1992 ; Vernon and Alles, 1994)
- in helping to identify the psychological characteristics of children and their families, and processes that help to identify those children most likely to gain from a cochlear implant (Quittner and Thompson, 1991; Kampfe et al., 1993)
- identifying the psychosocial consequences for the child's family but not for the child, to date (Downs et al., 1986; Quittner et al., 1991).

The ethical dilemmas are, firstly, that cochlear implants are of doubtful or unproven benefit in prelingually and perilingually deaf children; that encouraging parents to seek cochlear implantation serves to delay acceptance of deafness and the learning of sign language; that national organizations of deaf people have not been involved in decisions about the licensing of cochlear implants; and that it is unethical to submit children to irreversible, potentially life threatening surgery when its benefits are unproven (Anon., 1990). In contrast, advocates of cochlear programmes argue that any improvement in deaf children's ability to perceive sound, and so speech, is of benefit to them (Moog and Geers, 1991). In turn, critics point out that studies of the audiological, linguistic and psychosocial effects of cochlear implants are carried out almost exclusively by members of cochlear implant teams (Vernon and Alles, 1994). Those that are conducted by independent investigators suggest that the benefits offered by implants over conventional hearing aids are at best slight (Allen, Rawlings and Remington, 1993). Finally, they argue that the large amounts of money invested in implant programmes might be better spent on ensuring that appropriate conventional support – sign language tuition for families, acoustic or vibrotactile hearing aids, etc. – is offered to all children and families (Power and Hyde, 1992; Vernon and Alles, 1994).

As with the initial confirmation of deafness, assessment for implantation stirs up powerful feelings. Persistent difficulty in accepting a child's deafness may lead to inappropriate expectations about the benefits of a cochlear implant (Kampfe et al., 1993) and in turn intensify parental distress post-implantation (Quittner and Thompson Steck, 1991). Checklists of parental expectations may help professionals to identify parents with unrealistically high expectations and the provision of education and guidance about the effects of an implant, and counselling for parents can help to ensure that the parents of children entering an implant programme have as clear expectations as possible (Kampfe et al., 1993).

Educational and audiological support post-implantation are vital and are taxing for both child and family, as is the commitment and motivation of the child and family. It remains unclear whether the benefits seen with cochlear implants are primarily as a result of this level of commitment or the implants themselves (Vernon and Alles, 1994). It does appear that family stress and parental distress are no less for parents of children with implants than for families with deaf children generally (Quittner et al., 1991). However, the number of children in this study was small (n=29), the control population is not described and normative data from an unrelated study were used for at least one of their measures (the Impact of Childhood Hearing Loss). Quittner and Thompson Steck (1991) point out that to date no study has been conducted to examine the stress experienced by the children themselves nor of their psychosocial adjustment.

Conclusions

Deaf children and adolescents and their families offer a unique challenge to mental health professionals. In order to work effectively they must bridge the gap between the world of the deaf child and, for most deaf children, the world of his or her hearing family. They must work in families where there will often be substantial differences in communication and language use; where the growing child is entering a culture unfamiliar to his or her parents; and where many parents continue to experience real pain at the thought of having a deaf child. At the same time they must bear in mind the various additional impairments that deaf children may experience and how these will affect their development and presentation. Mental health professionals will also have to develop links with the wide variety of different professionals that deaf children will encounter in their lives, amongst whom controversy and disagreement about the needs of deaf children still occurs.

In order to accomplish this, services for deaf children and adolescents should contain these differences. That is, by an active policy of recruiting Deaf staff, multidisciplinary teams can reflect and understand the dilemmas that face deaf children and their families and so help to achieve resolution and growth. This should also apply to inpatient facilities. At present the UK lacks such facilities. If they are established they must surely aim to create a genuinely Deaf therapeutic milieu, with Deaf and hearing staff working together to meet the complex needs of deaf children, adolescents and their families.

References:

Ainsworth MDS, Bell SM (1970) Attachment, exploration and separation: illustrated by the behaviour of 1-year-olds in a strange situation. Child Development 41: 49–67.

Ainsworth MDS, Blehart MC, Waters E, Wall S (1978) Patterns of Attachment: a physiological study of the Strange Situation. Hillsdale, NJ: Erlbaum.

Allen T, Rawlings B, Remington E (1993) Demographic and audiological profiles of deaf children in Texas with cochlear implants. American Annals of the Deaf 138: 260–266.

Anon. (1990) Cochlear Implants in Children. Position Paper of the National Association of the Deaf (844, Thayer Ave. Silver Spring, MD, USA).

American Psychiatric Association (1994) Diagnostic and Statistical Manual of mental disorders: DSM-IV – 4th Ed. Washington DC: American Psychiatric Association.

Angold A (1994) Clinical Interviewing with Children and Adolescents. In Rutter M, Taylor E, Hersov L (eds) Modern Approaches to Child and Adolescent Psychiatry, third edition. Oxford: Blackwell Scientific.

Aplin DY (1985) Social and emotional adjustment of hearing–impaired children in special schools. Journal of the British Association of Teachers of the Deaf 9: 84–94.

Aplin DY (1987) Social and emotional adjustment of hearing–impaired children in ordinary and special schools. Educational Research Volume 29: 56–64.

Arnold D, Tremblay A (1979) Interaction of Deaf and Hearing Preschool Children. Journal of Communication Disorders 12: 245–251.

Balow IH, Brill RG (1972) An evaluation study of reading and academic achievement levels of 16 graduating classes of the California School for the Deaf, Riverside, California. Mimeo report, Contract # 4566 with the State of California, Department of Education.

Bonvillian JD, Folven RJ (1993) Sign language acquisition: developmental aspects. In Marschark M, Clark MD(eds) Psychological Perspectives on Deafness. London: Lawrence Erlbaum Associates.

Bracket D, Henniges M (1976) Communicative interaction of preschool hearing-impaired children in an integrated setting. Volta Review 78: 276–285.

Braden JP (1994) Deafness, Deprivation and IQ. New York: Plenum Press.

Burnes S, Seabolt D, Vreeland J (1992) Deaf culturally affirmative programming for children with emotional and behavioral problems. Journal of the American Deafness and Rehabilitation Association 26: 12–17.

Caselli C, Volterra V (1989) From communication to language in hearing and deaf children. In Volterra V, Erting CJ (eds) From Gesture to Language in Hearing and Deaf Children. New York: Springer-Verlag.

Chess S, Fernandez P (1980) Do deaf children have a typical personality? Journal of the American Academy of Child Psychiatry 19: 654–664.

Chess S, Korn SJ, Fernandez PB (1971) Psychiatric Disorders of Children with Congenital Rubella. New York: Brunner Mazel.

Cohn J, Tronick EZ (1983) Three month-old infants' reaction to simulated maternal depression. Child Development 54: 185–193.

Cole S, Edelman RJ (1991) Identity patterns and self- and teacher-perceptions of problems of deaf adolescents: a research note. Journal of Child Psychology and Psychiatry 32: 1159–1166.

Cox A (1994) Interviews with parents. In Rutter M, Taylor E, Hersov L (eds) Modern Approaches to Child and Adolescent Psychiatry, third edition. Oxford: Blackwell Scientific.

Desmond MM, Fisher ES, Vorderman AL, Schaffer HG, Andrew LP, Zion TE, Catlin FI (1978) The longitudinal course of congenital rubella encephalitis in non-retarded children. Journal of Pediatrics 93: 584–591.

Downs MP, Campos CT, Firemark R, Martin E, Myers W (1986) Psychosocial issues surrounding children receiving cochlear implants. Seminars in Hearing 7: 375–381.

Erting CJ (1987) Cultural conflict in a school for deaf children. In Higgins PC, Nash JE (eds) Understanding Deafness Socially. Springfield, IL: Charles C Thomas.

Erting CJ, Prezioso C, O'Grady Hynes M (1989) The interaction context of deaf mother–infant communication. In Volterra V, Erting CJ (eds) From Gesture to Language in Hearing and Deaf Children. Berlin: Springer-Verlag.

Evans JW, Elliot H (1981) Screening criteria for the diagnosis of schizophrenia in deaf patients. Archives of General Psychiatry 36: 787–790.

Feinstein CB (1983) Early adolescent deaf boys: a biopsychosocial approach. Adolescent Psychiatry 11: 147–162.

Feinstein CB, Lytle R (1987) Observations from clinical work with high school aged, deaf adolescents attending a residential school. Adolescent Psychiatry: Developmental and Clinical Studies 14: 461–477.

Forehand R, McMahon RJ (1981) Helping the Noncompliant Child: a clinician's guide to effective parent training. New York: Guilford Press.

Freeman RD, Malkin SF, Hastings JO (1975) Psychosocial problems of deaf children and their families: a comparative study. American Annals of the Deaf 120: 275–304.

Freud A (1946) The Psychoanalytic Treatment of Children. New York: International Universities Press.

Fundudis T, Kolvin I, Garside R (1979) Speech Retarded and Deaf Children: their psychosocial development. London: Academic Press.

Galenson EM, Miller R, Kaplan E, Rothstein A (1979) Assessment of development in the deaf child. Journal of the American Academy of Child Psychiatry 18: 128–142.

Goldin–Meadow S, Mylander C (1984) Gestural Communication in Deaf Children: the Effects and Noneffects of Parental Input on Early Language Development. Monographs of the Society for Research in Child Development. Serial no. 207 vol 49.

Goodman R (1994) Brain disorders. In Rutter M, Taylor E, Hersov L (eds) Modern Approaches to Child and Adolescent Psychiatry, third edition. Oxford: Blackwell Scientific.

Greenberg MT (1996) Personal communication.

Greenberg MT, Calderon R, Kusché CA (1984) Early intervention using simultaneous communication with deaf infants. The effect on communication development. Child Development 55: 607–616.

Greenberg MT, Kusché CA (1987) Cognitive, personal and social development of deaf children and adolescents. In Wang M, Reynolds M (eds) Handbook of Special Education: Research and Practice. Oxford: Pergamon Press.

Greenberg MT, Marvin RS (1979) Patterns of attachment in profoundly deaf preschool children. Merrill–Palmer Quarterly 25: 265–279.

Gregory S (1976) The Deaf Child and His Family. London: George Allen and Unwin.

Gregory S, Barlow S (1986) Interaction between deaf babies and their deaf and hearing mothers. Paper presented to the Language Development and Sign Language Workshop, Bristol.

Gregory S, Bishop J, Sheldon L (1995) Deaf People and their Families: Developing Understanding. Cambridge: Cambridge University Press.

Gregory S, Mogford K (1982) The development of symbolic play in young deaf children. In Rogers DR, Sloboda J (eds) The Acquisition of Symbolic Skills. London: Plenum Press.

Hall DMB (1989) Health for all children: a programme for child health surveillance; the report of the Joint Working Party on Child Health Surveillance. Oxford: Oxford University Press.

Harris M (1992) Language Experience and Early Language Development: From Input to Uptake. Hillsdale NJ: Lawrence Erlbaum Associates.

Harvey MA (1989) Psychotherapy with Deaf and Hard-of-Hearing Persons: A Systemic Model. Hillsdale NJ: Lawrence Erlbaum.

Heiling K (1995) The Development of Deaf Children:academic achievement levels and social processes. Hamburg: Signum.

Higgins PC (1987) Understanding Deafness Socially. Springfield, IL: Charles Thomas.

Hindley PA (1991) Signs of Feeling: a prevalence study of psychiatric disorder in deaf and partially hearing children and adolescents. London: Royal National Institute for the Deaf Research Report.

Hindley PA (1994) The Deaf Child and Family Team. Paper presented at the 3rd Congress of the European Society for Mental Health and Deafness, Paris, December 14–16.

Hindley PA (1997) Research review: psychiatric aspects of hearing impairment. Journal of Child Psychology and Psychiatry 38: 101–117.

Hindley PA, Hill PD and Bond D (1993) Interviewing deaf children, the interviewer effect. Journal of Child Psychology and Psychiatry 34: 1461–1468.

Hindley PA, Hill PD, McGuigan S, Kitson N (1994) Psychiatric disorder in deaf and hearing-impaired children and young people: a prevalence study. Journal of Child Psychiatry 35: 917–934.

Hoetink G, van Olst M, van Duyn W, Hilberink I (1994) Working with programmed activities in a child psychiatric inpatient unit. Paper presented at the 3rd Congress of the European Society for Mental Health and Deafness, Paris, December 14–16.

Hoyt MF, Siegelman EY, Schlesinger HS (1981) Special issues regarding psychotherapy with the deaf. American Journal of Psychiatry 138, 6, 807–811.

Jenkins H (1994) Family Interviewing: Issues of Theory and Practice. In Rutter M, Taylor E, Hersov L (eds) Modern Approaches to Child and Adolescent Psychiatry, third edition. Oxford: Blackwell Scientific.

Johnson R, Liddell S, Erting C (1989) Unlocking the curriculum: Principles for achieving access in deaf education. Gallaudet Research Institute Working Paper 89–8, Washington, DC: Gallaudet Research Institute.

Jordan IK, Karchmer MA (1986) Patterns of sign use among hearing impaired students. In Schildroth AN, Karchmer MA(eds), Deaf Children in America. San Diego, CA: College Hill Press.

Juré R, Rapin I, Tuchman RF (1991) Hearing impaired autistic children. Developmental Medicine and Child Neurology 33: 1062–1072.

Kampfe CM, Harrison M, Oettinger T, Ludington J, McDonald-Bell, Pilsbury Jr. III. (1993). Parental expectations as a factor in evaluating children for the multichannel cochlear implant. American Annals of the Deaf 138: 297–303

Kelly D, Forney J, Parker-Fisher S, Jones M (1993) The challenge of attention deficit disorder in children who are deaf or hard of hearing. American Annals of the Deaf 138: 343–348.

Kennedy P, Bruininks RH (1974) Social status of hearing impaired children in regular classrooms. Exceptional Children 40: 336–343.

Kennedy P, Northcott W, McCauley R, Williams SM (1976) Longitudinal sociometric and cross–sectional data on mainstreaming hearing–impaired students: implications for preschool programming. Volta Review 78: 71–81.

Kitson N, Fry R (1990) Prelingual deafness and psychiatry. British Journal of Hospital Medicine 44: 353–356.

Kitson N (1991) Personal communication.

Klein M (1932) The Psychoanalysis of Children. London: Hogarth Press.

Koester LS, Trim VM (1991) Face-to face interactions with deaf and hearing infants: do maternal or infant behaviours differ? Paper presented at the biennial meeting of the Society of Research in Child Development.

Ladd GW, Munson HL, Miller JK (1984) Social integration of deaf adolescents in secondary–level mainstream programs. Exceptional Children 50: 420–428.

Lazarus RS, Folkman S (1984) Stress, Appraisal and Coping. New York: Springer.

Lederberg AR (1984) Interaction between deaf preschoolers and unfamiliar hearing adults. Child Development 55: 598–606.

Lederberg AR (1993) The Impact of Deafness on Mother-Child and Peer Relationships.

In Marschark M, Clark MD (eds) Psychological Perspectives on Deafness. Hillsdale NJ: Lawrence Erlbaum Associates.

Lederberg AR, Ryan HB, Robbins BL (1986) Peer interaction in young deaf children: the effect of partner hearing status and familiarity. Developmental Psychology 22: 691–700.

Lesser SR, Easser BR (1972) Personality differences in the perceptually handicapped. Journal of the American Academy of Child Psychiatry 11: 458–466.

Levy-Schiff R, Hoffman MA (1985) Social behaviour of hearing-impaired and normally hearing children. British Journal of Educational Psychology 55: 111–118.

McCune N (1988) Deaf in a hearing unit: coping of staff and adolescents. Journal of Adolescence 11: 21–28.

Markides A (1989) Integration: the speech intelligibility, friendships and associations of hearing impaired children in secondary schools. Journal of the British Association of Teachers of the Deaf 13: 63–72.

Marschark M (1993) Psychological Development of Deaf Children. New York: Oxford University Press.

Meadow KP (1968a) Parental responses to the medical ambiguities of deafness. Journal of Health and Social Behaviour 9: 299–309.

Meadow KP (1968b) Early manual communication in relation to the deaf child's intellectual, social and communicative functioning. American Annals of the Deaf 113: 29–41.

Meadow KP, Greenberg MT, Erting C, Carmichael H (1981) Interactions of deaf mothers and deaf preschool children: comparisons with three other groups of deaf and hearing dyads. American Annals of the Deaf 126: 454–468.

Meadow KP, Greenberg MT, Erting C (1983) Attachment behavior of deaf children with deaf parents. Journal of the American Academy of Child Psychiatry 22: 23–28.

Meadow-Orlans KP, Erting E, Day PS, MacTurk R, Prezioso C, Gianino A (1987) Deaf and hearing mothers of deaf and hearing infants: interaction in the first year of life. Paper presented at the 10th World Congress of the World Federation of the Deaf, Helsinki.

Minuchin S (1974) Families and Family Therapy. London: Tavistock.

Moog JS, Geers AE (1991) Educational management of children with cochlear implants. American Annals of the Deaf 136: 69–76.

Newport E, Singleton J, Supalla S, Metley D, Coulton J (1996) The test battery for American Sign Language morphology and syntax. In press.

Pauls DL, Reymond CL, Stevenson JM, Leckman JF (1991) A family study of Gilles de la Tourette syndrome. American Journal of Human Genetics 48: 154–163.

Parry-Jones WL (1994) History of Child and Adolescent Psychiatry. In Rutter M, Taylor E, Hersov L. Modern Approaches to Child and Adolescent Psychiatry (third edition). Oxford: Blackwell Scientific.

Pettito LA, Marentette PF (1991) Babbling in the manual mode: evidence for the ontogeny of language. Science 251: 1397–1536.

Prior MR, Glazner J, Sanson A, Debelle G (1988) Research Note: Temperament and behavioural adjustment in hearing impaired children. Journal of Child Psychology and Psychiatry 29: 209–216.

Power DJ, Hyde MB (1992) The cochlear implant and the deaf community. Medical Journal of Australia 157: 421–422.

Quittner AL, Thompson Steck J (1991) Predictors of cochlear implant use in children. American Journal of Otology 12: Suppl. 89–94.

Quittner AL, Thompson Steck J, Rouiller RL (1991) Cochlear implants in children: a study of parental stress and adjustment. American Journal of Otology 12: Suppl. 95–104.

Rainer JD (1976) Some observations on affect induction and ego development in the deaf. International Review of Psychoanalysis 3: 121–128.

Rawlings BW, Jensema CJ (1977) Two Studies of the Families of Hearing Impaired Children. Office of Demographic Studies. Washington, DC: Gallaudet University.

Roberts C, Hindley PA (1999) Practitioner review: the assessment and treatment of deaf children with psychiatric disorders. Journal of Child Psychology and Psychiatry 40: 151–167.

Rutter M, Graham P, Yule W (1970) A neuropsychiatric study in childhood. Clinics in Developmental Medicine Nos. 35/36. London: Spastics International Medical Publications.

Rutter M, Tizard J, Whitmore K (eds) (1970) Education, Health and Behaviour. London, Longman.

Rutter M (1991) Autism as a genetic disorder. In McGuffin P, Murray RM (eds) The New Genetics of Mental Illness, Oxford: Butterworth-Heinemann, pp 225–244.

Schlesinger H (1988) Questions and answers in the development of deaf children. In M Strong (ed) Language Learning and Deafness. Cambridge: Cambridge University Press.

Schlesinger H, Meadow K (1972) Sound and Sign. Berkeley, CA: University of California Press.

Sinkkonen J (1994) Hearing Impairment, Communication and Personality Development. University of Helsinki, Department of Child Psychiatry.

Smith PK, Sharp S (1994) School Bullying: insights and perspectives. London: Routledge.

Snitzer Reilly J, McIntire ML: Bellugi U (1989) Faces: the relationship between language and affect. In Volterra V, Erting CJ (eds) From Gesture to Language in Hearing and Deaf Children. Berlin: Springer–Verlag.

Spencer PE, Deyo D, Grindstaff N (1990) Symbolic play behaviour of deaf and hearing toddlers. In Moores DF, Meadow–Orlans KP (eds) Educational and Developmental Aspects of Deafness. Washington DC: Gallaudet University Press.

Stansfield M, Veltri D (1987) Assessment from the perspective of the sign language interpreter. In Elliot H, Glass L, Evans JW, Mental Health Assessment of Deaf Clients: a Practical Manual. Boston: College–Hill Press.

Stokoe WC and Battison R (1975) Sign language, mental health and satisfactory interaction. Unpublished paper. Washington DC: Linguistics Research Laboratory, Gallaudet College.

Swisher MV (1984). Signed input of hearing mothers of deaf children. Language Learning 34: 69–85.

Vandell DL, Anderson LD, Ehrhardt G, Wilson KS (1982) Integrating hearing and deaf preschoolers: an attempt to enhance hearing children's interactions with deaf peers. Child Development 53: 1354–1363.

van Gent T, Hilberink S (1994) Psychiatric disorders in children and adolescents referred to the first psychiatric clinic for deaf and severely hard of hearing children and adolescents in Holland. Paper presented at the 3rd Congress of the European Society for Mental Health and Deafness, Paris, December 14-16.

Vernon M (1967) Characteristics associated with post-rubella children: psychological, educational and physical. Volta Review 69: 176–185.

Vernon M, Alles CD (1994) Issues in the use of cochlear implants with prelingually deaf children. American Annals of the Deaf 139: 485–491.

Williams CE (1970) Some psychiatric observations on a group of maladjusted deaf children. Journal of Child Psychology and Psychiatry 11: 1–18.

Winnicott DWW (1958) Collected Papers: Through Paediatrics to Psychoanalysis. London: Tavistock.

Woll B (1995) Personal communication.

Woll B, Herman R (1996) The Development of a Pilot Battery for the Assessment of British Sign Language. London: City University and North Thames Regional Health Authority.

Wood D, Wood H, Griffiths A, Howarth I (1986) Teaching and Talking with Deaf Children. Chichester: John Wiley.

World Health Organization (1992) The ICD-10 Classification of Mental and Behavioural Disorders: clinical descriptions and diagnostic guidelines. Geneva: World Health Organization.

Chapter 4
Adult Psychiatry

NICK KITSON AND ALICE THACKER

Introduction

The primary tool of the psychiatrist in both diagnosis and treatment is communication. The most substantial difference in assessing the psychiatric status of Deaf adults is their language. To achieve accurate assessment, its normal and abnormal meaning and form must be fully understood.

Adult mental health assessment

Health workers generally assess their patients before offering treatment. The medical approach undertaken by the psychiatrist starts with eliciting the story of events surrounding and related to the symptom, with relevant events in the patient's life history. Whenever the patient is unable to give a full accurate account, it may be necessary to take details from an informant. The mental state of the patient, as inferred from his or her behaviour, is observed during the interview. The initial formulation of the problem may lead to more specific questions and tests. If the presenting problem is thought to be caused by, associated with, or causing a physical change or illness, the patient may require a physical examination and investigations such as blood tests. The risks of treatment may also require general or specific physical examination or treatment.

Other mental health workers tend to focus on more specific areas of any problem. Traditionally, such workers pursued assessment after and at the request of the psychiatrist, as in the case of psychological testing. This led either to a relevant treatment package or to a contribution to the overall assessment. More recently other mental health workers have singly (or jointly with psychiatrists or others) initiated the assessment process. All these assessment activities lead to a formulation of the problem and a medical diagnosis. The assessment and diagnostic process is ongoing, with reviews depending on response to treatment or other changes in the patient or his or her environment.

Psychiatric diagnostic categories are broadly divided into psychoses, 'neuroses', personality disorders, addictive behaviours and learning disability, global or specific. Psychoses are further divided into functional and organic. A psychosis is a severe illness that includes loss of touch with reality. Sufferers are usually deluded. The functional psychoses tend to run in families, have a genetic component, start for no apparent psychological reason, have a course which is largely unresponsive to circumstances but responds to medication. There is research evidence of chemical and physiological changes in the brain and sometimes limited structural change, but these are poorly understood. The predominantly organic nature of psychoses is confused by evidence that stressful life events can cause or precipitate them. Most people whose mental disturbance is obvious to the lay person, will be suffering a functional psychosis. The prime subcategories are schizophrenia and manic depressive psychosis. Organic psychoses have a demonstrable physical cause and may be acute (e.g. delirium tremens following withdrawal from alcohol) or chronic progressive disorders (e.g. senile dementia). Their rapid diagnosis is essential as, if treated early, a few are reversible, but once established may be permanent.

Modern diagnostic systems, such as the ICD-10 (WHO, 1992), categorize disorders traditionally known as 'neuroses' less simply, but more comprehensively. For the sake of brevity, however, we shall use the term 'neuroses' for those disorders which are neither psychoses nor personality disorders. Although generally classified as mental illnesses, they are viewed as exaggerations or minor aberrations of normal behaviour or experience. Although they can be associated with bodily changes, in part be determined genetically, and respond to medication, neuroses are generally viewed as primarily psychological disturbances. Psychoanalysis views them as defensive patterns of behaviour, protecting against the pain and anxiety of past traumas and relationships and reminders in the present. Cognitive psychology views neuroses as disturbances of thought processes and behaviour. Patients suffering them are usually aware they have a problem, though often unaware of the causes both in the present and from their past experiences. Neuroses are usually responsive to circumstances and the range of psychotherapies is usually the treatment of choice, though many will improve without specific treatment.

Personality disorders, as the name implies, are part of the patient's personality. They can usually be understood in the light of the patient's development and are distinct from personality changes such as those occurring after a head injury. Personality disorders are persistent and pervasive, with a characteristically poor response to treatment. Making the diagnosis is a more subjective and less reliable process than for other categories of disorder, and can be abused with the purpose of rejecting patients.

Assessment of Deaf patients

Inadequate assessment may result in incorrect treatment and very prolonged hospitalization for Deaf patients (Denmark, 1966; Timmermans, 1989). Dickert (1988) presented identical case histories to mental health workers labelling them as deaf or hearing patients. Workers in both specialist Deaf services and general services rated 'deaf' cases as needing more supervision and medication despite rating the most mentally ill patients as less severe. The Deaf services' workers had more positive attitudes to deafness and recommended a comparatively lower dose for the least severely ill patients. Altshuler and Rainer (1970) found that experienced psychiatrists made negative assumptions with regard to the rehabilitation prospects of Deaf patients.

Specialist mental health workers for Deaf people cannot assume that the information given on referral is accurate or has been elicited appropriately. Misdiagnoses have been common. Mental illness may be missed because abnormal behaviour is attributed to the patient's deafness (Denmark and Eldridge, 1969). Alternatively, a Deaf patient's frustration in communication released as an 'explosive reaction' may be mistaken for evidence of mental illness (Denmark, 1966). It is important for mental health workers for Deaf people to report facts elicited and direct observations in a detailed and objective fashion. Inferences and conclusions should be recorded entirely separately. Non-specialist mental health workers are not likely to be able to elicit facts nor observe communication for themselves due to their own limited communication skills. For example, it is not uncommon for the observation to be made that a patient 'is paranoid'. This is not an observation but an inference. The behaviour leading to that inference — perhaps aggressive persistent accusations that people are plotting maliciously — as well as details of the circumstances and form in which such accusations occur, is more useful than a label to any subsequent mental health worker.

In mental health work for Deaf people it is particularly important that assessments are thorough (both broad and deep) as well as clearly recorded. Usually, most management of the patient's illness or problem will be carried out by non-specialists due to lack of resources or geographic necessity. The first priority for the specialist is to act as the servant of more local and available workers, who will find observations more useful than inferences when making their own judgements in changing circumstances. Clearly, where possible, specialists should, because of their knowledge of Deaf culture and the mental health care of Deaf people, be the ones making judgements in changing circumstances.

The mental health worker for Deaf people, although usually seen as a 'super specialist', actually needs to be a generalist, as the services of other specialists are generally not available to the patient because of communication differences. Doctors may be able to take an accurate story from the patient through an interpreter, though even those who understand the issues usually do not use an interpreter (Ebert and Heckerling, 1995). All except those fluent in sign language will be handicapped when examining mental states as most of this assessment relies on direct observation of the patient's behaviour, attitudes and emotions associated with the context and content of the interview. The attitudes and emotional responses of Deaf patients are easily misunderstood. The assessor needs to distinguish the patient's emotional expression and assumed attitudes that are merely part of storytelling in sign, including taking on the roles of others, from real 'here and now' emotional responses and attitudes. The story may recount emotions and attitudes of the past but stir 'here and now' emotions in the telling. Attention to this degree of subtlety is important for diagnoses of mental illness. It is also at the core of psychodynamic diagnostic processes and treatments.

Diagnostic categories are used to predict the future, thereby both directing treatment and advising patients on their prognosis. They are devised on the basis of clusters of symptoms and observed behaviours. For example, people with severely depressed mood have been noted also to suffer sleep loss (particularly in the early morning), loss of appetite and weight and worse symptoms in the early part of the day than later on. If a depressed person has one of these symptoms, it is a reasonable prediction that he or she will have others. Sufficient numbers and/or severity of symptoms leads to a diagnosis of major depression which, in turn, predicts a positive response to antidepressant medication in a fairly short period of time. Consistent antidepressant medication over several months predicts a lower probability of illness in the next few years, and so on. These predictions have been tested scientifically and form the basis of modern medical practice, including psychiatry.

The challenge facing psychiatrists for Deaf people is to know how the phenomena occur in Deaf people and whether they predict the same prognosis and responses to treatment as would be expected in the hearing population. Most mental health workers for Deaf people are hearing. They have traditionally assumed that hearing models of psychiatry are appropriate to Deaf people. Some authors have challenged this (Ridgeway and Checinski, 1991), recommending research methodologies designed by Deaf people. Although empirical science should yield the same result whoever is conducting the investigation, method and rigour are likely to be improved by the involvement of Deaf people with appropriate mental health experience. The European Society for Mental Health and Deafness attempted to gain a consensus of experts in the field (Swaans-Joha, Mol and Than 1990). Only one expert, a psychologist, was Deaf but all agreed the standard classifications of that time, ICD-9 (WHO, 1978) and DSM-III-R (American Psychiatric Association, 1988) were appropriate to Deaf people. Draft versions of ICD-10 (WHO, 1992) were also accepted.

The first difference in the assessment of Deaf patients is to recognize that referrals often originate from unusual sources. In Great Britain most referrals to mental health services are from local family doctors, and referrals to mental health sub-speciality services are from local psychiatrists or family doctors. In Deaf mental health services the majority of referrals have been from social workers for deaf people. Sophisticated Deaf people, who know their rights and the system, can gain access directly or via non-specialists through interpreters. However, a large minority or perhaps the majority of Deaf people who need mental health services do not have either the sophistication or the stamina needed to arrange interpreters for appointments with the family doctor, then (typically) the local general psychiatrist, following on to a service that can assess and treat them through sign language and appropriate cultural models. Deaf people with mental health problems (being such a geographically widespread small minority) cannot maintain expert mental health workers at the local level. Widely available sign language-using professionals, who have a broad general interest in health and social function, are therefore essential to enable Deaf people to gain access to all services, including mental health. In Great Britain these are the social workers for deaf people. They instigate most referrals to Deaf mental health services (Denmark and Eldridge, 1969; Denmark, 1985). With increasing sophistication of services and wider knowledge, referrals are increasingly made by psychiatrists — although most of *those* continue to be instigated by social workers.

Denmark (1985) found that the majority of those referred to a Deaf mental health service in the north of England did not have mental illness, but only nine of 250 patients had no psychiatric abnormality. Behavioural problems and maladjustment, which Denmark (1985) assumed to be due to deafness, accounted for over one-fifth of patients; developmental disorders of communication, one-fifth, whereas two-fifths had mental illness. In a similar study of 185 patients referred to the service in the south of England between 1986 and 1989, Hamblin and Kitson (1992) found that 18% of subjects had no psychiatric abnormality. Behavioural problems, including conduct disorder, and personality disorder accounted for 25%, and 31% for mental illness — of which 10% had 'neuroses'.

Physical examinations and investigations are particularly important in deaf patients to detect progressive disorders which have significance for mental function. Significant visual impairment and blindness is commonly associated with deafness. In Deaf people, particular attention needs to be paid to the effects of blindness in compounding mental state and communication problems. A congenitally blind child has greater difficulty learning the rules of communication with his mother through eye contact and responsive smiling. The concept of self may develop late, so that the 'I–You' distinction is delayed, to the extent that the individual may wrongly be labelled 'autistic'. In addition, representational play, in many respects the basis for symbolic language, develops much later than normal.

As a result, congenitally blind adults may have depersonalized relationships; they may seem unmotivated and 'schizoid'. Professionals are likely to underestimate mood, intelligence and personality in patients with reduced expressive behaviour. In Usher's syndrome (commonly referred to as retinitis pigmentosa, which is a progressive consequence), a genetic (usually autosomal recessive) disorder of early childhood deafness associated with later-onset progressive blindness through pigment deposits on the retina, has been said to be associated with a five-fold increase in the likelihood of schizophrenic-like psychosis (Halgren, 1958), though this is now being questioned. Sensorineural deafness is the most common complication of maternal rubella. Rubella causes multiple impairments by attacking specific cells in specific organs. Approximately 25% of Deaf people have impairments of organs other than those responsible for hearing; however, this figure rises to 37% in Deaf people with a history of maternal rubella. Rubella is associated with the late development of many other disorders. Sever, South and Shaver (1985), in a thorough review, report a prevalence of diabetes as high as 20% and a prevalence of thyroid disease (mostly reduced function) of 5%. Pendred's syndrome, an autosomal recessive genetic disorder, also associates congenital deafness with thyroid disease. Hypothyroidism may mimic depressive illness with slowness of all bodily and mental functions, yet if not appropriately treated can lead to dementia. Hyperthyroidism speeds up bodily functions and can mimic anxiety, mania or schizophrenia. Up to 10% of those with congenital rubella may suffer late-onset eye damage. Rarely, congenital rubella may lead to progressive rubella panencephalitis, a severe central nervous system disease caused by chronic infection of the brain with the rubella virus. It presents with learning problems and incoordination (ataxia), and progresses relentlessly. New behaviour disorders or epileptic phenomena can present late in congenital rubella, but without ataxia. In addition to the common physical disorders associated with the key causes of deafness there is a multitude of minor disorders associated with genetic syndromes and environmental causes of deafness, which will have a direct or indirect psychological effect on mental state. Assessors need to be wary of all the possibilities.

In the first instance, diagnosis and recommendations for management are based on the performance of the patient during the interview. Because the life experiences of Deaf people differ so widely, it is difficult to draw valid conclusions from any difficulties they may have in giving an account of themselves.

They may, for example, have serious difficulty in expressing time concepts. This may lead either to a lack of usable information, or to a distortion of events; for example, the patient may try to link the onset of symptoms to a major, memorable event, thus giving the false impression that he attributes causality to it. For remote events, in particular, the patient's inability to codify in language can have a profound effect on recall, leading to greater dependence on hearing informants. Informants are often family members who, because they cannot sign, place a greater emphasis on perceived behaviour problems than on the Deaf person's own feelings and thoughts.

Deaf people who have had inadequate communication models at home and school may suffer in interviews in several ways. Some adults of normal intellect and mental status may have difficulty with formal questions such as 'how?' and 'why?', even in sign language. This may be because they are accustomed to being *told* rather than *asked* (Thacker, 1991). A multiple choice question format may be required, taking care not to lead or limit the subject too far, by presenting concrete examples. As sign is directional, the pronouns for actor and object of action are relative; they do not have the stable values of 'you' and 'yourself'. The authors have seen subjects respond to the question '*You blame yourself?*' as though the interviewer had asked '*Do I blame you?*' Questions about control are particularly difficult (Thacker, 1994a). Too impoverished or rigid a vocabulary and concepts may masquerade as poverty of content, tangentiality, derailment, poor insight and social withdrawal (Thacker, 1991).

The assessment of cognitive level must be approached thoughtfully. An example of problematic assumptions would be the following: sequencing tasks presupposes that a subject will organize elements from left to right. This is an invalid expectation for many Deaf patients, who do badly on paper tasks but organize quite complex practical sequences very well, or who do well in activities requiring a high level of temporal or spatial organization but which are not dependent on this particular ordering. This effect may be due to the poor level of literacy achieved by many Deaf people, for whom reading and writing are not included in the central linguistic and cognitive constructs of the world.

Many researchers have found perceptual problems to be linked to schizophrenia in hearing people (Lancet (Editorial), 1981), and it is important to distinguish those symptoms from the central auditory imperception which is experienced by up to 50% of people with congenital rubella. This syndrome comprises an inability to respond to sound on a cortical level, regardless of hearing threshold. It results in deficits in localization of sound, figure/ground discrimination, and interpretation of sound. (The same problems, in fact, are routinely experienced by hearing aid users.) Again, this disorder often plays a role in the inappropriate diagnosis of autism in adults and children. These factors emphasize the need for a professional with expertise in language pathology and deafness.

Affective disorders

The affective disorders include depression, mania, the combination of the two, mixed affective states, and bipolar manic depression, with phases of both. Depressions not considered to be primarily functional psychoses, as described in the introduction to this chapter, were classified under the neuroses, with labels such as depressive neurosis or reactive depression. Most depression in community surveys is of this type. Unfortunately, the differentiation of psychotic and non-psychotic depression with or without biological features is not clear cut and remains controversial even in psychiatry for hearing people.

Up to the late 1980s most authors have reported less depressive illness in Deaf people. It has been said to appear differently as an agitated state (Altshuler, 1971). Only Robinson (1978) reported no difference qualitatively or quantitatively. Altshuler (1986) reported that psychomotor retardation was rare and guilt was almost absent in clinical presentations and argued consistency with psychoanalytic theory, through lack of superego development (i.e. internalized control) and therefore impaired development of guilt and of the 'lock' on rage. He noted that depressed children, similarly, rarely show psychomotor retardation. There is a problem when mental illnesses are claimed to present differently in Deaf people. How can such claims be tested? The diagnosis would have to predict the same consequences as the diagnosis in hearing people, but the consequences might also be different. Ultimately this can be tested only with a reliable biological marker, such as a blood test. These are currently not available for the main mental illnesses.

Previously low rates of depressive illness have been attributed to the delayed personality development of many Deaf people. It has been suggested that hearing is required for normal development of 'object relations'* and a conscience. Altshuler (1971) reminds us that Freud commented, 'the ego . . . wears an auditory lobe'. Similarly, it could be attributed to a failure to achieve Klein's depressive position. Melanie Klein, a child psychoanalyst, believed children go through three phases in the early childhood development of human relationships. The 'undifferentiated' phase is the earliest, there being no recognition of the difference between self and others. The next phase is the 'paranoid schizoid position' where the child, recognizing the difference between self and others, blames others for all that is bad or gives others credit for all that is good. It is only when children recognize some control and therefore some responsibility for their own environment, that they can start to feel guilty. They can then achieve the 'depressive position'. Morbid guilt or self-blame is a key feature of major depressive illness. In the most ill with psychotic features, it leads to abnormal beliefs that the depressively ill person has done some great harm that he or she cannot possibly have done. An example is that of a Deaf patient who wrung her hands in continuous anguish, complaining that she had caused a local rail crash, killing many.

*'Object relations' is a term used in psychoanalytic theory for the development of attitudes, emotions and behaviours that determine our relationships with other human beings.

The crash had, in fact, occurred while she was an inpatient under close observation due to suicidal risk.

In San Francisco, Evans and Elliot (1987) found depression fairly common — especially in patients seen in satellite clinics. In London, rates of referrals for depression have more than quadrupled over an approximately three-year period, see Figure 4.1. During the period there were four significant changes which might have accounted for the increase. The overall referral rate increased by about three times. Fifty per cent of patients were first assessed in their own residence compared to very rare home assessments previously. Deaf people had become established as mental health workers in the service and were involved in assessments. Psychotherapy services were developed. Access had improved in three ways and the fourth change might have altered perceptions of the service's target clientele. It seems likely that these factors accounted for the increase in depression, and it is unlikely that chance or other factors were significant. Community psychiatric research (Checinski, 1991) suggests that much more depression in the Deaf community exists than is referred to Deaf mental health services, although it is likely that this refers mostly to minor depression.

Whereas the previously noted relative lack of identification of Deaf people with depressive illness appears to have been due to a lack of services, it remains quite possible that delayed personality development and an agitated appearance masks the depressive illness process in some Deaf people. They might be misdiagnosed as having behaviour

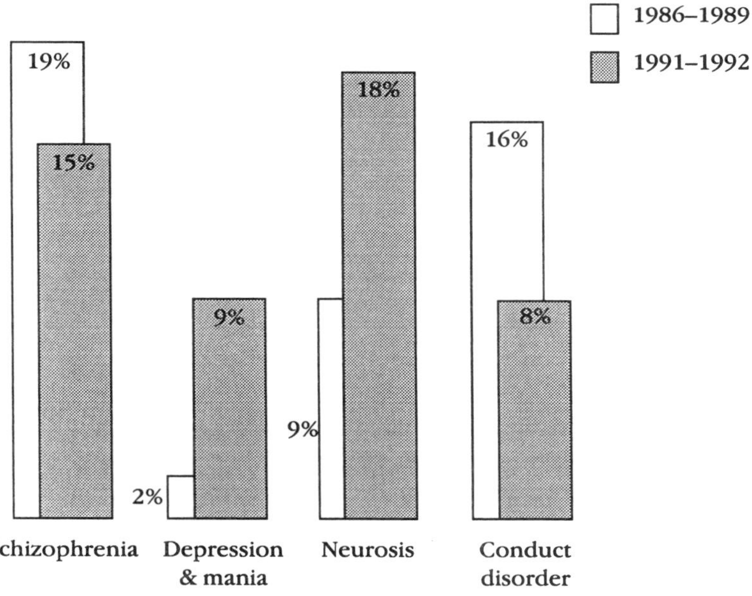

Figure 4.1 Increase in rates of depression in London 1986–1992.

disorder, when their behaviour is a response to an underlying and treatable depressive illness. The 'biological' symptoms of depressive illness, where present, may be useful, though some biological symptoms (loss of appetite, loss of weight, disinterest, poor concentration or slowed behaviour) are ordinarily responsive to mood. If they were consistently present and not responsive to day-to-day circumstances, they might indicate that the 'behaviour disorder' was in fact a response to major depressive illness. The depressive symptoms of early morning waking and feeling significantly worse in the mornings are less evidently a psychological reaction and therefore may be more diagnostically useful. Most of us when emotionally disturbed have more difficulty getting to sleep than waking early. The most significant features of depressive illness diagnostically are its phasic nature and relative lack of reactivity to circumstance. The common emotion of depression that we all feel is not depressive illness. We know the cause and our state can be improved by an improvement in circumstances. If the Deaf person has always had the behaviour problem, it is less likely to be secondary to a depressive illness. If there are long episodes of the behaviour problem, which come and go and are not responsive to circumstances, then an underlying depressive illness is more likely. Depressive illness or mania in the biological family should lead to a higher awareness of the possibility in the patient.

Markowitz and Nininger (1984), reporting a case of bipolar manic depression, commented that the literature describes bipolar disease as a rarity in Deaf people. Altshuler (1971) reported that in 15 years of experience there had been only one case with at least one truly depressive phase followed by a manic phase. In a two-year period the London Deaf service, which covers a general population base of up to 20 million, has diagnosed four cases — each with at least one truly manic and one truly depressed phase — and two further cases with only diagnoses of mania from new referrals. There were an additional six patients with unipolar mania on the long-term case load in 1994. Unipolar mania is also rare in hearing people and it is questionable whether it is merely chance that a depressive phase has not occurred.

Schizophrenia

Schizophrenia is a serious mental illness, most commonly starting in late adolescence or early adult life, which usually leads to a deterioration in emotional and social functioning. Kraepelin (1919) observed this pattern and termed it Dementia Praecox (precocious dementia). It usually starts with odd behaviour, which is secondary to the patient's suffering experiences and beliefs that are not appropriate in their culture. Bleuler (1950) described symptoms, which are remembered as the four As:

- Autism (withdrawal from social contact).
- Affective (inappropriate or blunted emotional response).
- Association (loose or bizarre associations).
- Ambivalence (doubtful or alternate contradictory thoughts or actions).

These are now amongst those referred to as the 'negative symptoms' of schizophrenia.

Schneider (1959) listed the 'first rank symptoms', the presence of any one of which he considered diagnostic (Chandrasena, 1987). They are now amongst those referred to as the 'positive symptoms' of schizophrenia. Some patients with manic depressive psychosis have since been observed to have Schneiderian First Rank Symptoms, though these are still a powerful tool in the diagnosis of schizophrenia.

The first rank symptoms of schizophrenia are (Mellor, 1970):

- Audible thoughts.
- Voices heard arguing (usually in the third person).
- Voices heard commenting on one's actions.
- The experience of influences playing on the body (somatic passivity experiences).
- Thought withdrawal, insertion and broadcasting of thoughts so others know them.
- All feelings, impulses and volitional acts that are experienced as the work or influence of others (passivity experiences).
- Delusional perception.

Delusional perception arises out of a normal perception to which special meaning is attributed. It is a variety of primary delusion, that is a delusion that arises 'out of the blue' from no understandable origin. All primary delusions are themselves now considered as if a first rank symptom. Schneider (1959) was of the view that 'when any one of these modes of experience is undeniably present, and no basic somatic illness can be found, we may make a decisive clinical diagnosis of schizophrenia.'

There is no evidence that schizophrenic psychoses are more common in Deaf people (Altshuler and Sarlin, 1963), though no reliable figures exist. Altshuler and Sarlin found a prevalence of schizophrenia in Deaf people of 2.5% from a hospital study. They recognized the flaws in their own study, attributed to increased lengths of stay for Deaf patients (Altshuler, 1986) and could not reliably say there was any greater prevalence of schizophrenia in Deaf people than the 1% found in the overall population. Subsequently, Altshuler and Sarlin (1963) studied schizophrenia in parents and siblings of Deaf patients with schizophrenia and found the rates of schizophrenia were similar to those found in studies of families of hearing patients with schizophrenia. Studies of referrals to Deaf mental health services (Denmark, 1985; Hamblin and Kitson, 1992) and

Checinski's (1991) community survey have not found any more Deaf people with schizophrenia than would have been expected. Adequate research requires reliable studies of representative samples. As Deaf people with serious mental health problems are managed so differently by our society from their hearing counterparts it is difficult for comparisons to be made. Once services for Deaf people, and Deaf and hearing people's awareness of the issues, have improved reliable research may be possible.

Observation of the content of speech and the form of language are the prime tools for diagnosing schizophrenia in hearing people. Deaf patients can be severely disadvantaged in this regard. The language of Deaf people should not be equated to any spoken language. Word for sign translations of sign language and the writings of many language-deprived Deaf people have been found to suggest thought disorder, their communications showing a fragmented, confused quality (Altshuler, Baroff and Rainer, 1963). Written samples can be used in diagnosis only by experienced mental health workers for Deaf people, and then only with caution. Comparing the patients' writings when well with those when they are suspected of being ill can be valid.

Deafness may arise from an aetiology causing an organic brain deficit, the effects of which must be distinguished from those of functional psychoses, such as schizophrenia (Vernon and Rothstein, 1968). Communication anomalies may erroneously suggest chronic schizophrenia or organic disorder as language-deprived Deaf people may talk in concrete terms (Basilier, 1964). Another potential cause of confusion is that many normal Deaf people do not signal topic changes in a way that is clear to hearing people, and the ongoing lack of feedback which results from this may lead to frustration and disrupted expression. It is quite typical in Deaf culture for the signer to take on the role of the subject in sentences. For example, a male client might well describe an event or picture featuring a woman by using just the verb. This may be seen as a problem with ego boundaries, abnormal self-reference or as a language disorder. Many Deaf people are said to perseverate abnormally when, in fact, they are using a strategy of rapidly repeating signs because they think their conversational partner has not understood them, or for emphasis. Studies of American Sign Language (ASL) have shown that repetition is also used routinely to distinguish nouns from verbs and for other grammatical and semantic functions. It is probable that British Sign Language (BSL) incorporates similar devices (Thacker, 1991, 1998). The second author has noted in her own practice and in interactions with colleagues that confirmation of known facts and long-held opinions through the use of repetition is much more highly valued by the Deaf community than by hearing peers. This repetition of themes may appear suspect to a hearing clinician unfamiliar with Deaf usage.

A patient's very insistence on communicating with the hearing professional may earn him or her an undeserved label of 'thought-disordered'.

Intrusions from spoken language may appear to be inappropriate or rhyming word choice, when in fact it may be choice based on cultural usage and the demands of the situation (Thacker, 1991).

A study was carried out on 30 schizophrenic and five manic-depressive Deaf patients, and a matched group of healthy Deaf controls (Thacker, 1994b). The sign language produced in the context of an interview was transcribed and analysed by the second author and a Deaf associate.

Some 31 error categories were developed. Some errors are as common in control subjects as in patients. Specific behaviours have been grouped into descriptive categories, as follows.

Cross-linguistic (BSL–English) contamination

These errors primarily take the form of a linking of a sign to the English word that sounds the same. For example:

> Interviewer: YOU SAY WOMAN INSIDE YOU HAVE? MEAN WHICH, BODY OR SOUL?
>
> Schizophrenic subject : SOUL (conventional sign) SOLE (pointing to bottom of foot) TWO FEET JUMP IN MY MOUTH.

Production errors

This descriptive category would include unusual, stereotyped handshapes for recognizable signs (Corina et al., 1990), and phenomena not directly comparable to a spoken language:

- Reversals. One schizophrenic woman fingerspelled backwards when acutely ill, others made the movements of actual signs backwards. This may not be as disordered as speech articulated backwards would be, as reversing movement does not have such a serious effect on intelligibility.
- Errors are frequently produced through substitution or omission of manual features: this aspect was particularly striking in one acutely schizophrenic woman who routinely made signs in the wrong location (for example she traced a circle around her face rather than over her palm to describe a JAR).

Attention to the shapes of signs rather than semantic relationships

This is similar to Andreasen's (1979) 'clang' category: 'A pattern of speech in which sounds (or in this case, sublexical handshapes) rather than meaningful relationships appear to govern word choice.' Both might indicate deficits in interpersonal communication and failure to suppress unhelpful language processes.

Case 1:
Examiner: PLEASE WRITE SENTENCE (using the patient's sign for 'sentence', which was a narrow horizontal rectangle made in the air in front of the signer. This request was in the context of a written picture description task. The client had been writing single words.)
Schizophrenic patient: YES, SENTENCE (plucks sign out of air and ties it around her waist).

Case 2:
Interviewer: (showing a picture of a fish) THIS WHAT? Schizophrenic patient who had been educated in Jamaican Sign Language but had been exposed to BSL for 15 years: FISH (spoken, and signed as follows: Jamaican sign — one hand flat, projecting out from chin, appears to correct to BSL sign of flat hand wriggling away from body; adds the other hand to produce a gesture resembling fluttering wings; quickly performs formal BSL sign for BIRD, i.e. thumb and forefinger tapping next to mouth) 'Bird!' (spoken while pointing at fish).

Topic switching/derailment

Interviewer; ALL POLICE WORLD DISAPPEAR . . . WHAT HAPPEN?
Subject: WHEN WORLD c.e.l.l. c.e.l.l. GROW SPREAD SPREAD LATER YOU KNOW d.o.n.o.s.a.u.r. WALK SIDEWAYS MONKEY RISE UP SLOW . . . [Interviewer indicates lack of comprehension, repeats question] SUPPOSE NAUGHTY STEAL FIGHT FIGHT NOSE BLEED . . .
(The subject apparently was diverted by the thought of Godzilla and King Kong taking over an unpoliced planet).

Perseveration

Sign/word level (e.g. WAIS Similarities)

Interviewer: EYE EAR SIMILAR HOW?
Subject: BEEF DEAF WRITE HOSPITAL
Interviewer: EGG SEED SAME HOW?
Subject: b.e.e.f. THERE b.e.e.f. THERE

Thematic perseveration

Interviewer: YOU FAMILY COMMUNICATE HOW?
Subject: MYSELF CLEVER MOUTH CLEVER SPEAK SIGN SPEAK MOUTH TEA FOOD SOME NURSE FOOD THERE BAD EAT HERE SAW c.h.e.s.t.n.u.t. NO DIFFERENT ME SAY NO BAD BOY SAY DIFFERENT w.a.l.n.u.t.

Echopraxia

Slavish imitation of the interviewer's signs.

Telescopage

Described by Lecours and Vanier-Clement (1976) as corresponding 'to a variety of phonemic paraphasia in which a deviant segment, used as a single word, borrows units from more than one conventional segment'.

> Manic-depressive subject, looking at a picture of a boy having a tantrum: BAD-BOY (simultaneously producing sign for BOY with index finger while protruding little finger, the conventional marker for BAD.)

Visual–spatial behaviours unique to signers

An example of this is the young woman, during her first schizophrenic episode, who assigned different personalities to her two hands, and vastly different locations and time lines to the two sides of her body.

Sign errors seen in signers without psychiatric history or symptoms

Mayberry (1992) has elicited semantic substitutions (e.g. FATHER for MOTHER) from healthy fluent signers who learned sign in early childhood; indeed, individuals with native competence substituted 10% of signs in a storytelling task. We have observed this as well, most notably in a control subject who told us that she is SHY QUIET PERSON I *ENCOURAGE* CROWDS LIKE SIT ALONE READ.

Of these, the following anomalies were significantly more common in the mentally ill groups (listed in order of statistical significance). The terms in bold print are those made ONLY by subjects suffering schizophrenia:

- **Incoherence.**
- Topic derailment.
- Perseveration of theme.
- **Visual–spatial anomalies.**
- Illogicality.
- Stereotypy.
- 'Clangs'
- Perseveration of signs.
- **Paraphasias.**

Thus it appears that Deaf signers in good mental health make errors which can be mistaken for schizophrenic anomalies, a tendency which can lead to inequities in diagnosis and treatment (Thacker, 1998).

Talking past the point is part of thought disorder, but is also a common defence by patients against poor receptive skills. The diagnostician should be wary of following suit in defence against their poor receptive skills of sign (Kitson and Fry, 1990).

Evans and Elliott (1981) found only nine of 15 of the usual symptoms of schizophrenia useful in diagnosing Deaf patients in America. The remaining six symptoms were common in Deaf patients with or without schizophrenia and therefore not helpful in diagnosing schizophrenia (Table 4.1).

Evans and Elliott (1981) argued that Schneider's first rank symptoms may discriminate for schizophrenia in this population, but were too dependent

Table 4.1: Useful symptoms for diagnosing schizophrenia

Discriminating for schizophrenia	Non-discriminating
Loss of ego boundaries	Poor insight
Delusional perception	Labile affect
Restricted affect	Poverty of content
Illogicality	Poor rapport
Abnormal explanations	Vagueness
Hallucinations	Inability to complete a course of action
Inappropriate affect	
Remoteness from reality	
Ambivalence	

on the use of sound. They also noted that abstract ego psychology terms were difficult to apply to Deaf patients. The term 'loss of ego boundaries' implies 'Specific problems in the areas of reality testing, object relationships, lack of differentiation of self and others and identity formation' (American Psychiatric Association, 1968). Fraunhofer and Kitson have challenged this as first rank symptoms can be clearly expressed in BSL and are commonly used in the psychiatric assessment of Deaf patients in the London service. Their study found loss of ego boundaries was amongst the most common primary symptoms found in Deaf people with schizophrenia. They compared 12 Deaf patients diagnosed as having schizophrenia with 12 patients without psychosis, looking for Evans' and Elliott's (1981) primary and secondary symptoms and Schneider's first rank symptoms (Fraunhofer and Kitson, 1991). As the study was by retrospective case note analysis, there was no observer bias and the information was from spontaneous written clinical comments. The diagnoses had been made clinically prior to the study according to ICD-9 (WHO, 1978) criteria. Anecdotally the authors can confirm, from their use of the PSE9 (Thacker, 1994a) on many of the patients studied by Fraunhofer and Kitson, a good correlation between their ICD-9 schizophrenia diagnoses and PSE9-ID-CATEGO research diagnosis nuclear schizophrenia (Wing and Stuart, 1978). Eight subjects from the schizophrenic population had shown a clear history of recent onset of behavioural problems accompanied by a marked decline in social or occupational functioning. Four patients with schizophrenia did not show a clear history of recent onset of illness and resembled the control group with a history of recent exacerbation of longstanding behavioural problems. Fraunhofer and Kitson (1991) found seven of 12 patients with schizophrenia had first rank symptoms, with more than four of Evans' and Elliott's (1981) primary symptoms. Five of the schizophrenic group scored between one and three primary symptoms but no first rank symptoms. Four patients from the control group also had either one or two primary symptoms. Their study did not support the findings of Evans and Elliott (1981) that primary symptoms alone are sufficiently discriminatory for schizophrenia, but supported Evans' and Elliott's (1981) view that their secondary symptoms were non-discriminating, finding them equally spread between the schizophrenic and control groups. Fraunhofer and Kitson (1991) concluded that Schneider's first rank symptoms can be a sufficient indicator of schizophrenia in Deaf patients and are therefore not too dependent on sound. The primary symptoms of Evans and Elliott (1981) appear to have a less definitive, but useful, diagnostic role. There were no guidelines in Evans' and Elliott's (1981) original study as to how many primary symptoms are necessary to indicate the diagnosis in Deaf patients. The results obtained by Fraunhofer and Kitson (1991) suggest that an ICD-9 (WHO, 1978) diagnosis of schizophrenia requires four or more primary symptoms. Less than four primary symptoms is suggestive of psychosis and indicates that the patient needs to be investigated further.

The use of the Present State Examination (PSE9) (Wing, Cooper and Sartorius, 1983) in BSL was pioneered by the authors, who had completed training in PSE administration together with Alex Cranwell, a Deaf native user of BSL and who has completed courses in sign linguistics (Thacker, 1994a). The PSE9 has been the standard research instrument for the diagnosis of schizophrenia. It comprises a semi-structured interview exploring in detail the symptoms of psychoses. It proved feasible to translate into sign language and was not in any way dependent on the use of sound. A guide BSL translation on video was developed, but the PSE can and should be adapted for individual patients as it has the advantage of relying on concepts rather than standard wordings. The developers examined each item, discussing its meaning, how it would be most accurately rendered in BSL, and whether it was psychologically valid within Deaf culture and experience. A videotape of the signed version was then translated back into English by a bilingual interpreter. Comparison of the back-translated English with the original yielded few instances in which the meaning was unclear or insufficiently close to the original concept to be valid. Deviations were corrected to produce greater accuracy and clarity. So far this version of the PSE has been administered to 23 individuals with clinical diagnoses of schizophrenia or manic-depression and to two healthy Deaf control subjects.

Two psychiatrists competent in BSL carried out an inter-rater reliability study of PSE ratings, utilizing the videotapes of these interviews. In each of the 30% of scores where there was disagreement, the less fluent and experienced rater had given a score with low confidence rating or had not assigned a diagnosis.

Kitson and Fry (1990) noted normal mumbling in sign can be misinterpreted as hallucinosis (Deaf people may mumble and dream in sign (Hurst, 1988)) and that apparently abnormal explanations or beliefs may be explainable by lack of vicarious learning or naïvety and not fit the criteria of a delusion. For example a Deaf patient understood a science fiction programme to be factual. He was not deluded, merely naïve, yet this had been thought to be a symptom of mental illness. Often close exploration of such phenomena is required, necessitating very accurate and detailed communication. Where television is experienced as talking about the patient, a diagnosis is more convincing. Idiosyncratic signs (those specific to individuals or small groups) may be misinterpreted as the inventions of people suffering schizophrenia called neologisms (Misiaszek et al., 1985). Regional signs can be similarly misinterpreted.

Deaf patients with schizophrenia do report auditory hallucinations. Critchley et al. (1981), reviewing such patients, found 'exact subjective experiences were difficult to determine'. Du Feu and McKenna (1996) found 10 of 16 profoundly prelingually deaf patients with research diagnoses of schizophrenia gave definite accounts of hearing voices. Our patients refer to voices in various ways — getting at them or talking to each other — but very rarely quote the content. One patient was able to tell us 'hearing children shouting fingerspelling in my head'. Another reported her sister 'Talking' (generic sign) in her abdomen, which was the part of the body where she did in reality perceive the vibrations of loud sounds (Thacker, 1994a). Fraunhofer and Kitson (unpublished) found patients were able to go into great detail concerning their experience of auditory hallucinations, but noted that whether the experience is akin to 'hearing' in the conventional sense is impossible to say. The authors are now involved in an in-depth survey of the characteristics of verbal auditory hallucinations in Deaf patients with schizophrenia. This involves the administration of a questionnaire in BSL, rather like the PSE (but much more detailed), including the source of the voice, where it is heard, the accent, etc. Preliminary data suggest that some Deaf patients are able to go into much detail concerning their voices, but it is no surprise that they are generally perplexed by their experiences. A Deaf definite hallucinator through her ears could identify the person who was 'talking' to her, but not the gender. This may imply that the experience of 'hearing' voices is not a true auditory experience, in that the 'voices' do not possess the correlates of vocal pitch and could not physically differentiate the sound. Alternatively, it may be an example of the illogicality of schizophrenia.

Those who do not experience voices may, for example, when asked if they experience the voices, reply, 'How should I know — I am Deaf!' Illogically, even some who do experience voices, stated by them to be through their ears, say the same. This again may be an illogicality of schizophrenia.

At first sight it is surprising that profoundly Deaf people suffering from schizophrenia should experience verbal auditory hallucinations, the more so as a lower prevalence of 'voices commenting' has been noted among other cultural minorities (Chandrasena, 1987). It has been taken to suggest that hallucinations come from a 'central organic base' (Altshuler, 1971). In other words, that schizophrenia is a physical disease of the brain rather than a purely psychological state. Kitson and Fry (1990) contest that view, pointing out that 90% of Deaf people have hearing parents who use their voices, possibly to criticize or even provide a running commentary. Facial expression, posture and gesture can be enough to give a Deaf person the quality, though not the exact content, of any spoken language.

They suggest that the complaint of hearing voices by Deaf mentally ill people is not so surprising, when it is understood that Deaf people have the concepts and have been exposed to the meaning of heard voices by others. It is only the sound to which they have not been exposed. Despite this, there is significant other evidence that schizophrenia originates from organic processes.

The status in Deaf people of verbal auditory hallucinations and phenomena that appear to be their visual equivalents, can now be explored further with the advent of functional imaging technology, which allows the activity of brain areas to be determined during particular brain states. It has been established that language areas of the brain are involved in verbal hallucinations in hearing people — especially the left frontal lobe (McGuire et al., 1993; Silversweig et al., 1995) and that healthy Deaf signers' 'silent sign' originates in this area (McGuire et al., 1997). We are also involved in studies designed to determine those areas involved in the hallucinations that Deaf people experience. Maybe these studies will go some way to answering the question, 'Can deaf people hear voices?' posed by Monteiro and Critchley (1994).

'Neuroses'

Neurotic disorders have rarely been reported by psychiatric services for Deaf people (Kitson and Fry, 1990), but are seen increasingly with the establishment of psychotherapy and improved psychology services for Deaf people (Figure 4.1). Like depressive illness, the apparent absence appears to have been an artifact of service provision. These clinical experiences are supported by recent research. In community studies Hindley et al. (1994) found significant emotional disorders in Deaf children, and Checinski (1991), in a preliminary report, found depression at about 20% and anxiety at about 10% prevalence in Deaf adults. Gerber (1983) noted 'problems in living' due to the discrimination of society against Deaf people, and organic disorders associated with deafness that may present as 'anxiety states, affective disturbances, conduct disorders, adjustment disorders, and marital, family or work problems'. Gerber (1983) added that due to communication difficulties 'behaviour disturbances are observed more often than problems of interpersonal concerns or neurotic symptoms'. Little is known about the prevalence of eating disorders, which rarely present to Deaf mental health services. The authors can recall only three primary diagnoses of eating disorder over about five years, during which referrals were at a rate of about 120 per year, though many patients have had secondary body image or eating problems. Hills, Rappold and Rendon (1991), in a study of 100 deaf college students, found the prevalence and distribution of bingeing and body image distortion to be essentially the same as in similar hearing populations, indicating a probable similar prevalence of clinical eating disorders. These authors suggest a greater awareness amongst professionals and prevention programmes.

Behaviour disorders

Psychiatrists for adults rarely use the terms 'behaviour' or 'conduct' disorder. Those referred to adult services with disturbances of behaviour tend to have behaviours that can be understood in the context of the patient's personal development, are of long standing, and can be predicted to be resistant to treatment. This is considered part of the patient's personality and labelled as 'personality disorder'. The diagnosis of personality types or disorders is notoriously unreliable.

Until recently it had been generally agreed by psychiatrists for Deaf people that Deaf people exhibit concrete thinking, rigidity, decreased empathy, projection of responsibility on to others, lack of insight or self-reproach, unrealistic views of their ability, increased demands and impulsivity with poor control of rage (Altshuler, 1971). The implication was that these behaviours were generally characteristic of Deaf people and their culture. For example, 'Egocentric and rigid behaviours, products of deaf enculturation, can be mistaken for personality disorders' (Misiaszek et al., 1985). Mental health workers with hearing people will recognize that such behaviours are not at all exclusive to Deaf people. Contact with Deaf people who did not have mental disorder appears not to have been common amongst mental health workers for Deaf people. Had there been more contact it is unlikely that such statements would have been written.

One cross-national study between America and Yugoslavia (Altshuler et al., 1976) found greater impulsivity in 'normal' Deaf people as well as in patients. Sarlin and Altshuler (1978) found a delay in the development of the relationship between cognition and affect which provides a potential model for impulsivity. When confronted with a challenge there is inability to trust the environment and a lack of practice at sequential responses through lack of imaginative play. The result is an inability to think out a sequential plan, and therefore an immediate response to feelings by impulsive actions. Similar patterns of behaviour to those in deaf children were found in deprived children, one presumably through neglect, the other through the problems imposed by deafness in a hearing family. An alternative or — more likely — concurrent model is that of organic brain damage, resulting in irritability. Chess and Fernandez (1981) found rubella children with deafness as an only sequela to suffer impulsivity, which resolved by age 13–14 years. Notably, more rubella children with deafness and additional sequelae were impulsive and this did not resolve. Altshuler (1986) compares deafness with other deprived groups and argues cogently that it is lack of audition, in other words the deprivation of Deaf people in a hearing world, that leads to impulsivity. The world of Deaf people is changing with recognition of sign language in schools and later life. Anecdotally it seems that along with these changes there is a general reduction in impulsivity in Deaf patients.

Research into the prevalence of behaviour disorders in Deaf people has mostly been conducted in children (see Chapter 3). It shows that such disorders are at least twice as common as in their hearing counterparts (Meadow 1981; Hindley et al., 1994), but they are not the norm. Basilier (1964) first highlighted the prevalence of behaviour disturbances in young Deaf people, emphasizing impulsive and aggressive behaviour. He also emphasized a better prognosis than for hearing subjects, a point that is generally agreed upon by psychiatrists for Deaf people. Deaf people presenting to psychiatric services with such behaviours often have personal histories and current behaviour which would result in the label of 'personality disorder', yet many have a much better prognosis. The ESMHD's attempted consensus of experts (Swaans-Joha et al., 1990) added a subtype to the ICD group 'emotional and behavioural disorders with onset usually occurring in childhood or adolescence', of 'emotional, behavioural and psycho-social adjustment disorders related to deafness in early life (Basilier-type)'. For pragmatic reasons the authors can accept this subclassification, if it is given the same diagnostic coding for statistical purposes as its parent classification. It seems enough to be aware that Deaf people with this disorder are likely to have a better prognosis, without inventing a new diagnosis. There are no valid studies to suggest the existence of such a disorder. The fact that hearing people can suffer a similar collection of behaviours for similar reasons, for example, hearing people brought up in institutions or those with organic brain disorders, suggests that the same mechanisms are operating. At the ESMHD's consensus meeting of experts (Swaans-Joha et al., 1990), there was considerable debate over the term 'surdophrenia' originated by Basilier (1964) to describe impulsive behaviour in Deaf people. One of the authors was present and had already argued against the term (Kitson and Fry, 1990) on the basis that its literal translation is 'deaf mind' implying it is the norm for Deaf people and its name has been confused with schizophrenia and its subcategories, most of which end in 'phrenia'. Although the compromise was to dispose of the term, we do not agree with the need for a separate category and suspect that, as a vestige of past practice, it will vanish in time.

There is little evidence that Deaf people are more or less prone to any particular personality disorder. Paranoid personality has been said to be common, although it appears that this is due to a lack of clarity between early childhood Deafness and later acquired deafness. In the latter case there is a greater sway of opinion, though even there its justification is questionable (see also Chapter 11). Vernon and Andrews (1990) suggest that any increased prevalence of paranoid personality traits is reality-based in Deaf people, as well as suggesting that 'schizoid' personality is more frequent in rubella and low-birthweight causes. Grinker, Werble and Dye (1977) claimed that a 'borderline' personality is not seen in a Deaf client group. However we have had experience of successfully treating deaf patients, who fit the diagnostic criteria for borderline personality disorder. Farrugia (1992) suggests that the diagnosis of borderline personality disorder is probably less common in a Deaf population, due to reduced access to mental health services. Farrugia (1992) also suggests that borderline personality disorders might be more common in deaf people due to frustrated relationships with parental figures in early life.

From clinical experience it appears that behaviour disorders are becoming less of a problem in Deaf patients. It may be that Gerber (1983) was right in noting that due to communication difficulties 'behaviour disturbances are observed more often than problems of interpersonal concerns or neurotic symptoms'. Now that the reaction of society towards Deaf people has improved, and mental health services are staffed by Deaf people, we may be better able to see the emotional problems previously hidden by behaviour disturbance and poor communication.

It is hoped that readers will realize from this review that the scientific base of mental health assessment of Deaf people is still in its infancy and more research and observations from practice are required. To avoid error and unintentional adverse labelling of Deaf people it is vital that Deaf people themselves become involved in the process.

References

Altshuler K (1971) Studies of the deaf: relevance to psychiatric theory. American Journal of Psychiatry 127: 1521–1526.

Altshuler KZ (1986) Perceptual handicap and mental illness, with special reference to early profound deafness. American Journal of Social Psychiatry 6: 125–128.

Altshuler K, Rainer J (1970) Observations on psychiatric services for the deaf. Mental Hygiene 54: 538.

Altshuler K, Sarlin MB (1963) Deafness and schizophrenia: a family study. In Rainer J, Altshuler M, Kallmann F, Deming E (eds) Family and Mental Health Problems in a Deaf Population. New York: Columbia University, pp 204–213.

Altshuler K, Baroff G, Rainer J (1963) Operational description of a pilot clinic. In Rainer J, Altshuler M, Kallmann F, Deming E (eds) Family and Mental Health Problems in a Deaf Population. New York: Columbia University, pp 155–166.

Altshuler KZ, Deming WE, Vollenweider J, Rainer JD, Tendler R (1976) Impulsivity and early profound deafness: cross-cultural inquiry. Amer. Ann. Deaf 121: 331–345.

American Psychiatric Association (1988) Diagnostic and Statistical Manual of Mental Disorders (second edition). Washington DC: American Psychiatric Association.

Andreasen NC (1979) Thought, language, and communication disorders, I and II. Archives of General Psychiatry, 36, 1315–1330.

Basilier T (1964) Surdophrenia: the psychic consequences of congenital or early acquired deafness. Acta Psychiatrica Scandinavica 40: 362–372.

Bleuler E (1950) Dementia Praecox or the Group of Schizophrenias (translated by J. Zinkin). New York: IUP.

Chandrasena R (1987) Schneider's First Rank symptoms: an international and inter-ethnic comparative study. Acta Psychiatrica Scandinavica 76: 574–578.

Checinski K (1991) Preliminary findings of the study of the prevalence of psychiatric disorder in prelingually deaf adults living in the community. Proceedings, Mental Health and Deafness conference. London: St George's Hospital Medical School.

Chess S, Fernandez P (1981) Do deaf children have a typical personality? Annual Progress in Child Psychiatry and Child Development, 19: 295–305.

Corina D, O'Grady Batch L, Norman F (1990) Spatial Language and Spatial Cognition in Left and Right Lesioned Signers. Paper presented at the Third International Conference on Theoretical Issues in Sign Language Research, May 17, 1990, Boston.

Critchley E, Denmark J, Warren F, Wilson K (1981) Hallucinatory experiences of prelingually profoundly deaf schizophrenics. British Journal of Psychiatry 138: 30–32.

Denmark J (1966) Mental illness and early profound deafness.British Journal of Medical Psychology 39: 117–124.

Denmark J (1985) A study of 250 patients referred to a department of psychiatry for the deaf. British Journal of Psychiatry 46: 282–286.

Denmark JC, Eldridge RW (1969) Psychiatric services for the deaf. Lancet II: 259–262.

Dickert J (1988) Examination of bias in mental health evaluation of deaf patients. Social Work 33: 273–274.

Du Feu M, McKenna PJ (1996) Auditory Hallucinations in profoundly deaf schizophrenic patients: a phenomenological analysis. Scientia 1: 5.

Ebert D, Heckerling P (1995) Communication with deaf patients: knowledge, beliefs, and practices of physicians. Journal of the American Medical Association 273: 227–229.

Evans J, Elliott H (1981) Screening criteria for the diagnosis of schizophrenia in deaf patients. Archives of General Psychiatry 38: 787–790.

Evans J W, Elliot H (1987) The mental status examination. In Elliot H, Glass L, Evans J W (eds) Mental Health Assessment of Deaf Clients: A Practical Manual. Boston, MA: Little, Brown and Co.

Farrugia D (1992) Borderline personality disorder and deafness. Journal of the American Deafness and Rehabilitation Association 25: 8–15.

Fraunhofer N, Kitson N (1991) 'A study of Evan's and Elliot's Criteria in Mental State Assessment of Schizophrenia in the Prelingually Profoundly Deaf' Proceedings, Mental Health and Deafness Conference. London: St George's Hospital Medical School, pp 54–56.

Gerber BM 1983 A communication minority: deaf people and mental health care'. American Journal of Social Psychiatry 3: 50–57.

Grinker RR, Werble B, Dye R (1977) The Borderline Syndrome, New York: Basic Books.

Halgren B (1958) Retinitis pigmentosa in combination with congenital deafness and vestibulocerebellar ataxia; with psychiatric abnormality in some cases. A clinical and genetic study. Acta Genetica 8: 97–104.

Hamblin L, Kitson N (1992) Springfield supra-regional deaf unit: a retrospective case note survey. Abstracts, Royal College of Psychiatrists Annual Meeting, p 73.

Hills CG, Rappold ES, Rendon ME (1991) Binge eating and body image in a sample of the deaf college population. Journal of the American Deafness and Rehabilitation Association 25: 20–28.

Hindley P, Hill P, McGuigan S, Kitson N (1994) Psychiatric disorder in deaf and hearing impaired children and young people: a prevalence study. Journal of Child Psycholology and Psychiatry 55: 917–934.

Hurst J (1988) Metaphors of communication in the dreams of deaf people. Psychiatric Journal of the University of Ottawa 13: 75–78.

Kitson N, Fry R (1990) Prelingual deafness and psychiatry. British Journal of Hospital Medicine 244: 353–356.

Kitson N, Klein H (1995) Deaf services by Deaf people? Proceedings, third international congress, European society for mental health and deafness, in press.

Kraepelin E (1919) Dementia Praecox and Paraphrenia. Barclay RM (trans.), Edinburgh: E&S Livingstone Co.

Lancet (Editorial) (1981) Hearing loss and perceptual dysfunction in schizophrenia. Lancet 2: 848–849.

Lecours A, Vanier-Clement M (1976) Schizophasia and jargonphasia. Brain and Language, 3, 516–565.

McGuire PK, Shah GMS, Murray RM (1993) Increased blood flow in Broca's area during auditory hallucinations in schizophrenia. Lancet 342: 703–706.

McGuire PK, Robertson D, Thacker A, David AS, Kitson N, Frackowiak RSJ, Frith CD (1997) Neural correlates of thinking in sign language. Neuroreport 8: 695–698.

Markowitz JC, Nininger JE (1984) A case report of mania and congenital deafness. American Journal of Psychiatry 141: 894–895.

Mayberry R (1992) Mental Phonology in Sign Language. paper presented at the Fourth International Conference on Theoretical Issues in Sign Language Research, San Diego.

Meadow K (1981) Studies of behaviour problems of deaf children. In Stein L, Mindel E, Jabaley T (eds) Deafness and Mental Health. New York: Grune & Stratton, pp 3–22.

Mellor C (1970) First rank symptoms of schizophrenia. I. The frequency in schizophrenics on admission to hospital. II. Differences between individual first rank symptoms. British Journal of Psychiatry 117: 15–23.

Misiaszek J, Dooling J, Gieseke A, Melman H, Misiaszek JG, Jorgensen K (1985) Diagnostic considerations in deaf patients. Comprehensive Psychiatry 26: 513–521.

Monteiro B, Critchley EMR (1994) Deafness and communication. In Critchley EMR (ed) Neurological Boundaries of Reality. London: Farrand Press, pp 55–65.

Ridgeway S, Checinski K (1991) Mental health research methodology with deaf people. Proceedings, Second International Congress, European Society of Mental Health and Deafness, La Bastide, Avenue Vauban, 8, b-5000, Namur, Belgium, pp 208–211.

Robinson L (1978) Sound minds in a soundless world. DHEW Publication No ADM77-560, Washington DC: US Government Printing Office.

Sarlin MB, Altshuler KZ (1978) On the inter-relationship of cognition and affect: fantasies of deaf children. Child Psychiatry and Development 9: 95–103.

Schneider K (1959) Clinical Psychopathology (fifth edition). New York: Grune & Stratton.

Sever JL, South MA, Shaver KA (1985) Delayed manifestations of congenital rubella. Reviews of Infectious Diseases 7 (Supplement 1): 164–169.

Silversweig DA, Stern E, Frith C, Cahill C, Holmes A, Grootoonk S, Seaward J, McKenna P, Chua SE, Schnorr L et al. (1995) A functional neuroanatomy of hallucinations in schizophrenia. Nature 378: 176–179.

Swaans-Joha D, Mol I, Than P (1990) On Terminology: Mental Health Problems among Deaf People and Mental Health Care. University of Amsterdam.

Thacker A (1991) Communication: disorder, deprivation, or discrimination? Proceedings of the Inaugural Conference of the British Society on Mental Health and Deafness. London: St George's Hospital Medical School, November, 1991.

Thacker A (1994a) A sign language version of the Present State Examination. CIDI-SCAN. International Journal of Research in Psychiatry 3:204–205.

Thacker A (1994b) Formal communication disorder: sign language in deaf people with schizophrenia. British Journal of Psychiatry 165: 818–823.

Thacker AJ (1998) The Manifestation of Schizophrenic Formal Communication Disorder in Sign Language. Doctoral Dissertation, Department of Psychiatry, St George's Hospital Medical School.

Timmermans L (1989) Research project European society for mental health and deafness. Proceedings, European Congress on Mental Health and Deafness. Utrecht, pp 87–91.

Vernon McC, Andrews JF (1990) The Psychology of Deafness. New York and London. Longman.

Vernon McC, Rothstein DA (1968) Prelingual deafness an experiment of nature. Archives General Psychiatry 19: 361–369.

Wing J, Stuart E (1978) The PSE-ID-CATEGO system. Supplementary manual. London: Institute of Psychiatry.

Wing JK, Cooper JE and Sartorius N (1983) The Measurement and Classification of Psychiatric Symptoms. Cambridge University Press, Cambridge.

World Health Organization (1978) Mental Disorders: Glossary and Guide to their Classification in Accordance with the Ninth Revision of the International Classification of Diseases (ICD-9). Geneva: WHO.

World Health Organization (1992) The ICD-10 Classification of Mental and Behavioural Disorders: Clinical Descriptions and Diagnostic Guidelines. Geneva: WHO.

Chapter 5
Deafness and Intellectual Impairment: Double Jeopardy?

CHRIS WILLIAMS AND SALLY AUSTEN

Definitions and theoretical aspects

Deafness

Defining deafness is fraught with difficulties. Although precise audiological measurements of frequency and pitch can be made, hearing remains a subjective experience of the listener. If listeners can reliably report their experience of sound at differing frequencies and pitch then an objective audiogram reflecting their hearing capability can be constructed. This requires considerable co-operation and understanding on behalf of the individual. For some people, whose intellectual capabilities are impaired, producing an audiogram can pose difficulties for the examiner. Fortunately these are not insurmountable and a variety of free-field, evoked responses and operant techniques have evolved to aid the audiologist. In most cases a general classification of levels of hearing impairment can be generated and an individual may be assigned to a particular level of hearing impairment, from mild to profound. The generally agreed boundaries within this continuum of impairment are:

- Mild hearing loss 25–40 dB.
- Moderate 41–70 dB.
- Severe 71–95 dB.
- Profound > 96 dB.

However, this audiogram refers only to intensity or loudness and ignores pitch or frequency. In general, higher frequencies are more susceptible to loss than lower frequencies. The implication of this is that female voices may become progressively more difficult to hear than male voices as hearing is lost through disease or ageing. This can lead to added difficulties as most carers for individuals with mental retardation are female, and this should be considered when developing an understanding of potential communication difficulties for these individuals. Hearing is not simply a mechanical process of responding to sound, there is an environmental component that can enhance or hinder the social application of hearing in communication. This interaction between biology and environment forms part of the concept of 'double jeopardy' whereby difficulties are compounded to be more than the sum of their parts. This concept is explored more fully later in the chapter.

Intellectual impairment or mental retardation

Similarly, intellectual impairment or mental retardation can present difficulties in definition. A broad working definition might take the form:

> mental retardation is a delay in the development of a range of cognitive and behavioural characteristics for an individual compared with those characteristics that are considered normative for his or her age during the developmental period conventionally considered to be up to the age of 18 years.

In addition to developmental delay as one of the defining characteristics there also exists in some individuals behaviour that is socially and culturally maladaptive in a normative environment.

Hence, a definition of mental retardation has three primary elements:

- Significant under-functioning in some or all cognitive skills.
- Dysfunctional social behaviour either through limited development of social competence or excess development of maladaptive behaviours.
- Manifesting during the developmental period of 0–16 years.

More recently there has been an active debate over definition towards a greater recognition of the interaction. This concept underpins the revised American Association on Mental Retardation (AAMR) definition, which encourages flexibility in interpreting IQ cut-off scores and enlarging the concept of adaptive behaviour to ten specific adaptive skills, including communication, social and leisure skills (Reiss, 1994).

Cognitive skills

The traditional approach to assessing cognitive skills has been to use normative referenced psychometric scales. This assumes the existence of an underpinning 'general' factor in intelligence in conjunction with a range of additional factors having greater variability within individuals.

This is the primary rationale of generating a single figure for an intelligence quotient from the summation of sub-scales using standardized tests. A further assumption is made to constrain the design of intelligence tests to fit the normal distribution. This mathematical model has attractive statistical properties relating to the distribution of variables within a population, and most contemporary intelligence tests are constructed to map on to this distribution. Hence, the items selected are determined by their fit to a mathematical model. It is this which determines the statistical frequency of intellectual impairment in a population. The most widely used psychometric tests for this purpose are the Wechsler scales (Mittler, 1970). Three batteries of tests have been developed to cover a wide age range. They are constructed so that a score of IQ 100 divides the population neatly in two — 50% scoring above and 50% scoring below. This then forms the 'average IQ' of a population. The tests are further constrained to produce a standard deviation score of 15 IQ points to equate with the variability in cognitive competence within a population. By manipulating the difficulty of items in the tests and meticulous standardization studies, an instrument is produced which, when used by trained psychometric administrators, produces a reliable measure of the position of any individual on a normal distribution curve having a mean of 100 and standard deviation of 15. The AAMR classification system for mental retardation defines categories of retardation by reference to this distribution. This system is also adopted by the ICD-10 and DSM-IV classification systems. Mental retardation is defined as any score beyond two standard deviations below the mean. Hence, a table of levels of mental retardation, associated IQ measures and statistical distribution can be constructed (Table 5.1).

These figures deal with population groups and conceal individual variation, particularly when sensory difficulties may impede the development and manifestation of the cognitive skills sampled in formal intelligence tests. It is therefore necessary to be cautious in allocating individuals to categories based upon IQ assessment alone. Additional features must include elements of social competence, which are much more difficult to assess using a normative model. A range of assessment strategies has been developed to investigate adaptive behaviour. Most are based upon performance criteria derived from observational studies of normative behaviour (Williams, 1986; Hogg and Raynes, 1987).

Interpretation of scores obtained from these kinds of instrument is very much more subjective. Their main use is as descriptive data and as baselines from which to judge improvement following educational

Table 5.1 Mental retardation, associated IQ measures and statistical distribution

Level of mental retardation	Range of IQ measure	Estimated population frequency
Mild	50–70	30/1000
Moderate	35–49	3.0/1000 (Moderate and Severe combined)
Severe	20–34	
Profound	< 20	0.5/1000

programmes. Repeated measures can indicate change over time as a result of intervention, although they are subject to greater measurement error than formal psychometric instruments. Nevertheless, taken together it is possible to identify those individuals deemed to be mentally retarded for the purpose of educational or care provision. Recent aspects of UK legislation have highlighted the necessity to have such operational definitions in helping to determine services under the Mental Health Act 1983 and with respect to the sexuality and fiscal laws of the UK (Ashton and Ward, 1992).

However, despite apparent precision, the above assessment procedures attempt to categorize from a continuum. This must necessarily be arbitrary and the 'true' prevalence of retardation in any community rests upon criteria unrelated to the needs of those so labelled. A better system exists following the publication of the World Health Organization (WHO, 1980) classification of impairments, disabilities and handicaps. This system identifies three elements:

- *Impairment:* any disturbance of the normal structure and functioning of the body, including the systems of mental function.
- *Disability:* the loss or reduction of functional ability and activity consequent upon impairment.
- *Handicap:* the disadvantage experienced as a result of impairment or disability. Handicap thus represents the social and environmental consequences of impairments and disabilities.

This system of classification reveals important distinctions in the perception of disability, ranging from the biological to the socio-psychological.

Impairment

At this level we can identify a range of dysfunctions in the individual which have an organic origin, only some of which are presently identified. The most frequently occurring of these in mental retardation are the chromosome abnormalities of trisomy 21 and Fragile-X syndrome, making up approximately 30% of the known causes of intellectual impairment. A much smaller proportion of intellectually impaired individuals have identifiable genetic disorders leading to inborn errors of metabolism or morphological abnormalities. The remaining causative factors include perinatal brain damage, epilepsy, maternal infections and environmental toxins. There still remains a further 30% for whom no causative factor has yet been identified, apart from ascribing polygenic variation and/or environmental deprivation (Craft, Bicknell and Hollins, 1985).

Of these causative factors, trisomy 21 has most relevance in studies of hearing impairment in individuals with intellectual impairments. Cunningham (1982) reported a prevalence of 80–95% of hearing loss in Down syndrome children. Since the majority of these children had conductive or mixed hearing loss, the importance of early detection and otological and audiological management was stressed in order to minimize subsequent disabilities in communication arising solely from untreated and unrecognized hearing impairment. The importance of identifying biological causative factors is highlighted by the virtual elimination of maternal rubella infection as a causative agent for congenital hearing loss, visual impairment and learning disability, following active immunization programmes (Tookey, 1994). Other viral agents are recognized with increasing frequency as causing similar congenital impairments, with cytomegalovirus (CMV) assuming the role of the rubella virus (Kropka and Williams, 1986). Finally, the condition of otitis media with effusion (OME) has become accepted as a common causative factor in hearing impairment (Ballantyne, 1977) and has been found to be associated with learning disabilities (Masters and Marsh, 1978).

By identifying the causative agents, the first link in the chain of impairment–disability–handicap can be broken in a substantial number of cases. In spite of this, however, many still slip through the preventive net and present with significant disability as a consequence of the hearing–intellectual impairment.

Disability

The primary disability of a hearing impairment is one of communication. Both receptive and expressive skills are compromised. Hearing people live in an aural–oral culture and use speech as their main mode of communication. Hearing-impaired people, especially pre-lingually deaf individuals, are excluded from this culture and create a separate culture known by some as the 'Deaf world' (Sacks, 1990; Firth, 1992). Herein lies the **handicap** of deafness imposed by the dominant hearing culture — to be discussed later. The disability starts from communication problems and extends into socialization, education and, ultimately, occupation (Medoff, 1980; Lillemor, Hallberg and Carlsson, 1993).

When the hearing impairment is in addition to an intellectual impairment there is a compounding effect referred to as 'double jeopardy' by Williams (1993). This compounding effect has been implicated in the underestimation of intellectual competence in hearing-impaired individuals, who may find themselves identified with intellectually impaired people more than with hearing-impaired people, thus partly accounting for the increased incidence of hearing difficulties in groups of intellectually impaired people. Yeates (1991) reported an incidence of hearing loss within a sample of 300 adults with severe learning disabilities approaching 40% of her study group. Kropka (1979) reported data to show an overall incidence of 10% hearing impairment in a hospitalized population of adults, including mild and moderate learning disabilities, of whom 1.5% were not intellectually impaired on formal psychometric assessment.

This hidden population of hearing-impaired individuals must have been considerable when hospitalization was the major residential provision apart from remaining within the parental home. Fortunately this is no longer the case in the UK and 'care in the community' has dramatically altered service provision from institutional to an 'ordinary life' provision. In addition to this historical discrimination, disadvantages arising from dual impairments in hearing and intellect can be significantly disabling, particularly in a hearing–speaking community into which hearing–intellectually-impaired people are expected to integrate. Without the skills of the dominant culture the individual is at risk of segregation, social isolation and financial disadvantage.

Historical aspects of 'double jeopardy'

Formerly, the dual disability of deafness and intellectual impairment would have been likely to lead to institutionalization to provide life-long care with only limited emphasis on remedial action to overcome the communication disability. Those born deaf, and deafened adults, could be found in mental handicap hospitals displaying many characteristics of 'behaviour disturbance' solely due to misunderstood attempts at communication between themselves and staff or other patients. This is well demonstrated by the case of Mr A, who was admitted as a patient to the former Royal Western Counties Hospital in Devon, UK in 1949, at the age of 12 years, following action by the police as a result of his stealing a few apples. Mr A was born deaf, as was his mother and three of his brothers. On admission, the clinical notes indicated that Mr A was to be detained under the Mental Deficiency Act of 1913 and referred to him as:

> . . . deaf and dumb and formal testing is impossible. He is extremely simple and childish and does not respond to training. He is incapable of benefiting from training and education even in a special school for the deaf. His comprehension is limited and he cannot tell the time or point to his eyes or ears. His moral sense is poorly developed and he is a pilferer. He is a feeble-minded grade. He is apathetic without initiative and seems to be content to play with a toy rabbit. He needs care, supervision and training.

Unfortunately, it would appear that Mr A received very little in the form of training, for five years later in his file is noted:

> . . . is a bully and makes vicious attacks on other patients. He appears to delight in causing pain. He is in need of constant supervision in his own interest and for the protection of others.

At that time Mr A's IQ was quoted as being 45, but no further details given as to how this was calculated. For the next 24 years of Mr A's life in hospital he was to acquire a reputation of 'challenging behaviour', necessitating a variety of pharmacological and environmental controls to curb his activity. He eventually became settled as a 'pot boy' in the hospital kitchens where he befriended two similarly deaf men with Down syndrome. The three individuals developed an idiosyncratic signing system known only to themselves. Towards the end of the 1980s a rehabilitation programme was being developed at the hospital where Mr A lived, using 'ordinary' housing. Mr A and his two colleagues were among the first to be accepted for the training for which he had been admitted to the hospital some 30 years previously! During this period of rehabilitation Mr A received help in learning social, domestic and communication skills and in 12 months he rapidly achieved 100% success in all three areas as measured by his social training achievement record (STAR) (Williams, 1986).

Communication training was implemented by use of an adapted version of British Sign Language (BSL) using a graduated vocabulary of functional signs. Mr A's two colleagues were similarly instructed and all three gentlemen successfully moved to live in a warden-assisted flat in a local town, where Mr A gained part-time employment in the catering trade. He regained contact with his family and lives a virtually independent community life in spite of his earlier handicaps. The most recent formal assessment of his IQ indicated a level of functioning within the average range for non-verbal items.

That this gentleman had survived for 30 years in a hospital before having the opportunity to develop, in 12 months of specialized individual help, sufficiently to live independently is a measure of the double jeopardy of deafness and supposed intellectual impairment. It was the acquisition of a signed communication system that was critical to Mr A's liberation.

Signing

The natural language of people born deaf is a visual language expressed by whole-body, face, hand and finger movements using a conventional system of iconic and symbolic signs. It is received visually and in some cases by touch. It has a vocabulary and a syntax, which, although differing from that of spoken English, is nevertheless systematic, lawful and legitimate. Competent signers have no problem conveying all of the nuances and abstractions previously thought to be the exclusive property of vocal communication (Kyle and Woll, 1985). The myth of signing as a second-class language has hindered its acceptability among traditional teachers of the deaf. This myth has been exposed and the greater efficacy of sign and gesture communication has gained wide acceptance, with total communication being advocated for all individuals with multiple sensory and intellectual disabilities (Downing, 1993).

That this should have taken so long to come about is an indication of the self-appointed supremacy of speaking service providers in maintaining a virtual oral-manual apartheid and the imposition of vocal language on deaf people, as if to speak was to become like a hearing person and somehow 'better'. As long ago as the 1940s Heider and Heider (1941) reported on their observational studies of children born deaf showing evidence of 'language development' using gestures that demonstrated syntactical constructions. In contrast, Myklebust (1960) had argued that people born deaf could act as a form of 'natural preparation' of language-less individuals whose cognitive skills would consequently be severely limited as a direct result of having no language. He developed the thesis that, since deaf people are lacking in language, they should perform poorly in problem-solving, thinking and other cognitive tasks. However, this was subsequently shown not to be so, by Furth and Youniss (1975) demonstrating competence in cognitive functioning of a non-vocal nature in so-called 'language-less born deaf' individuals.

One exception to this has been the demonstration of difficulties in sequential tasks for pre-lingually deaf individuals (Tomlinson-Keasey and Smith Winberry, 1990). The authors have similarly noticed during clinical assessment of pre-lingually deaf adolescents attending a vocational skills training course that, although performing within the average range on all other non-verbal sub-tests of the WAIS-R, significant difficulties were experienced with the picture arrangement subtest. This test requires the individual to rearrange a random placement of visual stimuli depicting a cartoon story into the correct temporal sequence to tell a logical story. Pre-lingually deaf individuals would understand the task but not be able to generate the solution. They would rearrange the random order and, when asked to tell the story would describe the content of each card independently. This suggests that visuospatial languages have a different internal representation from spoken languages when dealing with temporal sequencing and interpretations of causal events that are chronologically sequential.

Since, by its nature of production, a spoken language can only be conveyed item by item, whereas a signed language can convey simultaneous as well as sequential information, there exists an intrinsic difficulty in trying to convey a linear language in its visual form through writing to users of a language that has different internal syntax and possibly internal parallel processing. Conrad (1979) has shown the significant disadvantage suffered by pupils with pre-lingual deafness when learning traditional orthographic reading, and the written language of sign communicators takes skill to interpret as it is generally written in signed rather than spoken word order, leading the unwary to underestimate the intellectual competence of the writer who cannot write English in the correct word order. Worldsign (Orcutt, 1985) was a valiant attempt to utilize a combination of visual graphics and signs to generate a language that could bridge this gap and overcome the difficulty that a child born deaf has in learning a written language based upon sound rather than sign. Unfortunately, it does not appear to have gained the acceptance its underlying intention warranted.

It is becoming increasingly accepted that sign language should be taught by, and experienced with, natural sign language users. And since natural sign language users are almost exclusively deaf themselves this gives a unique enhancing role for Deaf workers in rehabilitation services that has yet to be implemented widely. In contrast to this natural approach using the skills and competencies of the Deaf world, a form of communication intervention has been described which appears, initially, to have demonstrated phenomenal intellectual prowess in individuals hitherto considered as uncommunicating, largely through autism as their primary disability (Biklen, 1990, 1992, 1993). The very seductiveness of the reported success is likely to lead to its implementation in helping hearing-impaired learning-disabled individuals express themselves without the toil of having to be taught a manual language largely by non-manual language users. This method is known as 'facilitated communication' and is a technique that involves physically assisting an individual to point to letters to spell out messages. That extraordinary 'messages' have been spelled out seems to have convinced many users of facilitated communication that the underlying disability does not exist, only that the proper tools for expression have yet to be employed. Biklen has described apparent communications from severely disabled individuals that contain a usage of vocabulary, syntax and reasoning more akin to graduates than might be expected from intellectually impaired individuals. This should not be at all surprising since it is usually graduates who are enlisted to facilitate such communications by placing their hands over the hands of the disabled individual to enable messages to be tapped out on keyboards or by letter pointing.

That this is reminiscent of table-turning and Ouija board messages seems to have eluded Biklen and his devotees, and the uncritical enthusiasm with which such methods are accepted necessitates the recent critical comment by Thompson (1993) and empirical demonstration of facilitator guiding (Simon, Toll and Whitehair, 1994) to avoid widespread advocacy of a method of communication that is likely to convey more from the facilitator than the communicator. That such 'innovations' can achieve this level of enthusiasm is an indication of the hunger for an easy route to communication with those who, on the surface, can appear alien to the dominant culture of the speaking–hearing population. It is essential that we are not seduced by apparently easy solutions such as suggested by 'facilitated communication', and proper consideration should be given to empirically and ecologically established communication systems emanating from a world that knows how to convey messages without speech.

Double jeopardy for client or therapist?

Clinical aspects of work with intellectually impaired Deaf people

In the second part of this chapter the focus is on the double jeopardy of the therapist who has to adapt treatment techniques not once, as for a

Deaf client, but twice for a client who is Deaf and has an intellectual impairment. The Deaf–intellectually impaired client may present for treatment with the same disorders as other more able clients: depression, psychotic illness, behaviour problems and so on, as well as others related to intellectual impairment, such as the practical difficulties of daily living skills and learning. On presentation the intellectual impairment may be known or suspected. Clinicians working with Deaf people or with those with intellectual impairments will have their own style of assessment and treatment. Here, some of the differences in assessment and treatment of Deaf people with intellectual impairments are suggested.

Assessment

Assessment of people with intellectual impairments has often been associated with cognitive assessment or 'IQ testing' (see above). This may be important in judging whether someone is achieving full potential — or being given the opportunity to achieve this. It can also be useful when previous treatments have been unsuccessful and there is a query about whether the level of intellect required to make use of the treatment has been pitched too high. However, it can also be misleading. If a person with multiple disabilities is suspected of being depressed then it is important not to be side-tracked by the level of intellectual impairment, but initially to treat the depression.

Neurological impairment is often associated with intellectual impairment and perhaps more so in Deaf people with intellectual impairment. The cause of deafness and the cause of the intellectual impairment may often be identical: an assault on the brain. This may occur congenitally as with rubella, or Rhesus incompatibility; be perinatal, such as prematurity; or post-natal, such as meningitis. Neurological damage may bring with it specific problems, such as epilepsy, or more subtle difficulties, such as impulse control problems and attention deficits. Psychometric assessment for neurological conditions is difficult due to lack of appropriate test material and lack of Deaf norms, therefore much of the assessment will need to be via observational methods.

Treatment

Treatment plans should be devised carefully after consideration of the following:

- The various presenting problems — deafness, intellectual impairment, depression, challenging behaviour and so on.
- The prospects of improving any of these problems — the deafness and intellectual impairment are unlikely to change, whilst the depression and challenging behaviour may do so.

- Who is the client? Will intervention involve attempting to change something in the client, in the environment, or in the people involved in the client's life?
- Resources — every service has limits and, whilst the client's needs should be recorded genuinely, treatment plans should be realistic and achievable goals set.

Each model of therapy has its own treatment techniques, all of which are equally appropriate for both the understanding and treatment of the presenting problems of Deaf people with intellectual impairments. The ease with which the various treatment techniques are adapted and applied may vary, however, and some areas that must be considered are described here.

Empowerment and directiveness

Many of the most able Deaf people experience disempowerment, and come to therapy expecting to have something done *to* them by the therapist. With the most linguistically able clients this can be explored through therapy and the balance redressed. With the less able client the therapist needs to consider the position more thoroughly.

The therapist must make a conscious decision about the part played by informants such as carers or families in the assessment and treatment of the client. For example, the therapist should compare the relative importance of maintaining the client's confidentiality, thus reinforcing his independence as an adult, with gaining and having access to the family in order to gain background information to aid the assessment or change the way in which family members interact with the client.

If clients are not able to set their own goals for therapy it may be necessary to provide very clear, directive statements about what is and is not acceptable behaviour. These rules could be renegotiated if the client becomes able. For example, a therapist may say to a client with challenging behaviour, '*It is OK to be angry and it is OK to shout but it is not OK to hit or kick.*' The therapist must ensure that others working and living with the client follow the same guidelines. Therapists must also ensure that if clients are not able to renegotiate guidelines for themselves, they do not thereby seriously restrict their clients' human rights.

Psychological articulation

People vary in their ability to articulate their thoughts and feelings, dependent on their language skills, cognitive skills and past experience. Feelings, even positive ones, can be distressing and difficult to cope with if you do not know what you are experiencing. For example, imagine you felt excitement for the first time ever and you did not know what it was;

you would probably appraise this situation as quite unpleasant. Feelings are infinitely more manageable if they have a name, their duration is to some extent predictable, and they are considered normal by people who are significant in your life.

Without labels and measures of feelings it is also very difficult to assess when one is feeling better (or worse). During treatment it is useful to get a baseline measure at the start and to measure improvement throughout. To be able to measure, the labels should first be in place. The therapist will need to check the client's psychological vocabulary and, if it is not sufficient for the purposes of therapy, provide a means of education.

Labelling

The emotions most needed to be discussed in therapy need to be labelled. This could be by a sign, a word, a picture or even a colour. More able clients could devise or choose the label themselves, whilst for some clients the therapist will have to create the label after thorough observation of the client. The more disabled the client, the more pro-active the therapist needs to be. To create labels on behalf of clients it is best to observe them in a range of situations over time, including the perceptions of those people who know them best, until the therapist is fairly confident of what behaviour or facial expressions represent what emotion. From then on, each time the client seems to be feeling an emotion the therapist and the carers can present the appropriate label. The aim of this is, firstly, for clients to feel that their feelings are being contained and validated by significant others and, secondly, to enable clients eventually to internalize the labelling process.

Later on, we provide case histories in which emotions are labelled by cartoon pictures of words, signs and colours.

Measuring

Once the emotions are labelled, a measuring system is required so that the emotion can be shown to be containable, and its course predictable. Painful emotions are less distressing when you know they will end eventually. Thus, time should be spent helping clients to articulate when things are worse and when they are better; that feelings are different before, during and after particular situations and that feelings come in different forms, speeds and sizes. Measures should be devised and implemented within the capabilities of clients to represent the properties of feelings. Able clients may benefit from use of a 10-point Likert scale; less able clients may be able to use a similar scale with three points. For example, a client labelling *Fear* could measure it by the words 'no Fear', 'bit Fear' and 'big Fear' or could measure it by a picture of a frightened person — in various sizes.

Measuring, at its simplest, can become a matter of Yes/No: did the feeling occur or not. This must be recorded over time.

Semantically, the concept of measuring is slightly incorrect as one could claim to **label** a feeling as, for example, 'big Fear'. For the purpose of this exercise, educating clients that the same feeling can have a variety of presentations depending on speed, size, etc., it is advisable to separate the concepts firmly: the feeling is labelled '*Fear*' and measured 'big Fear'.

From the knowledge that emotions are to some extent predictable comes the knowledge that they are therefore controllable and that clients have the power to alter their feelings, either by changing something in themselves or in their environment.

Normalizing

By working on the labelling and measuring of feelings, the therapist is also normalizing those feelings. Many clients with additional disabilities will have been disempowered generally and, specifically, may have experienced disapproval of some emotions, such as anger, and scorn at others, such as fear. Because of the negative reactions of others to their emotions, clients may have developed unpleasant feelings secondary to the original emotion. For example, a client may feel frightened after he has felt angry because he expects to be rebuked or he may be ashamed after he has felt frightened because he expects scorn. By allowing and normalizing the original emotion the therapist can rapidly desensitize clients to these secondary emotions.

Clients of all abilities who experience unpleasant feelings often believe that they are unique in feeling this: either that the extremity of their feeling is unique or that it is unique to experience this feeling in this situation. By overtly labelling and measuring feelings in a medium that is comprehensible to clients, they can change that belief to one of, . . . '*if we talk about it and there are measures for it, it must be to some extent normal and manageable*'.

A further benefit of working on accepting feelings is that you can create a non-punitive context for rejecting certain behaviours resulting from the feeling, such as: anger is good, hitting people is not; fear is good, avoiding going out of the house is not.

Language

If the client is Deaf and has a known or suspected intellectual impairment there is a high chance that he will also have language disorder or language delay. He will probably be fluent neither in BSL nor in spoken or lip-read English. He may have developed idiosyncratic signing or no formal language at all.

In this situation the therapist must be prepared to develop and use a wide range of communication skills involving mime, sign, role play and drawing. Consulting rooms should have paper and pens as a matter of course. Access to video equipment becomes extremely important as an option for providing feedback to the client, giving homework or helping him to remember the contents of the sessions.

Therapists who work with Deaf people need communication skills that are inversely proportional to the communication skill of the client. That is, the poorer the signing skills of the client the more skilled the signing skills of the therapist need to be. The therapist must take into account that clients may, for example, be echolalic or echopraxic, may not have the skills necessary to judge whether the receiver has understood, or may have grammatical difficulties with time, placement or pronouns. Deaf therapists, who will not of course be exempt from such problems, may have an advantage, as one can generally be more flexible in one's own first language. A hearing therapist may want to consider working with a Deaf member of staff: depending on skills and qualifications, a Deaf member of staff could observe the hearing person's work and feedback their comments; could be a co-therapist; could work directly with the client under the supervision of the hearing therapist; or could have the whole case delegated to him or her.

Memory

Therapists should remember that people with intellectual impairments are likely to have memory problems. There is very little empirical evidence in this area even with hearing intellectually impaired people. A rule of thumb, however, could be that the more severe the intellectual impairment the more severe the memory difficulties to be expected. With Deaf intellectually impaired people the statistical relationship may not be a clear linear one. If brain damage has occurred then the effect on memory could be more unpredictable and it is not uncommon to meet people whose intellectual impairment is only mild but whose memory problem is more severe (Hogg, Sebba and Lambe, 1990).

Furthermore, people with limited language who do not have these types of brain damage may still have practical difficulties with remembering if they have not developed sufficient strategies to compensate for their poor verbal memory. Recording information into a visual form, not just into sign language, will be necessary and therapists should be aware that not only must they *use* such strategies but they may need to *model* them to clients.

Reading

Written material is currently used with great success in a variety of mental health assessment and treatment approaches used with hearing people.

- Leaflets and posters in the community and in primary care services are used to inform people about some of the most common problems, and the help that is available. This has a secondary benefit of reducing stigma to the mental health problem.

- Once in treatment, clients may receive education handouts describing either the problem more fully or the type of therapy. For some clients, fully understanding their condition, learning that it will not kill them, or that it does not mean they are losing control of their minds, is enough to make the problem remit spontaneously. This is commonly experienced in the treatment of anxiety disorders.
- Written measures of feeling or experience are used either before treatment to assist in the diagnosis or at intervals throughout treatment to facilitate clients' awareness of their own state and to measure improvement. For example, the *Beck Depression Inventory* (BDI), the *Hospital Anxiety and Depression Scale* (HAD) and/or the *Minnesota Multiphasic Personality Inventory* (MMPI).
- Homework tasks, such as diaries to label, measure and explore feelings and thoughts, are useful and emphasize the clients' role in their own treatment.

The average reading age of Deaf adults is only 8.75 years (Conrad, 1979). Much of the written material commonly used in both assessment and treatment may therefore be inaccessible to many Deaf clients. In addition, if the client has a known or suspected intellectual impairment then the written word must be virtually eliminated. The concepts held within the words are still valuable. Alternatives must be found, therefore, by use of drawing or videos.

Visual behaviour

Although each psychological model of therapy can be used in the understanding of the client's problems, treatment may often need to be in the form of a behavioural translation. People with limited language will learn mainly from modelling.

This should be considered both in hypothesizing which behaviours have been learned and can therefore be unlearned, and in designing therapeutic interventions. Role play and modelling should be considered as visual alternatives to 'verbal' therapies. By using interventions *in situ* the therapist can control the environment to some extent, may be seen to condone feelings, can be on hand to help with labelling and measuring feelings and can model coping strategies. Some people with intellectual impairments or brain damage find learning very difficult. This may be for a variety of reasons, such as memory problems, attention difficulties or fear of new situations. In this case, new material must be repeated many times. For this a video of the therapy session or a summary will be invaluable. Thus, therapy may not always take place in the consulting room.

Case-studies

We now present two examples with a brief formulation and a description of how treatment was adapted for use with the specific clients.

> Example 1: John, aged 35
> John has a profound prelingual hearing impairment. He is cared for by his uncle, his parents having both died of heart conditions. John talks about heart attacks regularly but is not thought by his doctor to be of increased risk of one himself. John's language is limited. He manages with a few signs and gestures and a few written words, although on testing he is found to have only a very mild intellectual impairment. He has severe agoraphobia which seriously affects the quality of his life and restricts the likelihood of his achieving the independence that would otherwise be expected of him, given his deafness and mild intellectual impairment. Members of his family, including his late father, are reported to have had anxiety disorders.

Formulation

Systemic, psychodynamic and cognitive–behavioural models could all be considered. Given the need to alleviate the symptoms as soon as possible, a cognitive–behavioural model was chosen, drawing on family systems theories in order to remove secondary reinforcement of anxiety behaviours.

John probably learned anxiety behaviours from his parents and this developed into an acute anxiety state on their death. His anxiety is maintained by a fear that his own anxiety symptoms, such as palpitations, may cause his own death. By avoiding anxiety-provoking situations he cannot desensitize himself to anxiety and is perpetuating the agoraphobia. His language limitations mean that 'verbal' therapies are not accessible to him and visual adaptations are required.

Treatment

Anxiety education is used to explain how anxiety serves an important purpose in our lives by keeping us safe, that it is completely normal but that sometimes the amount of the person's anxiety is disproportional to the situation. Anxiety has three main components: the physiological, the cognitive and the behavioural. All of this information is conveyed in cartoon form with some supporting words, signs and role play.

Some cartoons may be used with a number of different clients. Others have to be unique to specific clients. For example, for John the physiological symptom of palpitations is represented as shown in Figure 5.1.

The cognitive symptom '*I think I'm going crazy*' is represented as shown in Figure 5.2.

The behaviour symptom of avoidance or running away from situations is represented as shown in Figure 5.3

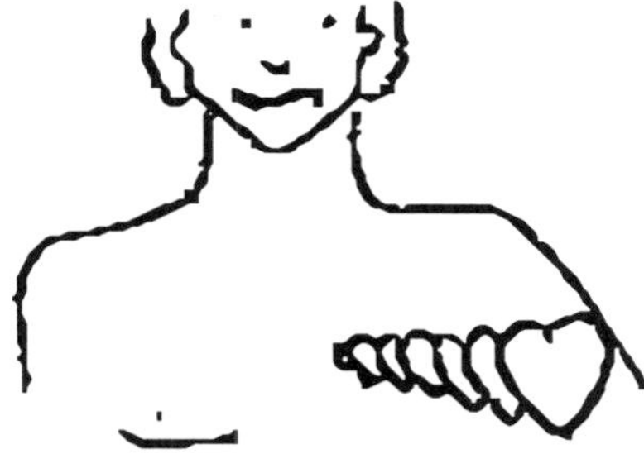

Figure 5.1 Representation of John's physiological symptom of palpitations.

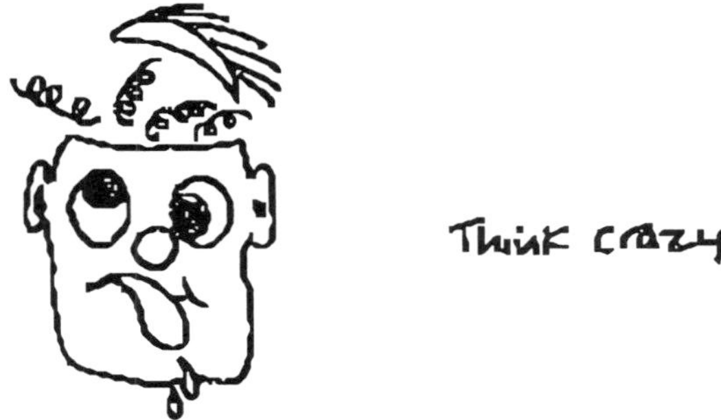

Figure 5.2 Representation of John's cognitive symptom 'I think I'm going crazy'.

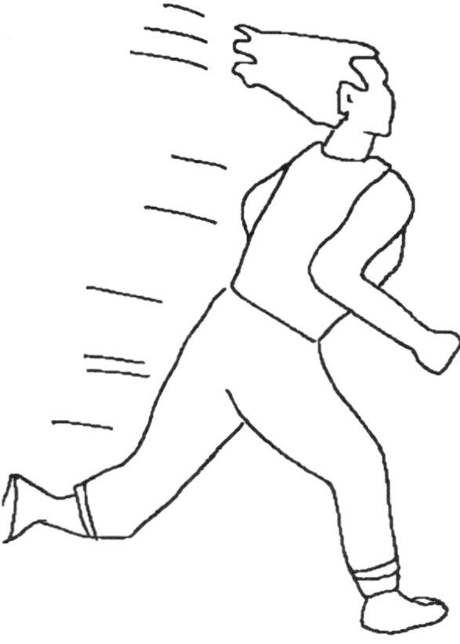

Figure 5.3 Representation of the behaviour of John's avoidance or running away from situations.

Labelling

The whole family is involved and all members are encouraged to talk about their fears and symptoms of anxiety. Games are played using flash-cards of the symptom pictures. This increases the relevant vocabulary in both sign and pictures. It also has the effect of normalizing the experiences for the client and his family and removing the stigma. Games include 'Snap', and 'Charades'.

John recognizes his most distressing symptom as palpitations, and since the BSL sign for general anxiety is fingers pounding the left side of the chest as in a palpitation, this was the picture he chose to represent '*fear*'.

Measuring

John could manage a Likert scale of three points. Measures were implemented daily, at first measuring only '*Fear*'.

When John became adept at this, the measures were expanded to include a variety of physiological and cognitive symptoms. John had difficulty in grasping that anxiety will always eventually dissipate as he had difficulty with the concept of 'before and after'. John was very skilled, however, at dates and times so for a few occasions he was required to record his anxiety every 10 minutes for two hours, starting at a time when he was very anxious, to experience how it could improve over time.

Intervention

Physiological symptoms

Relaxation and controlled breathing were used to combat the effects of hyperventilation. Hyperventilation causes raised adrenalin levels in the blood which, in turn, cause unpleasant physical sensations such as palpitations, sweaty hands and feeling sick.

This was practised every day. John's uncle was encouraged to model the use of relaxation and breathing techniques as a strategy for coping with anxiety. This was augmented by a videotape presentation of relaxation training.

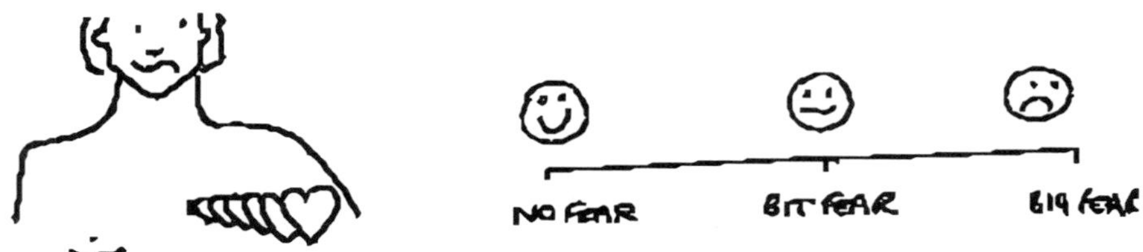

Figure 5.4 John's Likert scale of three points.

Cognitive symptoms

Anxious people commonly experience negative thoughts rushing through their minds, such as *'I'm going to choke'*, *'I'm going to faint'* *'Everyone is looking at me'*. Reassurance by others does not usually help anxious people in the long run as they just require ever-increasing amounts of reassurance. Disproving the doubts for themselves is useful. Thus, after John had been anxious he was asked, *'Have you died?'* *'Did you faint just then?'* By answering in the negative he was disproving his negative beliefs and reassuring himself.

Specific to John's case was the history of family heart problems and the hypothesis that John considered himself likely to die from a heart attack. Given John's language problems it was likely that John had never understood the results of the doctor's investigations revealing that he was not at increased risk of a heart attack and that his life expectancy was normal. With the doctor's agreement John was briefly examined again and the examination and the explanation of the results videoed. This was then translated into a linguistic form that John could understand (basic sign, picture and writing) and videoed on to the same tape. By replaying it John could challenge some of his negative thoughts and reassure himself.

Behavioural symptoms

The individual is encouraged to put himself deliberately in anxiety-provoking situations and to stay in the situation until the anxiety fades. When a 0–10 Likert scale measure of anxiety is used, individuals should aim to put themselves into situations of approximately 5 out of 10 anxiety. Since John was using a three-point Likert scale he was placed initially in low anxiety-provoking situations. If too severe a situation had been chosen he might have become so anxious that he would have left the situation, which would reinforce the belief that the only way to cope with anxiety is to escape from the situation. Anxiety has a natural lifespan. It can last only a matter of minutes because the body adjusts to the amount of adrenalin in the bloodstream and eventually all the physiological mechanisms diminish.

To John, who has linguistic difficulties and is therefore better at concrete interpretations, the idea of deliberately doing the thing which most frightened him — going out of the house — seemed a bizarre suggestion. Repeated role play was necessary to convince him to try the intervention. A small distance was chosen and role play was used in the living room to show what would happen using a third person to play John's role. Every step was role-played: leaving the house, walking to the identified place, standing still, feeling the anxiety with the therapist reminding John to breathe slowly and relax various muscles in the body, waiting, breathing slowly until the anxiety had gone, walking slowly home, where he got a pat on the back and a cup of tea. John was then required to role play himself a number of times in the living room before actually trying it himself.

Sufficiently small goals should be used to ensure success. The task should be practised twice a day for a week before increasing the target length. At each stage, target plans were drawn out and measures of anxiety before, during, and after the task are recorded. Gradually, as his confidence grew, John was able to take over deciding future goals and can now do the desensitization unaccompanied. Success is a reward in itself but it was still important to have a 'significant other', encouraging and congratulating him.

It is important when treating agoraphobia to tackle all the things that make the client anxious. Rarely is the problem only open spaces, but will usually include enclosed spaces too: anywhere away from the safety of home. Once John had accomplished various distances outside, some of his other fears, such as crowded restaurants, were worked on in the same way, starting with an empty café and building up gradually to larger and busier ones.

Desensitization can be used for most fears, but it must be done very slowly and methodically. Families and carers should be reminded to be patient. Articulate people with fairly new avoidance behaviours can improve dramatically in a matter of weeks, whereas those with long established avoidance behaviours and additional disabilities must be allowed much longer. John's treatment took approximately one year and required a commitment of one hour a week from the therapist using approximately half of this time in face-to-face work with him and the other half in the preparation of drawings and video materials.

Example 2: Martin, aged 30 years
Martin also has a profound, prelingual hearing impairment. His upbringing was unsettled. He was the victim of much rejection and violence and was excluded from a series of schools for aggressive behaviour towards others. At 15 years of age he was admitted to a psychiatric hospital and experienced temporary success in a rehabilitation and training setting. However, an attempt at independent living when he was 19 years old ended with him being charged on two occasions with assault, the second of which resulted in him being treated in a secure hospital for a number of years. Martin was diagnosed as having a psychopathic personality disorder and a mild intellectual impairment.

Formulation

Intellectual impairments

On meeting Martin a number of discrepancies were apparent. Firstly, his skills in practical areas such as self-care and problem-solving seemed very advanced, whereas his language and memory for facts seemed poor. His deafness had not been diagnosed until the age of 6 years and he had no access to sign language until the age of 15. His comparative weakness may have been related to this lack of early opportunities, or may have reflected a global intellectual impairment.

A cognitive assessment was carried out and it was established that Martin's IQ was in the low average range at least, and that his memory was intact. It was therefore more likely that his problems stemmed from poor language development and lack of information. This would also negatively affect his ability to memorize verbal information. In effect, Martin did not have a global intellectual impairment but did have areas of specific learning difficulty which would need to be considered in attempting to treat his aggression problem.

Aggression

The scientist practitioner model promotes the use of hypotheses for formulation and treatment planning.

The diagnosis of psychopathic personality disorder implies an element of untreatability. However, the first hypothesis was that, if due to an impoverished environment his presentation had led to the incorrect labelling of him having global rather than specific learning disabilities — a result of his learning environment rather than organicity or personality — then the same could be possible of his aggression: that his aggression is a learned behaviour and may be unlearned.

Secondly, it was observed that, far from having poor anger control, Martin was overcontrolled and was almost constantly angry and controlling himself. In effect, his outbursts of aggression were the result of 'the last straw that broke the camel's back'. This is not a helpful method as it has a saturation point at which outbursts are virtually a requirement. Thus, it was hypothesized that by expressing his anger regularly, as it occurred, the build-up of anger would be avoided and the need for catastrophic outbursts would thereby reduce.

A further observation was that anxiety was maintaining Martin's maladaptive method of anger control as he held a catastrophic belief that his anger was uncontrollable. Thus, intervention would also need to desensitize him to his own anger.

The formulation plan would therefore need to encompass these three hypotheses, which would be either proven or provide information from which to reformulate the hypotheses.

Therapists

This example requires the clinical skills of a clinical psychologist but the signing skills of a native BSL user. There is no Deaf clinical psychologist in the UK at the moment. Therefore, the need for a clinical psychologist and native signer was met by using two therapists. A hearing clinical psychologist supervised a Deaf counsellor who did the face-to-face work with Martin. He therefore had access to the appropriately skilled clinician and the appropriate cultural and linguistic process.

Treatment

Martin had a very limited vocabulary for emotions. He was particularly limited in the language that associated emotions with anger as he felt all his anger was bad and unmentionable. He seemed to panic and be unable to discuss the subject. The first task was to label his emotions. A Likert scale of 0–10 was used, with 0 being not at all angry and 10 being the most angry imaginable so that he would be totally out of control. Martin and his therapist started by labelling such emotions by numbers and then added names, first in sign and then in written English. To name these emotions required meticulous negotiation between the Deaf counsellor and Martin to choose words and signs that they both knew and which would become their standard. The supervisor had the numbers as a guide when the words chosen seemed unorthodox. These are the English words chosen to represent the stage of anger:

1. Happy
2. OK/Fine
3. Calm
4. Fairly
5. Sad
6. Fed up
7. Depressed
8. Ready to be angry
9. Blow up angry, nervous
10. Hit

This labelling process gave Martin the language with which to express his emotions. They illustrate the importance of using a native BSL user when the client's language is limited, and of tailoring interventions to the individual. They are not the usual words of an English-speaking clinical psychologist.

Measuring

Martin was then asked to plot his anger on a graph three times daily. He discussed this graph weekly with his therapist, who would ask about the situations that had preceded a rise or fall. Thus, the discussion and the reinforcement of his own answers would create a greater sophistication in his awareness. For example, Martin may be asked, '*What happened just before your anger rose from 3 to 7?*' He may answer, '*The nurses were talking about me and I got more angry*'. This increases his awareness of cause and effect. (To hear or see oneself giving a piece of information is much more powerful and reassuring than being told the same thing, as it represents empowerment and self-control rather than providing external control, so it was important for Martin to be asked, not told.)

Thus, Martin's measuring became more sophisticated than that of John. It became a measurement of incidence, antecedents and consequences.

Normalizing

The other effect of the graph is to normalize and allow the emotions. Whilst the labelling process often has this role, Martin was so convinced that his emotions were bad that he was not reassured until his therapist required him to plot them on the graph and then discuss them.

Formulation

The 'unmentionable' anger was made mentionable and mentioned three times daily. Martin was initially anxious about all of his anger, hence his use of the bottling-up method. This was redefined and we said that Martin should be anxious about anger only when it was at 8 or above. He was encouraged to show anger in the 0–7 range more often. In real terms this meant that Martin was allowed to shout, throw things and push people for the first nine months but not to hit or injure people. (This had to be agreed with the whole team first, particularly the nursing staff.) Thus, success was measured by Martin's graph reading, for example, 1–7–4 rather than 3–3–3. It was a day of celebration when Martin threw his anger management diary at the therapist. He had expressed anger, his anger had not escalated out of his control, and the therapist was able to feed this back to him. Furthermore, at the time when he was angry he could still be aware that there was such a thing as anger management.

Decatastrophising anger

Catastrophic beliefs are often challenged or explored by use of a verbal therapy such as cognitive, behavioural or analytic psychotherapy. Given Martin's limited language, the visual behaviourism took precedence. Role play was used to allow Martin to practise being angry. By pretending to be an angry person he was, by definition, not himself an angry person. This was a novel situation for him and he found the irony humorous. He could also experience being on the receiving end of anger in a controlled situation. He learned that to a large extent anger is controllable and not a catastrophe, and can even be funny. Assertiveness training was then introduced using role play to find solutions which used negotiation and assertion rather than aggression or passivity.

Linking awareness and control

Having decided to encourage the expression of anger between 0 and 7 we had to work at controlling anger between 8 and 10. This was achieved using a visual analogy. The analogy of 'RED' was chosen at the point around 8 on the scale at which anger starts to become dangerous. 'RED' was then used in a variety of situations as a cognitive cue. Given that Martin's language and verbal memory was poor, at a time of heightened arousal it is likely to be at its poorest. But, in only the split second required to say/sign/point 'RED' or use a red flash card, Martin was able to communicate something as complex as '*I am becoming uncontrollably angry; either help me or get out of my way*' or the therapist is able to say, '*It looks like you are becoming uncontrollably angry; leave the building now and walk until you feel better*'. A red poster in his bedroom reminded Martin to use this for communication when in trouble, and reinforced that the 0–7 band is acceptable. He need worry only about the red area of 8 and upwards.

Having covered the 0–7 and the 8–10 categories, the next task was to encourage Martin to use his awareness of the former to prevent the latter. The analogy of a car radiator dial as the engine gets hotter was used to show the importance of anger awareness and seeking help before reaching the red zone (Figure 5.5).

The red poster in Martin's bedroom took on the additional role of reminding him to be aware of his anger and to seek help before it reached the red zone.

Improving control

The first nine months' work covered only labelling, measuring and normalizing of anger. We worked with the knowledge that anger at the 9 or 10 level might be uncontainable and that if staff were at risk Martin would have to be moved to alternative accommodation. However, we

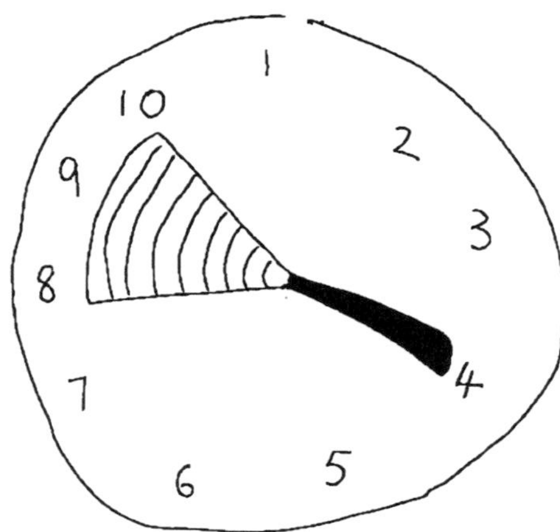

Figure 5.5 The analogy of a car radiator dial ... before reaching the red zone.

fought against any desire to tell him to control his anger as it would reinforce his belief that his anger was catastrophic and maintain his unhelpful bottling-up method. After nine months Martin had gained a conceptual understanding of our teachings so that we could impose some rules to cover his weak areas. As his language and verbal memory was still weak (though improving) these were chosen carefully. We wanted only three rules so as not to overload his verbal memory.

- When you are nearing the red zone and you may become violent GET OUT. (He would go to his bed area or outside.)
- If you think people are talking about you, ask for help. Find out what the truth is.
- When you are being teased learn to let comments bounce off you rather than absorb them. (This was presented visually to indicate that absorbing insults can create a 'hot' situation; bouncing comments away will cool you down.) (Figure 5.6)

In BSL, signs for thoughts are usually generated from the head, whereas signs for emotions are generated from the chest.

Visually it is important that teasing, which creates negative cognitions, enters through the head and is absorbed into the torso, where the BSL sign for 'angry' is initiated. Thus, it shows how an unchallenged thought can lead to an emotion.

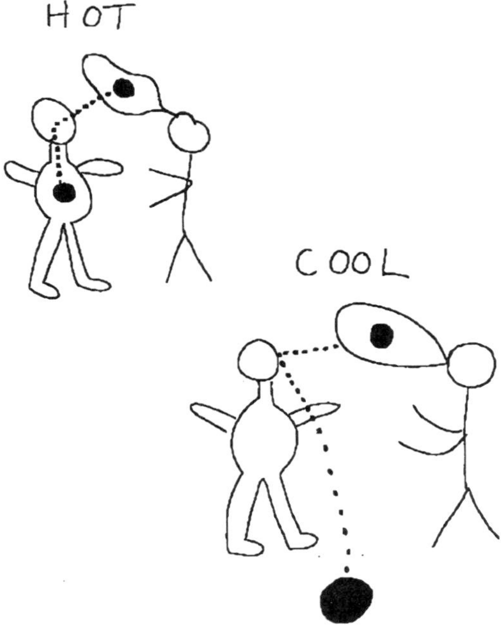

Figure 5.6 '... bouncing comments away will cool you down.'

After 12 months it was time to stress or test the new control system and show the benefits of the better control. A reward-based behaviour programme was introduced. In return for curbing the residual threatening or aggressive behaviour (such as pushing or finger wagging) Martin could earn time away from the hospital. After 18 months he was discharged from hospital. The targets set were well within his reach but the stress of being monitored in this way was difficult for him at first. However, after failing to achieve his free time for the first two weeks Martin then went on to succeed consistently.

Resources

As with the previous case-study, this treatment requires a commitment of resources. The treatment lasted for 18 months and each week involved one hour of Deaf counsellor time and one-and-a-half hours of supervision between the clinical psychologist and the Deaf counsellor. This is a commitment of four hours staff time weekly for 18 months. But when you consider the various options for the accommodation of people who have been labelled as having a psychopathic personality disorder, it is a bargain!

Conclusion

All people deserve the right to equal treatment provision. Our rehabilitation and treatment imperatives must be two-fold. Firstly, to ensure that all Deaf–intellectually impaired people have full access to appropriate audiological support and to language and communication. For Deaf people this must be sign, and increasing the awareness and understanding of sign in the wider population will limit the social handicap imposed by a dominant hearing culture. Secondly, this extends to psychological services provided for Deaf–intellectually impaired people. If people have difficulties which make our traditional treatment approaches ineffective then there are things we must do to adapt. Much work is already being done by Deaf specialists to adapt treatment to be culturally and linguistically appropriate. In working with Deaf people who have global or specific intellectual impairments this needs to be expanded to be cognitively appropriate. These adaptations represent the double-jeopardy, not of the client so much as of the therapist.

The challenge of adapting therapies can be daunting but also rewarding. In the words of Hutton (1977, unreferenced):

> 'It is only when we as professionals can reduce our irrational wish to do such a good and complete piece of work that the client will never again need help, that we can begin to see what limited, but worthwhile, intervention is possible.'

References

Ashton G, Ward A (1992) Mental Handicap and the Law. London: Sweet & Maxwell.

Ballantyne J (1977) Deafness (third edition). London: Churchill Livingstone.

Biklen D (1990) Communication unbound: autism and praxis. Harvard Educational Review 60: 291–314.

Biklen D (1992) Typing to talk: facilitated communication. American Journal of Speech and Language Pathology 2: 15–17, 21–22.

Biklen D (1993) Communication Unbound. New York: Teachers College Press.

Conrad R (1979) The Deaf School Child. London: Harper & Row.

Craft M, Bicknell J, Hollins S (1985) Mental Handicap: A Multi-disciplinary Approach. London: Baillière Tindall.

Cunningham C (1982) Down's syndrome: An Introduction for Parents: London: Souvenir Press.

Downing JE (1993) Communication intervention for individuals with dual sensory and intellectual impairments. Clinics in Communication Disorders 3: 31–42.

Firth GF (1992) Chosen Vessels. Exeter: Private publication.

Furth HG, Youniss J (1975) Congenital deafness and the development of thinking. In Lennenberg EH, Lennenberg E (eds) Foundations of Language Development. London: Academic Press.

Hogg J, Raynes N (1987) Assessment — Mental Handicap: A Guide to Assessment Practices, Tests and Checklists. London: Croom Helm.

Heider F, Heider GM (1941) Studies in the psychology of the deaf. Psychology Monographs 53: 1–56.

Hogg J, Sebba J, Lambe L (1990) Profound Retardation and Multiple Impairment. Vol.1: Development and Learning. London: Chapman & Hall.

Kropka BL (1979) A Study of the Deaf and Partially Hearing Population in the Mental Handicap Hospitals of Devon. Report to the RNID: London.

Kropka BI, Williams C (1986) The epidemiology of hearing impairment in people with a mental handicap. In Ellis E (ed) Sensory Impairments in Mentally Handicapped People. London: Croom Helm pp 35–60.

Kyle JG, Woll B (1985) Sign Language. Cambridge: Cambridge University Press.

Lillemor RM, Hallberg, Carlsson SG (1993). A qualitative study of situations turning a hearing disability into a handicap. Disability, Handicap and Society 8: 71–85.

Masters L, Marsh CE (1978) Middle ear pathology as a factor in learning disabilities. Journal of Learning Disabilities 11: 54–57.

Medoff M (1980) Children of a Lesser God. New Jersey: James T White & Co.

Mittler P (ed) (1970). The Psychological Assessments of Mental and Physical Handicaps. London: Tavistock.

Myklebust ER (1960) The psychological effects of deafness. American Annals of the Deaf 105: 372–385.

Orcutt D (1985) Worldsign: a new multi-sensory language. Human Communication Canada 9: 11–12.

Reiss S (1994) Issues in defining mental retardation. American Journal of Mental Retardation 99: 1–7.

Sacks O (1990) Seeing Voices. London: Pan Books.

Simon EW, Toll T, Whitehair PM (1994) A naturalistic approach to the validation of facilitated communication. Journal of Autism and Developmental Disorders 24: 647–657.

Thompson T (1993) Book review, American Journal of Mental Retardation 98: 670–673.

Tomlinson-Keasey C, Smith-Winberry C (1990) Cognitive consequences of congenital deafness. Journal of Genetic Psychology 151: 103–115.
Tookey P (1994) Personal communication.
Williams C (1993) Hearing Impairment and Learning Disability: Double Jeopardy. Paper presented to the Annual Conference of the British Institute of Learning Disability, Devon, UK.
Williams C (1986) Social Training Achievement Record: STAR. Kidderminster: British Institute of Learning Disability.
World Health Organization. (1980) International Classification of Impairments, Disabilities and Handicaps. WHO: Geneva.
Yeates S (1991) Hearing loss in adults with learning disabilities. British Medical Journal 303: 427–428.

Chapter 6
Mental Health in Children who are Deaf and Have Multiple Disabilities

DAVID E. BOND

Introduction

Severe to profound deafness in school-aged children has an estimated prevalence of approximately 1 to 1.2 per thousand. Severe to profound mental handicap or learning difficulties has an estimated prevalence of approximately 3 to 4 per thousand of the population (Wing, 1971), with approximately 30 to 40 per thousand having lesser degrees of handicap. Links between mental handicap and sensory disabilities often remain unrecognized, despite a body of research evidence which indicates quite clearly that with certain causes of mental handicap, the association with auditory and vision impairment is well recognized (for example, in the case of cytomegalovirus, rubella, and in other traumatic* causes of multiple handicap, and in a variety of genetic defects which are responsible for over one-third of all causes of mental handicap). Up to one-half of the causes of blindness, and at least a third of the causes of deafness (Fraser, 1964; Holland, 1986) arise through genetic anomalies which may also be responsible for mental disabilities. In other conditions, such as Down's syndrome, sensory handicaps may occur as a result of genetic anomaly, as well as structural anomalies of the eyes and ears combined with a predisposition to infection. In a 1966 survey an incidence of more than 35% of hearing impairment was found in mentally handicapped people who lived in a hospital environment for the mentally handicapped (Parsons et al., 1966). Approximately 12–15% of inmates had severe to profound hearing impairments, whilst the remainder had mild to moderate hearing impairments.

Recognition of sensory impairments in multiple handicap is often easily overlooked. This is particularly the case in conditions such as Down's syndrome, where learning and communicational disorders were often attributed to the nature of Down's syndrome, rather than as

*The author uses 'traumatic' to refer to causes of deafness that are associated with specific or generalized brain damage, such as congenital rubella syndrome and cytomegalovirus.

overlooked sensory disabilities. Balkanay (1980), Bond (1991) and others indicated quite clearly that anomalies of the ear, and of hearing, occur in almost every Down's syndrome child. This research has been replicated by others, with very similar results, and yet other research studies which investigated the information-processing and linguistic capabilities of people with Down's syndrome sometimes suggest that they have temporal sequential processing difficulties arising through some cognitive difference. The researchers showed no awareness of the effects of hearing loss on people with Down's syndrome. Hearing loss shows a high correlation with temporal sequential processing difficulties (Bond, 1970; 1991).

The incidence of hearing impairment among people with learning difficulties or mental handicaps is substantially higher than sensory impairments occurring in other populations. As indicated above, there are common genetic causes which occur in sensory impairment as well as in learning difficulties or mental handicaps. Anoxia and prematurity or low birthweight as well as infections during pregnancy (e.g. cytomegalovirus and rubella) may also contribute to multisensory disabilities.

For a smaller group of the population, genetic causes combining hearing loss and other disabilities (such as in Usher's syndrome — retinitis pigmentosa plus hearing loss) also have a higher level of incidence. Deaf–blind children (using the definition that the child's hearing loss is such that the visually impaired child needs special provision as a hearing-impaired* individual, and the visual impairment is such that the hearing-impaired child requires special treatment as a visually impaired individual), occurs in approximately 1/10 000 school-aged children. However, in view of genetic factors and traumatic causes of mental handicaps or learning difficulties, the incidence of dual sensory impairment or multisensory disability is substantially higher amongst people who have mental handicaps or learning difficulties.

Hearing-impaired children born to parents who are hearing (at least 90%), have more traumatic aetiologies or causes of their hearing loss (such as rubella, anoxia, prematurity, low birthweight, mumps or cytomegalovirus) compared with hearing-impaired children born to parents who are deaf. Most of the traumatic aetiologies, and a number of genetic anomalies, contribute to other handicaps, including brain disorders (Van Dijk, 1982). People who are brain damaged are significantly more likely to have psychiatric disorders than people who are not brain damaged. This was shown by Graham and Rutter (1968) who reported that 58.3% of children with brain damage also showed psychiatric problems.

Vernon (1969), in a study of deaf children at Riverside School for the deaf in California, reported that 10% of the children who had hereditary factors

*The terms 'hearing-impaired' and 'deaf' have been used throughout this chapter to describe those who are affected by hearing loss. Some people who have severe to profound hearing loss may prefer to be called deaf rather than hearing-impaired.

as the cause of their hearing problems, 27% of the premature, and 31% of rubella-damaged children, had emotional and or behavioural problems in addition to their hearing impairment. These children showed higher levels of restless, hyperactive, distractible and involuntary behaviours than other children. This study clearly indicates the likelihood of deaf children with multiple disabilities showing a substantially higher level of emotional and behavioural problems than other groups of hearing-impaired children.

Despite the evidence that there is a higher incidence of emotional and behavioural disturbance among deaf children with additional disabilities, there has been little, if any, clear epidemiological data since the Vernon (1969) study. What factors contribute to mental health disabilities in children with multisensory impairments?

Hearing impairment and its consequent effects on communication, learning and interaction often go unrecognized by those working with children who have learning and other disabilities, unless they are specially trained to recognize sensory impairments and understand their consequences.

The behavioural and emotional difficulties of hearing-impaired children often reflect difficulties which they face in environments where they are unable to communicate effectively, or where their needs as a hearing-impaired child are not met appropriately. From clinical observation and parent reporting, but not from an organized survey, it appears that hearing-impaired children with multiple disabilities, placed in inappropriate environments (where their communication initiatives are not recognized and where those working with them are unable to communicate effectively), show substantially higher levels of maladaptive behaviour and suffer significantly higher emotional disturbance than hearing-impaired children with multiple disabilities who are placed in an environment where their needs as deaf children are recognized and catered for appropriately.

Although it is difficult to obtain objective data detailing incidence of mental health problems in deaf students with multiple disabilities, various comments have been made about the behaviour and adjustment of deaf children. Schlesinger and Meadow (1972) found 11.6% of their sample of deaf children and 2.4% of the hearing sample were severely disturbed, whereas 19.6% and 7.3% of the deaf and hearing samples, respectively, had behavioural problems. In a survey of 516 hearing-impaired students. Vernon (1969) in a study of 413 deaf students showed that 22.5% had severe emotional problems and 5.1% had psychotic behaviours. Vernon (1969) also indicated that children who were deaf showed between three and five times the level of emotional disturbance compared to children with normal hearing.

Whilst surveys and clinical/medical information may provide a baseline to indicate the potential frequency of mental health problems among people who are multisensorially deprived, or deaf with additional disabilities, there is a need to look at reasons why surveyed information is so variable, why some groups of multisensorially disabled children thrive and make progress, whereas others with similar aetiologies or causes for their disabilities fail and demonstrate significant mental health problems.

We also need to know what factors might contribute to mental health problems. How predictable is the development of mental health problems and at what stage of development? How do we treat or prevent mental health problems that are treatable or preventable, and how do we manage mental health problems which do not appear to respond to treatment?

Factors which may contribute to mental health problems in children with sensory impairments

In experiments with students who had no significant handicaps, Bexton, Heron and Scott (1954) experimentally and temporarily deprived students of sensory input. In the follow-up experiments these students showed a diminished ability to solve problems. They had inaccuracies of perceptual responses and their emotional status showed indication of disturbance. Writers such as Goetzinger (1972) reported a correlation between hearing loss and social emotional behavioural difficulties among the deaf. These ranged from mild confusions and some mild emotional behaviour disturbance with mild to moderate hearing losses (20–40 dB), to a substantially higher level of incidence of emotional, behavioural and social skill problems among those with severe to profound hearing losses. Although correlations of this nature do not always occur (for example Williams, 1970; Hindley et al., 1994), hearing loss may also result in differences in communication needs and differences in behaviour. These differences are sometimes used by educators to assist in identifying children who may have a hearing loss. The child who is hearing impaired may be more attentive to body language, gesture, mime, etc., than to aural-oral communication. He may copy other children's behaviour instead of attending to the teacher, show poor attention in class until her voice is raised (Bond, 1993). Hearing impairment is not the *cause* of behaviours which are commonly attributed to people who are deaf (such as egocentricity, possessive, rigid, impulsive behaviours). These are not exclusive to the deaf, and hearing people may show similar patterns of behaviour. We could say, therefore, that whilst deafness or hearing difficulties may contribute to behavioural differences, hearing impairment is not the primary cause of emotional and social behavioural problems. It is also important to remember that not all deaf or multisensorially deprived children show disturbed or disturbing behaviours. Most can be — and are — emotionally and behaviourally adjusted, so whilst there may be a higher level of incidence of disturbed or disturbing behaviour associated with hearing loss or multisensory deprivation, sensory loss is not the only contributor to mental health anomalies. There is obviously a variety of other causative or contributory factors.

Communication and interaction factors

For the child who is multiply handicapped or multisensorially deprived there may be no reassuring or warning background sounds, no consistent auditory input and no consistent visual images. For the hearing child who has intact vision, auditory warnings and reassuring background sounds, further reinforced by familiar smells, bodily warmth and tactile or touch input, provide a consistency of receptive information which is reinforced by each of the sensory systems (Bond, 1981). Although very few children are totally deaf and totally blind, dual sensory impairment or multisensory deprivation is more a multiplication of disabling factors than it is of one handicap adding to another. For many of these children even the slightest combination of visual and hearing problems can totally disrupt their early perceptions of the world. This, in turn, may result in the child being somewhat unresponsive to traditional reinforcers such as food, warmth, love, affection, communication, interaction and self-actualization. From the child's viewpoint the apparent lack of consistency and input results in difficulties in predicting what is going to occur and consequently difficulties in exerting any influence or control over interaction, communication or behaviours of others. When the child has learning difficulties and visual problems in addition to a hearing loss, the problems of interpreting spasmodic and seemingly unrelated information are compounded — creating confusing, disorganized and discordant perceptions of the environment. In this apparently non-responsive, non-communicational and inconsistent interactional environment, in which adults fail to recognize or to respond to initiatives in communication from the child, the adult, in turn, may find the lack of responsiveness from the child unrewarding, and consequently fail to respond to unusual or different initiatives from the child other than those which indicate distress or discomfort. Adults may then use controlling responses and behaviours and negative reactions to the child's communication initiatives. It is known that when an interaction is pleasurable, rewarding or provides reciprocal benefits, it tends to increase. When the interaction ceases to be pleasurable it tends to decrease (Bond, 1991, 1993). Attention to negative behaviours or distress or discomfort behaviours, at the expense of attention to positive behaviours, usually results in an increase in the negative or other behaviours.

As the communication initiatives of children with multisensory disabilities are rejected, ignored or overlooked, the child often seeks alternative forms of consistent stimulation in order to exert some control over his environment, to counteract the effect of apparent rejection of communication initiatives and to provide some form of stimulation.

Different patterns or *modes* of behaviour which emerge from breakdowns in these early stages of communication appear to take several forms, for example:

- Attention-demanding behaviours, such as self-abuse, temper tantrums, refusal to co-operate (e.g. refusal to eat, toileting and other elimination problems).
- Self-stimulatory problems: eye-poking, or eye-pulling, rocking, self-abuse (tissue damage), tapping, rubbing and flicking bodily areas, etc.
- Withdrawal from social contact — non-responsiveness to external stimuli.

For many multiply handicapped sensorially impaired children, the inaccessibility or non-availability of a responsive communicational interactive context places behavioural and emotional development at risk, and the child's inappropriate (to us) patterns of behaviour and communication become habituated from a very early age. As children sometimes find inappropriate behaviours a successful way of controlling interactions and the attention of other people, they become reinforced and, eventually, develop into a repertoire of communicative attention-demanding behaviours available to the child.

For multiply handicapped children who show difficult patterns of behaviour, breakdowns in relationships may be further associated with further rejection and failure of the environment arising through the mental, marital or relationship breakdowns of their carers. When these children are placed in care their long-term outcomes often involve a history of repeated rejection and failure in relationships, with the child having no trust or faith in relationships, difficulties in sustaining any form of relationship, and the development of hostile, anxious, depressive or anti-social behaviours (Bond, 1993).

When communication and interaction processes are inadequate, inappropriate, non-responsive or non-reciprocal, behavioural and emotional development is placed at risk. Interactive and communicational behaviours are inextricably linked with behaviours that are crucial for social development and mental health. Some of the behaviours which are involved in an interactive communicational context are shown in Table 6.1.

Social cultural factors

A variety of social cultural issues may contribute to mental health problems in children who are multiply disabled, or in deaf children with additional disabilities. Approximately 90% of children who are deaf are born to hearing parents. The estimated frequency of dominant deafness is approximately 6–7.5% (Nance, 1976). Vernon (1969) indicates that approximately 10% of deaf children of deaf parents show behavioural

Table 6.1 Some behaviours in interaction-communication

Turn Taking
- Awareness of start and finish of others' contributions
- Understanding of others' contributions: awareness of others' body language, language, etc.
- Responsiveness to others' interactions: acknowledging and reinforcing acceptable responses
- Developing and modifying initiatives in response to the reactions of others
- Sharing skills, ideas and negotiating

Learning
- Association of information, generalization, classification, sequencing — organizational skills
- Recognition, identification and recall of information
- New rules — linguistic (grammatical construction, syntax, vocabulary) and social
- Acquiring and using new information

Establishing roles
- Identifying more or less skilled contributors
- Development of regard, understanding, appreciation of others
- Development of ideas, comparison of self with others, status and social group
- Formation of roles with others, developing relationships
- Modelling, and imitating others, customs, fashions
- Developing bonding and trust
- Development of assertive/submissive behaviours, etc.

(Bond, 1991; 1993)

disturbance, in comparison with 18–30% of deaf children of hearing parents. Deaf parents are also less likely to have additionally disabled or multiply disabled deaf children, as traumatic aetiologies (viral infections, such as cytomegalovirus and rubella, and other traumatic causes, such as anoxia, low birthweight, Rhesus negative, mumps, measles, chickenpox, etc.) occur significantly less among deaf children of deaf parents, but probably at the same or at a similar overall level of incidence in the hearing population. Most traumatic aetiologies contribute to other handicaps, including brain damage. People who have brain damage are significantly more likely to suffer from psychiatric disorders (Graham and Rutter, 1968).

There appears to be very little in the literature about deaf parents' management of deaf multiply handicapped children, but deaf mothers of deaf children are more likely to respond to their children's non-verbal initiatives at a much earlier stage than the hearing parents of deaf children and, therefore, are more likely to establish a responsive learning environment with their child at a very early stage in development. When this does occur, it reduces the prospect of rejection of the child's communicative initiatives and consequently increases the probability of socially appropriate attention-seeking and controlling behavioural responses (Bond, 1993). Hearing parents of deaf children may take some time before they start to understand their child's hearing loss and, consequently, may not respond to the child's needs whilst they go through processes of denial, guilt, anger, rejection and medical solution-seeking. The hearing parent of a deaf child may have difficulty developing acceptance and understanding of their child's needs, thereby delaying responding appropriately to the child's communications. Delays in responding to the child's communicative attempts and initiatives may start a pattern of different behavioural responses which require much more intensive work if long-term behavioural emotional difficulties and damage are to be avoided.

Cultural prejudices about multiple disability may occur in deaf or hearing cultural groups. As with any area of disability, social prejudices may adversely affect the way parents develop their communication and interaction with the multiply disabled child — and consequently further damage may occur through rejection, failure to bond with the child, and failure to provide a consistent, positive, interactive and stimulating environment. This is particularly relevant in some developing societies in which the disabled child is regarded very negatively. In some subsistence economies, belief systems may have encouraged the members of the cultural group to view the disabled child as a parasite, or as a reflection of the parents' 'sins'. Some of these prejudices can be socially transmitted to affect later generations and their management of children with disabilities, albeit at a deeper emotional level of rejection and guilt than an obvious surface level one. In some cultures, conditions such as head-banging, encopresis or enuresis are regarded as misbehaviour (Dutt, 1991). Whilst these problems may arise through environmental learning and developmental differences, and not emotional-behaviour disturbance, the methods of management and parental response may contribute to mental health difficulties.

Physiological conditions which may contribute to mental health problems

As indicated previously in this chapter, genetic conditions which have association with other sensory impairments or learning difficulties may also contribute to the learning and behavioural problems of multisensorially disabled or multiply handicapped deaf people. Deteriorating conditions such as Usher's syndrome (progressive retinitis pigmentosa or deterioration of the visual field in association with hearing loss) may be associated with increasing mental health problems. For example, Bond (1993) reported a case in which a young girl became depressed, withdrawn and non-communicative following transfer to a residential school for deaf children. In addition to an ataxia (an impairment of motor movement) her visual field had also deteriorated. In counselling sessions, the girl eventually wrote that she thought she was going to die in 1988. As she repeated this idea, further investigations revealed that she had recent experiences of close friends dying. With counselling and guidance, and once the date of October 1988 was passed, there was a gradual improvement in her condition. When last seen she was a confident pleasantly assertive young lady, and she had developed very positive ways of managing herself and her restricted visual field.

Cases have been reported (Bond, 1985, 1991, 1993) in which deaf children with multiple handicaps who showed a high level of involuntary behaviour (e.g. 'tics'), in association with atopic disorders such as eczema and asthma, were placed on a diet to eliminate known allergens from their diet. In one case a pupil (aetiology; rubella) with a psoriasis-like condition, severe asthmatic attacks and very severely disturbed behaviour (for example, he destroyed his clothing, broke items of plastic and had difficulties in relationships with others) showed a marked improvement in behaviour when placed on a diet free from cow's milk, and later on an additive-free diet. Admissions to hospital for asthma decreased, and his skin condition (which was previously treated with steroid cream) cleared up almost completely. On the occasions on which cow's milk was accidentally re-introduced to his diet, or when he was returned to normal foods, there were immediate deteriorations in the youngster's behavioural condition, and his skin condition and asthmatic attacks, which had previously been eliminated, returned.

Diabetes in deaf children, where there is marked variation in blood sugar levels, may also contribute to significant changes in patterns of behaviour in which the child may become irrational, sometimes violent, and show levels of inappropriate attention-demanding behaviours. In several cases known to the author, children manipulated their diet, taking inappropriate foodstuffs and causing blood sugar levels to become high. This resulted in excessively overactive and sometimes aggressive behaviour in which there appeared to be an element of enjoyment of the excitation and attention gained. Management of this behaviour was extremely difficult — and was eventually attained by a combination of operant conditioning (token economy), training to self-isolate, relaxation and giving greater responsibility for self-management.

Cases of behavioural emotional disturbance amongst deaf children, in which premenstrual tension was a significant factor in the behavioural difficulties, have been reported. In one case (Bond, 1979, 1993) a client showed extreme disturbances of behaviour at monthly intervals. Unfortunately, the pattern was not acknowledged by some of the professionals dealing with the case, and it took some considerable time to encourage recognition of this condition. When a lady gynaecologist investigated and diagnosed the condition and recommended treatment, a degree of control was finally achieved, but the establishment of the pattern of behaviour over a period of time proved extremely difficult to change.

For some multiply handicapped deaf children, life-threatening conditions in infancy have meant that very high levels of attention have been paid to every aspect of their behaviour. Consequently, many inappropriate behaviours may well have been reinforced through very high levels of attention from professionals and parents. 'Fading' high levels of attention in order to encourage greater levels of independence cannot always be easily achieved in life-threatening conditions, nor in interactional situations in which communication and an understanding of the world around them require very positive adult:child ratios; for example, deaf-blind children or physically disabled deaf children who have additional learning difficulties who need almost one-to-one or higher levels of management. The skill of the intervenor in these situations may assist the development of more acceptable behaviours. However, on many occasions we are placed in a 'catch 22' situation, i.e. if we do not provide the child with high levels of intervention, communication, interaction, learning and behaviour (and life, in some cases) may be placed at risk. If we do provide high levels of attention, the child becomes more attention-demanding, and learning and behaviour are placed at risk.

Environmental conditions

George, a deaf-blind boy who showed autistic features of behaviour, was placed in a school in which every effort was made to cater for his very complex learning and sensory disabilities. Over the course of one morning he would see his educational assistant, teacher, speech and language therapist, occupational therapist, advisory teacher for the deaf, and advisory teacher for the visually impaired. Over the course of the week he saw 14 different people. He was referred to the author because of an increase in autistic features of behaviour, which included an increase in finger regard, stroboscopic stimulation (flapping his fingers in front of his eyes), self-abusive behaviours, and withdrawal from interaction with others. When the number of people dealing with him was reduced to two, one for the morning and one for the afternoon, the difficult patterns of behaviour decreased and there was a gradual increase in George's attempts at communicating. All the specialists worked through the two intervenors, who then linked closely to work being done at home.

David, an 8-year-old boy, was profoundly deaf with mild learning difficulties and also showed most autistic features of behaviour. He was unable to communicate by spoken language. Assessed by professionals who did not have a background in working with deaf children with other learning difficulties, David was placed in a school for autistic children. All the other pupils communicated through spoken language (albeit limited in view of their autistic behaviour). David's behaviour became increasingly isolated and more bizarre until his parents requested specialist assessment. Placed in a school for deaf environment in which there was provision for deaf children with additional difficulties, and staff experienced in working with deaf children who had autistic behaviours, David made very good progress. In the environment of children who were autistic, David imitated their behaviours. He thought that this was the acceptable way of behaving. In the school for deaf, his behaviours changed; he became more communicative and interactive when he was provided with signed communication which was appropriate to his needs. For David, positive interaction with his peer group, and with supervising adults, provided him with the base of developing his communication, and developing positive controls over what was happening to him.

Lack of consistency in management, changes in environment without explanation, changes of communicators and key people within the environment, too much movement, lack of security of space and known familiar territory, can all tend to contribute towards disturbed or disturbing behaviour in the child who is deaf with additional handicaps.

Frederick, deaf-blind from birth, with a profound hearing loss and minimal residual vision showed normal non-verbal development until he was aged approximately $2^1/_2$ when he then suffered from a series of substantial epileptic fits. He placed an exceptionally high level of demand on adult attention, and whilst he showed marked improvements in his communication and relationship with others at school and home, when he was placed in a respite care programme where no one knew him he withdrew totally, covering his head with clothes, and showed a very high level of self-abusive behaviour. On return to school it took some weeks to re-establish Frederick's confidence in the people who worked with him, until he very gradually emerged from his 'cocoon' of clothing. Whenever changes occurred in Frederick's life he very quickly reverted to high levels of self-abusive behaviour and to his 'cocoon'. He established a pattern of behaviour which requires extremely careful management to avoid 'Fred' reverting to this withdrawal behaviour whenever faced with changes in environment, in the personnel interacting with him, or in learning demands.

Age and development

Some of the most disturbing behaviours that occur with multiply handicapped and multisensorially deprived children are those that emerge during adolescence. Very often work has encouraged more appropriate social behaviours, and extinguished masturbatory, self-stimulatory, self-abusive, physically aggressive challenging behaviours, and other aspects of behavioural difficulties whilst the child is pre-adolescent, only to see the patterns of behaviour re-emerge in adolescence. As the child is then older, physically stronger, and more skilful at identifying ways in which attention can be obtained, many of the re-emerging behavioural difficulties become much more difficult to control, and then develop into more habitual and challenging patterns of behaviour. Hormonal changes, as indicated previously in females as well as males, accompanying sexual arousal particularly in complex situations, present some of the most difficult and challenging behaviours. With increasing levels of sexual arousal we have often seen extremely difficult challenging behaviours emerge — behaviours which mirror those of infancy but which are substantially magnified.

Summary: contributory factors in mental health problems in children who are multisensorially disabled or deaf with additional handicaps

In an article about the mental health of children who are hearing impaired (Bond, 1993), it was reported that a sad feature of many hearing-impaired people who have mental health problems is that they and their families have often had early histories of inappropriate assessment, advice, communication, provision and support, and consequent failure in communication in the early stages of their education and development. Despite later identification of their needs, and appropriate treatment, many of those who did not have adequate or appropriate communication and support continue to show patterns of behaviour which are indicative of rejection in interaction and communication, long after they have left educational facilities for deaf children and students.

Although this chapter attempts to outline some factors which might contribute towards mental health problems in deaf people with additional handicaps, in most cases mental health problems arise through a combination of several factors. Table 6.2 lists factors which appear to contribute to mental health problems in deaf people.

It has been found that mental health problems appear to increase when any of the factors outlined in the last four groups in Table 6.2 occur. The more frequently any of these factors occur in an individual's development, the greater the probability of mental health problems (Bond, 1993). Children who are deaf may become victims of abuse, partly because of the assumption of abusers that the victims are unable to identify them or to report the abuse. Other significant factors in the abuse cycle appear to relate to differences in communication, i.e. where the hearing child may control most of their conversation at three years of age (Wood, Griffiths and Howard, 1986), communication with the deaf child is often more controlling and may be more physical, consequently desensitizing the child to inappropriate or abusive behaviour by other people. Although deaf children may not always be able to report abusive behaviour immediately, changes in behaviour, and reporting as communication develops, assist in the identification of abusers. Social skills training programmes, counselling and guidance and appropriate communication are essential to encourage positive self-confidence and assertion in order to prevent abuse or to facilitate reporting of abuse.

Table 6.2 Factors which appear to contribute to mental health problems

Physiological

Traumatic causes of deafness (such as accidents, infections, anoxia)
Additional handicaps
Allergic conditions which may affect behaviour
Brain/neurological damage; hyperkinesis or hyperactivity
Deteriorating physical conditions (e.g. Usher's syndrome, Refsum's disease, muscular dystrophy)
Physiological imbalances e.g. high blood sugar levels, hormonal imbalances
Developmental delays
Genetic anomalies associated with learning difficulties and mental handicaps

Psychological

Psychiatric or emotional behavioural conditions which might arise through exactly the same causes as for people who are not multiply handicapped, multisensorially impaired or hearing impaired. These conditions may be exacerbated by hearing impairment and by any of the other factors outlined here.

Specific learning difficulties

Information-processing difficulties, particularly impairments involving short-term memory, sequencing, analogous, associative, generalization, and classificatory reasoning
Attention deficits or disorders
Marked variations between different areas of ability (e.g. very capable on practical visual perceptual tasks, but marked difficulties in processing information)

Communication and interactional

Rejection and failure in communication and interaction
Rejection through inappropriate communication
Rejection through isolation or non-availability of a peer or social group with whom the child can identify or relate
Cultural and experiential differences, rejection and failure
Non-availability of peers with whom the child can interact on equal terms
Significant differences in function, capability and communication between the child and the class or peer group
Failure in tasks/and or communication — inadequate structuring of communication, curriculum, and the environment, to enable the child to succeed

Professional issues

Professional focus on particular issues rather than on client need
Inadequate or inappropriately trained and inexperienced professionals
Use of inappropriate tests and methods of assessment
Failure to investigate client needs fully and objectively; thorough comprehensive analysis and appraisal of the client and all aspects of his or her environment is essential
Inappropriate knowledge or awareness about problems and needs linked to hearing impairment
Inappropriate communication skills
Inappropriate educational and environmental management, placement and support

Other

Child abuse (physical, social, emotional, sexual)

Intervention

Assessment

Assessment at all stages of the intervention process is critical in determining appropriate plans for prevention, action or treatment.

Early identification and diagnosis of the needs of the multiply disabled child and the needs of the family is essential as a preventive measure. For the child, access or early communication through auditory input, sign, body language or visual symbols is critical in prevention of the establishment of habitual patterns of behaviour. Support, assistance and guidance by professionals working as partners, with the development of parental understanding of their child's disabilities, and assistance in the development of positive strategies which enable families to work constructively with the child, are crucial in prevention of development of habitual disorders and in the development of positive interactive and learning behaviours.

Various authors have discussed the assessment process in greater detail (e.g. Vernon, 1967; Levine, 1981; Bond, 1986, 1991, 1993). Features which these and other writers have identified as crucial in the proper assessment and identification of needs include the need to carry out an unbiased, objective and valid assessment which is reliable and accurate. Factors which need to be taken into account include background, aetiology of deafness and additional problems, the combination of impairments (including time of onset, nature and degree) and the child's aided and unaided responses to sound and speech. Communication is an essential factor that should be explored through the preferred mode, the optimum mode and the context in which it is most effective. Exploration of developmental, cognitive and intellectual functioning should include an evaluation in different contexts, as well as the identification of areas of specific learning difficulties, such as those in attentional and short-term memory areas. Verbal educational development, whether through sign communication or through other systems, may be crucial, with other information about cognitive function, in identifying the level at which intervention involving communication may occur most effectively. Behavioural and emotional functions in development should cover a range of personal social skills, views and behaviours, as well as work habits and skills. Sometimes overlooked is an appraisal of the environment in which the individual is functioning. In this aspect of analysis the interactive context, the attitudes and behaviours of others in the environment, understanding of individual needs by peers and supervising adults, and the appropriateness of support available, are crucial human features which require evaluation. In addition, frequency of movement, numbers of people in the child's environment, changes of personnel, consistency of management, appropriate levels of communication, models and behaviours available through other people, can all affect the child's self-perceptions, and perceptions of the world around him. Physical environmental factors are also very important. With the visually impaired deaf child, lack of clear definition in surfaces and surrounds, confusions created by too much visual information, too much movement, inappropriate lighting, lack of clearly defined spaces to work in, lack of security (e.g. extremely large rooms or claustrophobic rooms with many people in them) may all contribute to problems. It is essential that all these areas are investigated.

Communication

Improvements in the early identification of hearing loss, improving awareness of appropriate communication to meet individual needs, appropriate fitting of hearing aids, and the development of an early interactional context between the family and the child, are crucial factors in enabling positive mental health.

A context in which the child achieves equality of control, in which the child's initiatives in communication are identified and responded to, and in which the child shows awareness of and responsiveness to adults and peers' communicative initiatives and responses are some of the essential features of successful early interaction (Wood et al., 1986; Bond, 1993).

When a responsive communicational interactional context is not available, the child's development is placed at risk.

Most children who are hearing impaired, with early diagnosis and appropriate intervention through speech and/or sign, develop successful communication. Some deaf children (including those with additional disabilities) whose aided responses to sound indicate function within the severe to profound range of hearing loss, do not have adequate access to communication appropriate to their needs. For these children, visual or tactile/haptic (touch) communications systems become essential in order to enable them to have consistent access to an enabling interactive communicational environment. The needs of these children require special consideration and provision if the family or carers are unable to sign. Development of compatible, acceptable communication systems that can be used by all members of the family is a critical issue. For many deaf children, auditory input may be confusing, uncomfortable and unpleasant to listen to (Bond, 1981). For some deaf children, visual and tactile communication systems may provide a foundation of language, and understanding to develop receptive and expressive communication. Many deaf and multiply disabled children who are also prelingually severely to profoundly deaf will need visual communication systems throughout their lives. For some multiply handicapped or multisensorially impaired children, signed communication in the form of native sign language of their country may not assist them to access communication and interaction. They may require a different type of approach. There are different stages of communication which need to be built up slowly and carefully.

Earlier stages should be retained so that the child can use these for the basis of control in interaction with other people while developing expressive and receptive understanding and communication through the next stage.

These stages include:

- Body movement.
- Body language (e.g. to indicate discomfort, hunger or other needs, or wanting repetition of adult behaviours). For some children this may be shown by the most minute movements e.g. eye-pointing, eyelid fluttering, minute changes in body language, etc.
- Responsiveness/awareness to an adult signal (e.g. for the deaf-blind child a light tap on the back to indicate a child is being picked up, a child responds with a change in behaviour such as arm reaching).
- Consistent response to an object e.g. an object of reference such as a spoon or bottle to indicate feeding.
- Use of gesture or eye-pointing to indicate choice or response to environmental stimuli, visual stimuli, etc.
- Indication of an object or use of an object to gain attention (by eye-pointing, finger-pointing, touching etc.).
- Objects of reference, positive response to or use of objects to show understanding or gain attention e.g. fetching coat or car keys indicates a wish to go out.
- Basic sign — simple sequences of sign.
- Complex natural sign language.
- Sign combined with speech, symbol recognition, print recognition, etc..

A key factor in intervention with multisensorially disabled or multiply handicapped hearing-impaired children is providing them with access to communication to enable them to interact with and share control with others. Sharing of control needs to occur as early as possible in the child's development. Wood, Griffiths and Howard (1986) indicated that an ordinary child controls approximately 75% of interactions with adults at the age of three years. The importance of this interaction is also highlighted by Glynn, (1987) and Bond (1991, 1993).

Environmental intervention

For most multisensorially disabled or multiply handicapped hearing-impaired children, placement in an environment in which they can be successful can prevent or substantially reduce mental health difficulties and deviant behaviours.

Case-studies

Consider the case of David — significantly visually impaired with moderate to severe hearing loss and moderate learning difficulties. In a class of eight children with severe learning difficulties in a special school, where the other children communicated orally/aurally. Although the teacher attempted occasionally to sign to David, who could not understand speech, she was unable to keep up a flow of communication equivalent to the auditory/oral communication she was providing and responding to with the other children. David paid little attention, engaged in a high level of self-destructive (tissue damage) and self-stimulatory behaviours. Consideration was being given to placing him in a class for profoundly multiply handicapped severely learning-disabled hearing children. After assessment, David was transferred to a school for deaf children where he was placed in a small class for deaf children with additional disabilities. In the total communication environment of the school, where his initiatives and communication were recognized, David's behaviours and interaction changed substantially, showing he was capable of working on task for periods of up to two hours, and his level of non-verbal functioning improved to the moderate to mild range of learning difficulty.

John, a deaf visually impaired child at a school for severe learning difficulties, showed an increase in stroboscopic stimulation, temper tantrums, and had no apparent awareness of communication, despite his teachers' attempts to use a visual pictorial communication system. He engaged in a high level of abusive behaviour, and also abused (pinching, scratching, biting) staff working with him. Lighting in the room was poor. The room was part of an open plan classroom through which there was a high level of 'traffic' and movement. There were frequent staff changes, and changes in the people looking after him. John moved to a class where he had his own area, improved lighting, staff were able to communicate effectively using basic BSL or British Signs Supporting English (BSSE), and objects of reference and picture symbols were combined with a high level of positive reinforcement of appropriate behaviours. His behaviour stabilized over a two-month period, and the self-abusive behaviour decreased, as did his abuse of other people.

Cases have been previously reported in which monitoring and managing diet may result in substantial changes in behaviour of multiply disabled and sensorially impaired children. Managing behaviour through diet is not always effective, and as individuals tend to vary in their reactions to different foodstuffs, the outcomes are not always predictable. However, cases have been seen where substantial improvements in behaviour have been effected through changes in diet (Bond, 1985, 1991, 1993) and sometimes through changes in medication where an alteration or reduction in medication (originally prescribed to control behaviour) has resulted in a substantial change in behaviour and emotional state.

Case-study

Amanda was admitted to a school for the deaf, having previously attended another school for the deaf where her behaviour was reported to be unstable. She had been integrated into ordinary classes despite her moderate learning difficulties and the marked difficulties which she had in understanding spoken communication (even at a very basic level where sentence length exceeded three words). In a total communication environment (BSSE and basic BSL) there was initially no significant change in Amanda's behaviour or adjustment, despite communication being presented at a two- to four-word level, which was within her comprehension capabilities. When attending the previous school, Amanda had been placed on carbamazepine in order to control her behaviour and suspected epileptic fits. In consultation with her doctors, the carbamazepine was gradually decreased; with the decrease in medication her behaviour steadily improved. When the medication was eventually removed altogether her behaviour showed substantial improvements. Amanda's communication, work habits concentration and learning improved substantially.

Changes in the physical environment through improvements in comfort, diet, space, security of areas, lighting, visual-auditory conditions, enhancing the visual and personal appearance of the child, and innumerable other physical factors, have all assisted in improvements in the behaviour and adjustment of multisensorially disabled or multiply handicapped hearing-impaired children. At the same time, inappropriate environments where there are significant differences between the child who is deaf and children who are not deaf, are often permanently damaging to all aspects of the development of the deaf child and may result in substantially higher levels of emotional and behavioural disturbance. This observation would also appear to be supported in research with deaf children attending unit classes for deaf children where placement is not necessarily appropriate to the children's needs (Hindley et al., 1994). Improvements in the social, communicational and cultural elements of the environment are also crucial. Enabling pupils to identify and communicate with others on equal terms is a crucial factor in positive mental health. Placement in an environment in which differences are always negative and significant must have an adverse effect on self-concept — with consequent damage to mental health.

Positive management of behaviour

Positive management and 'engineering' opportunities for success for multiply disabled children is a key factor in the prevention and management of mental health and behavioural difficulties at home and at school. Concrete rewards, token economies, behavioural contracts, operant conditioning and other positive management techniques which were in use in the 1960s play a small part in the overall framework of a modern behaviour management system for multisensorially disabled or multiply handicapped hearing-impaired children today. Assessment and task analysis can provide information, which can then assist management. This includes the level at which information and material is presented to the child to enable opportunities for success, developing the positive regard of those working with the child, engineering success levels through enabling the child to succeed at a 90% plus level, and providing increased opportunities for awareness of self, awareness of the consequences of behaviours, and developing responsibility for behaviours. Home and school learning and social emotional discussions should include development of personal social skills to enable children to understand and deal with different social settings, providing greater opportunity for independence and providing meaningful activities in personal care and personal development. A broad and balanced curriculum with age-appropriate activities suitable for pupils' needs and interests, combined with placement and environments in which the multisensorially impaired child or multiply handicapped hearing-impaired child is empowered to compete, interact and communicate on equal terms with his peers, and with adults who are able to respond to and encourage and develop initiatives in communication, are all important to the way children view themselves.

The use of techniques to mirror (imitate) or videotape unacceptable behaviour to feed back information to the child can assist in reducing unacceptable behaviour. Photographs have also been used successfully — and photographic books and social training help the professionals and the parents to develop their children's self-confidence, achievements, and their understanding of their and others' feelings and emotions.

An important area for action includes increasing the awareness of those working with the child — 'putting them in the child's shoes', simulating the child's disabilities to gain an artificial view of how the child sees the world. When a videotape is made of an adult showing anger in correcting a child, the playback without sound may appear exceedingly amusing — for the deaf child the anger may be reinforcing, interesting visually, and sometimes very entertaining. It may also follow long periods of 'anger' being a significant attention factor in the child's early life, combined with adult control and adult anxiety. When these behaviours become a significant source of attention for the child, children sometimes increase their inappropriate behaviours in order to evoke these behaviours from supervising adults. An awareness of our own responses of anger, anxiety, consistency or positiveness can assist in improving management skills. With careful use of body language we may avoid confrontations and reduce difficult patterns of behaviour by:

- Reinforcement via eye contact when behaviour is acceptable, otherwise look slightly away.
- Smiling and increasing proximity when behaviour is acceptable (different reactions for different children are necessary, as the child who is autistic may regard this as a threat).
- Diverting — distracting — making a joke — a sense of humour is essential.

- Looking for very small improvements/positive changes in behaviours, smiling and nodding indicate acceptance. Try to show approval of small improvements (but do not overly reinforce easily achievable behaviours) through positive social approval — body language rather than overuse of concrete reinforcement.
- Trying to avoid teaching or giving eye contact when anxious or when non-harmful provocation occurs.
- Not taking personally the actions or behaviours of multisensorially disabled children. They are not trying to get at you. They may be reacting to something that has happened, perceiving it or the environment in a totally different way from you.
- Using videotape, audiotape and behaviour analysis techniques to provide baselines to enable examination of our, and the child's, behaviour in a more objective and systematic manner.

Parents and professionals using these and other objective techniques may identify causes of, or contributory factors to, behaviour and can become successful agents for behaviour change. Other techniques which might be incorporated into an overall behaviourally engineered environment for success include:

- Careful monitoring of TV and video to ensure that films that include violence or explicit sexual scenes are avoided. Deaf children appear to be easily desensitized and consequently need careful preparation and discussion about material viewed on television screens.
- Ensuring ample opportunity for constructive rewarding occupation of leisure time.
- Social skills — moral training, training in recognizing their own and others' emotions, what to do and how to do it in different social settings.
- Use of puppets, role play and drama as part of social awareness — social skills training.
- Relaxation training via breathing, massage, aromatherapy.
- Management of communication via alternative systems (e.g. use of pictures, symbols or photos to identify and express feelings).

Summary

Intervention in assisting multiply handicapped sensorially impaired children to develop more positive patterns of behaviour has gradually shifted from a controlling model of 'corrective rehabilitation' to one in which positive communicational, interactive contexts play a major role in enabling multisensorially disabled children to have their needs recognized. Increased opportunities for them to develop choice, communication, personal social skills, appropriate behaviour and responsibility for their behaviour on equal terms with their peers, can enable children previously regarded as severely multiply disabled, to achieve at substantially higher levels than may have previously been recognized as being possible.

Key factors in the preventive and treatment processes include early identification, comprehensive assessment by professionals who are well trained and experienced in identifying and providing for the needs of these children, and use of a range of intervention techniques which are appropriate to needs and ability, are creative, constructive and enabling.

One of the most difficult areas for professionals who work with these children is the child who does not respond to preventive or educational behavioural treatment, and shows little responsiveness to medical or other treatments. By use of more open-minded methods we are sometimes able to overcome some of these difficulties, but the problem remains that, for some children, despite team working with medical and other colleagues, significant mental health problems continue to affect the lives of some multisensorially disabled or multiply handicapped hearing-impaired children. Very often these mental health problems are similar to those experienced in other children or in adults who do not have sensory disability.

Our greatest concern remains for those sensorially impaired children whose mental health problems may be prevented or treated appropriately through recognition of their needs as a sensorially disabled person, and through provision of the right of access to appropriate communication, interaction and education. Unfortunately, we continue to see children who are deaf and whose mental health has been damaged because of inappropriate assessment and provision. It is hoped that the movement towards increasing awareness of mental health and deafness will improve assessment, communication and provision for all children who are deaf.

References

Balkanay TJ (1980) Otologic aspects of Down's syndrome. Seminars in Speech Language and Hearing 1: 39–48.

Bexton WH, Herron W, Scott TH (1954) Effects of decreased variation in the sensory environment. Canadian Journal of Psychology 8: 70–76.

Bond DE (1970) Some Aspects of Immediate Memory for Visually Presented Stimuli. A Comparison of Hearing and Hearing Handicapped Children. Unpublished MA Thesis, University of Auckland, NZ.

Bond DE (1979) Aspects of psycho-educational assessment of hearing impaired children with additional handicaps. Journal of The British Association of Teachers of the Deaf 3: 76–79.

Bond DE (1981) Hearing loss, language, cognition, personality and social development. In Jackson A (ed) Ways and Means III: Hearing Impairment. Globe Educational, pp 19–24.

Bond DE (1985) Managing Behaviour: Alternative Diet? Paper presented to the International Conference for Educators of the Deaf, Manchester.

Bond DE (1986) Psychological assessment of the hearing impaired, additionally impaired, and multi handicapped deaf. In Ellis D (ed) Sensory Impairments in Mentally Handicapped People. Beckenham: Croom Helm, pp 297–318.

Bond DE (1991) The Hearing Impaired Child with Additional Handicaps. Unit 17: Distance Learning Course for Teachers of Hearing Impaired Children. University of Birmingham, School of Education.

Bond DE (1993) Mental heath in children who are hearing impaired. In Varma V (ed) Coping with Unhappy Children. London: Cassell, pp 31–51.

Dutt GC (1991) How cultural beliefs hamper psychiatric treatment. ODA News Review 2: 14.

Fraser GR (1964) Profound childhood deafness. Journal of Medical Genetics 1: 118–151.

Glynn T (1987) Contexts for independent learning for children with special needs. Journal of the Association for Behavioural Approaches with Children 11: 5–16.

Goetzinger CO (1972) The psychology of hearing impairment. In Katz J, Handbook of Clinical Audiology. Baltimore, MD: Williams and Wilkins, pp 666–693.

Graham P, Rutter M (1968) Organic brain dysfunction and child psychiatric disorder. British Medical Journal 3: 695–700.

Hindley P, Hill P, McGuigan S, Kitson N (1994) Psychiatric disorder in deaf and hearing impaired children and young people: a prevalence study. Journal of Child Psychiatry and Psychology 35: 917–934.

Holland A (1986) Genetic aspects of visual and auditory impairment in mentally handicapped people. In Ellis D (ed) Sensory Impairments in Mentally Handicapped People. Beckenham: Croom Helm, pp 149–166.

Levine ES (1981) The Ecology of Early Deafness. New York: Columbia University Press.

Nance W (1976) Studies of hereditary deafness present, past and future. In Fresina R (ed) A Bicentennial Monograph on Hearing Impairment. Trends in the USA. Volta Review 78: 6–11.

Parsons MB et al. (11 students, of whom the writer was one) (1966) Hearing Impairment in Mentally Handicapped People. Unpublished paper. Education of the Deaf Course, Christchurch Teachers College, Canterbury, New Zealand.

Schlesinger H, Meadow K (1972) Sound and Sign, Childhood Deafness and Mental Health. Los Angeles, CA, University of California Press.

Tucker IG, Noland M (1984) Educational Audiology. Beckenham: Croom Helm.

Van Dijk J (1982) Rubella handicapped Children: The Effect of Bilateral Cataract and or Hearing Impairment on Behaviour and Learning. Lisse: Swets and Zeitlinger.

Vernon M (1969) Multiply Handicapped Deaf Children: Medical, Educational and Psychological Considerations. Washington Research Monograph for Council for Exceptional Children.

Williams C (1970) Some psychiatric observations on a group of maladjusted deaf children. Journal of Child Psychology and Psychiatry 2: 1–18.

Wing L (1971) Severely retarded children in a London area: prevalence and provision of services. Journal of Psychological Medicine 1: 405–415.

Wood D, Wood H, Griffiths A, Howarth I (1986) Teaching and Talking with Deaf Children. Chichester: John Wiley.

Chapter 7
Maltreatment of Deaf and Hard of Hearing Children

PATRICIA SULLIVAN, PATRICK BROOKHOUSER AND JOHN SCANLAN

Introduction

Children who are deaf or hard of hearing, as well as children with other types of disabilities, are at increased risk of maltreatment, including neglect, physical, sexual or emotional abuse, or any combination thereof. Given this increased risk, medical professionals providing diagnosis and treatment services to children with hearing impairments must be acquainted with maltreatment risk factors and perpetrator characteristics associated with this population. This chapter reviews available literature on maltreatment of children with disabilities and presents data about maltreatment characteristics, risk factors and perpetrator characteristics regarding children who are deaf or hard of hearing, derived from an epidemiological study utilizing the patient database at the Boys Town National Research Hospital (BTNRH). Maltreatment dynamics and safety factors in residential placements for children with hearing impairments are discussed and appropriate interviewing and therapeutic techniques for use with children with hearing impairments who are suspected victims of sexual abuse are reviewed.

Boys Town National Research Hospital

The Boys Town National Institute for Communication Disorders in Children was established as a division of Father Flanagan's Boys' Home (Boys Town) in 1972 to provide evaluation and treatment of children with communication disorders and to carry out research in related areas. In 1989, the name was changed to Boys Town National Research Hospital (BTNRH), better to reflect the clinical aspects of the programme. BTNRH is located near the campus of Creighton University adjoining St Joseph Hospital, the primary teaching hospital for the Creighton University School of Medicine. BTNRH is a department within Father Flanagan's Boys' Home and also functions as the Department of Otolaryngology and

Human Communication of the Creighton University School of Medicine, where all members of the professional staff hold faculty appointments.

BTNRH is in its twenty-sixth year as an active clinical and research centre. A broad research programme is conducted there, consistent with the range of clinical services, which includes basic and applied work in areas of hearing, deafness, speech and language, psychology, and child abuse and neglect. The clinical caseload at the Research Hospital and satellite paediatric clinics is currently more than 120,000 visits per year. About half of the patients come from within 200 miles of BTNRH, but referrals are received from all 50 states and several foreign countries. The Center for Abused Children with Disabilities is one of six divisions within BTNRH and provides clinical services to abused children with disabilities and their families, and conducts clinical research on the epidemiology of abuse and neglect and psychotherapy outcome studies.

Maltreatment defined

Maltreatment is a generic term for child abuse and neglect, and encompasses neglect, physical abuse, sexual abuse, and psychological or emotional abuse. In this chapter definitions will be employed which are commonly used in the USA.

Neglect is an act or acts or omission on the part of the caregiver responsible for the physical, emotional, intellectual and social well-being of the child. Recognition must be given to the fact that neglect may exist in many gradations, ranging from incipient stages to truly gross proportions. Along this continuum, neglect is classified as:

- Failure to educate a child or follow medical recommendations.
- Non-life-threatening lack of supervision or follow-through.
- Lack of adequate food, housing, and/or medical care.
- Life-threatening lack of adequate food, housing, and/or medical care.

Among deaf and hard-of-hearing children, some professionals argue that failure to communicate with a given child in his preferred communication mode, to provide an educational environment that gives instruction in the child's preferred mode, or parents who do not learn to communicate with the child in the preferred mode, constitutes neglect (Kennedy, 1989, 1990).

Physical abuse is defined as the consequences of events or acts of commission which:

- Are potentially injurious to the child.
- Encompass a tissue-damaging event or involve harmful restraint or control.
- Entail a serious physical injury requiring medical or dental services.
- Cause a fatality or life-threatening physical event.

An act of commission essentially means that the caregiver had the intention to harm, injure, maim, or murder the child.

Sexual abuse is the exploitation of a child for any sexual gratification and includes rape, incest, fondling of the genitals, exhibitionism, and voyeurism. Sexual abuse is considered to be:

- Witnessing sexual activity between adults, adults and children, and sexual abuse of other children.
- Fondling.
- Oral, genital, or digital penetration or genital abuse without penetration.
- Anal or vaginal intercourse or penetration.

Emotional or **psychological abuse** is difficult to define and document. It is considered to occur when parents or caretakers verbally abuse children or place excessive and/or inappropriate demands on their emotional, social, and physical capabilities.

In this chapter, perpetrators classified as intrafamilial include parents, grandparents, siblings, and adopted, step or foster parents or siblings. Extended family members such as spouses, uncles, aunts, and cousins are also considered intrafamilial. All other perpetrators are classified as extrafamilial and have no familial contact with the child.

Review of research

Professionals, including child protection workers and educators, believe children with disabilities are at high risk of being abused and that some disabilities are caused or exacerbated by such maltreatment (Schilling, Kirkham and Schinke, 1986; Sobsey and Varnhagen, 1988; Sobsey, 1994). However, there is a surprising paucity of methodologically sound research in the field of child abuse and disability (Knutson, 1988; Ammerman, 1991; Knutson and Schartz, 1994). Many children with disabilities exhibit behavioural characteristics such as tantrums, aggressiveness and non-compliance that affect parents and other caregivers negatively, increasing their risk for abuse (Solomons, 1979).

Impediments to recognizing signs and symptoms of maltreatment in children with disabilities have also been described. Communication problems inherent in many disabilities render children unable to understand and/or verbalize episodes of maltreatment (Brookhouser et al., 1986; Morgan, 1987). Such children are unable to report their victimization, and, in the absence of an eyewitness or a confession, incidents of abuse among disabled individuals do not readily come to the attention of child protective service or law enforcement personnel. Further, non-verbal children are at increased risk of maltreatment, as are children with disabilities limiting their speech and language skills (Sobsey and Varnhagen,

1988). Children with disabilities and their families often display characteristics associated with abuse in non-disabled populations, including poverty, poor coping abilities and parental history of abuse (Friedrich and Boriskin, 1978; Frodi, 1981).

The hypothesis that a child's disability plays some process role in maltreatment has yet to be tested empirically. Certain disabilities may constitute greater risk factors than others, while interactions between specific disabilities and caretaking roles could also enhance risk. Finkelhor et al. (1988) found that most daycare abuse occurs around toileting, suggesting that disabilities enhancing the need for toileting assistance may be associated with increased risk of sexual abuse. Sullivan, Vernon and Scanlan (1987) found that, in deaf youth, sexual abuse tended to occur in bathrooms, bedrooms and specialized transportation vehicles. Such data, together with highly publicized episodes of abuse at residential facilities, suggest that current educational practices (i.e. inadequate sex education and condoned physical interventions which can escalate to abuse) could play contributory roles in maltreatment of children and youth with disabilities.

Problems in existing evidence

The existing controversy (Starr et al., 1984; Ammerman, Van Hasselt and Hersen, 1988; Ammerman, 1991) with respect to the role of disabilities in cases of abuse can be attributed to a dearth of empirically based studies. Deficiencies in existing studies include differing operational definitions of maltreatment, poorly defined heterogeneous populations with disabilities, and questionable validation procedures for determining disabilities (Knutson, 1988; Ammerman, Van Hasselt and Hersen, 1988; Knutson and Schartz, 1994). Central registries of child abuse and neglect do not provide definitive answers because abuse records of children are not systematically entered among states, and disability data are not routinely included. Many incidents of maltreatment known to professionals and lay persons are not reported to appropriate agencies, leading to underestimates of true levels of maltreatment (Knutson, 1988). It is likely that children with disabilities are over-represented among unreported abuse incidents, and summary reports of child maltreatment may include an unknown number of children who are the subjects of multiple reports, thereby overestimating some rates of maltreatment (American Humane Association, 1988). More stringent methodological efforts are required to establish the prevalence of child maltreatment, within both populations with disabilities and appropriate comparison groups.

Disabilities can render children difficult to manage, cognitively impaired, communicatively limited, or limited in mobility and can be conceptualized as chronic stressors for caregivers while also disrupting the attachment process. Nearly all disabling conditions or their behavioural manifestations can also be occasioned by physical abuse or neglect (Sangrund, Gaines and Green, 1974; Solomons, 1979; Jaudes and Diamond, 1985). In specific instances, it is often impossible to determine whether the disability contributes to the occurrence of abuse or whether it is a consequence of abuse.

Other lines of indirect evidence argue that it is premature to discard the possible link between disabilities and abuse (Garbarino, Brookhouser and Authier, 1987). For example, recent research with communicatively impaired and hearing-impaired children has suggested hearing impairment as a risk factor in physical and sexual abuse (Sullivan et al., 1991; Knutson and Sullivan, 1993). Moreover, related data have suggested that parents of deaf children are more likely to use physical coercion than are parents of hearing children (Schlesinger and Meadow, 1972). Additionally, evidence from residential placement facilities suggest that sensorially impaired children may be at greater risk of maltreatment (Brookhouser, 1987; Whittaker, 1987).

Current state of knowledge

Incidence studies

There have been several studies of the incidence of abuse and neglect among samples of disabled children and adults referred to treatment centres. Sullivan et al. (1991) investigated patterns of abuse among a sample of 482 consecutively referred maltreated children with disabilities in a hospital setting. Results indicated that sexual abuse or a combination of sexual and physical abuse were the most common forms of maltreatment endured by the referred children with disabilities. The majority of the subjects had communication disorders, including speech and/or hearing impairments, learning disabilities and cleft lip and/or palate. Males with disabilities were more likely to be victims of sexual abuse than males in the general population and placement in a residential school was identified as a major risk factor for sexual abuse among disabled youngsters. The results were replicated in a five-year retrospective study of 4340 maltreated children who were patients in a paediatric hospital in which the majority were victims of sexual abuse (68%) while 32% were victims of physical abuse (Willging, Bower and Cotton, 1992). Studies in the UK (Westcott, 1991), Australia (Turk and Brown, 1992) and Canada (Sobsey and Doe, 1991) have also found that sexual abuse is the most prevalent form of maltreatment among children with disabilities. However, the major limitations of this research are subject selection biases, in that most subjects were obtained from hospital, medical treatment centres, or institutions for the disabled, which inherently have large numbers of abused individuals seeking treatment. Accordingly, they may miss large cohorts of neglected children who are typically not referred for treatment.

Prevalence estimate

The Boys Town National Research Hospital conducted a prevalence study in which hospital records over a 10-year period (i.e. 1981 – 1991) were merged with Nebraska Central Registry (NDSS) and Foster Care Review Board (FCRB) records from the same time period to identify cases of intrafamilial abuse (Sullivan and Knutson, 1998a). An important feature of this study was an additional merger with police records to identify cases of extrafamilial abuse. Out of a total of 39 352 records, almost 9000 matches were made between hospital and agency records, indicating an overall base rate of abuse of 21% for this hospital sample. A random sample of 3001 abused children was drawn from the total sample and a control group of 880 non-abused children was randomly selected from the hospital records. These 3881 records were then subjected to a detailed review to ascertain the presence of disabilities and the circumstances of maltreatment. Such a high prevalence rate of maltreatment in a hospital population that focuses on children with disabilities provides supporting evidence that disabilities can be a risk factor for maltreatment.

In the sample of 3001 maltreated children whose records were examined, there were 183 deaf and hard-of-hearing children. A total of 66 deaf and hard-of-hearing children were in the non-abused control group of 880 children. In the total data analyses, certain types of disabilities were found to be at risk for certain types of abuse. Deaf and hard-of-hearing children, alongside children with behavioural disorders and mental retardation, were at increased risk of physical abuse. For sexual abuse, children with attention deficit disorder, behaviour disorders, learning disabilities, and mental retardation were at increased risk. Children with mental retardation, speech language impairments, behaviour disorders, learning disabilities and orthopaedic impairments were at increased risk of neglect. Children with behaviour disorders and mental retardation were found to be at increased risk for all three forms of maltreatment. Children with speech and language impairments and learning disabilities were at increased risk of neglect and sexual abuse.

Another important finding revealed that 72% of extrafamilial sexual abuse was identified through the merger with law enforcement records. Previous prevalence studies have regularly noted that the maltreatment is predominantly intrafamilial. The results of our analyses also support the largely intrafamilial nature of abuse. Yet, a large number of maltreated children experience sexual abuse in an extrafamilial context. If investigators hope to understand disability as a risk factor in maltreatment, in data merger studies it is critical to use information only available through law enforcement agencies.

Behaviour disorders, speech and language disorders, mental retardation and hearing impairment were the most common types of disabilities found among the abused children in the sample. Abused children were 2.2 times more likely to have a disability than non-abused children. Children with disabilities were at greater risk of intrafamilial abuse than children without disabilities. Children with disabilities are 1.8 times more likely to endure neglect, 1.6 times more likely to be physically abused, and 2.2 times more likely to be victims of sexual abuse than non-disabled children. The perpetrators of this abuse were primarily parents and extended family members, including step and foster parents, grandparents, aunts, uncles and live-in companions of parents. However, extrafamilial abuse accounted for some 40% of the sexual abuse and perpetrators included baby sitters, clergy, van drivers, care attendants, older students, peers, neighbours, teachers and houseparents. Strangers accounted for only 7% of extrafamilial sexual abuse.

This epidemiological study indicated that almost one-quarter (22%) of children referred to a paediatric hospital in the USA had verified records of child maltreatment in social service and/or police records, strongly suggesting that the rate of referral of maltreated children to medical facilities is quite high. It further indicates that child maltreatment is a significant public health issue and its detection and prevention should be an integral part of primary care, particularly for infants, toddlers, and preschoolers less than 5 years of age. Healthcare professionals should be aware of the increased incidence of maltreatment among children referred to them for care and treatment and, accordingly, need to screen for histories of maltreatment and be alert for signs and symptoms of abuse and neglect. Given the increased percentage of children with disabilities among maltreated children, healthcare professionals also need to screen routinely for disabilities to provide this information to law enforcement and social service personnel during the conduct of maltreatment investigations. A model protocol for interviewing deaf and hard-of-hearing children who are suspected victims of child sexual abuse is given in Appendix A.

Maltreatment characteristics of deaf and hard-of-hearing children

A sample of 312 deaf and hard-of-hearing children evaluated at the BTNRH from 1984 to 1994 was reviewed to determine the maltreatment characteristics of a consecutively referred population of children with disabilities. These 312 children included 198 males and 114 females who comprised five groups:

- 123 children (73 M; 50 F) who were abuse victims (ABUSED).
- 58 abuse victims (46 M; 12 F) known to be perpetrators of abuse (APERP).
- Seven (3 M; 4 F) who were abuse victims with identified alcohol or chemical dependency problems (ACD).
- 23 (20 M; 3 F) who were abuse victims, known perpetrators, and had identified alcohol or chemical dependency problems (APERCD).
- A non-abused control group of 56 males and 45 females.

The mean age at the time of initial visit to BTNEH was 13 years (*SD* = 3.48) for the four abused groups and 8 years (*SD* = 3.75) for the non-abused control group. Both groups of deaf children ranged in age from 4 to 18 years. The children were referred from 24 states and one Canadian province. Referral was made for routine three-year evaluations mandated by Public Law 94–42 for the non-abused control group and for psychological evaluation and treatment for the abused groups. BTNRH is a national referral source for deaf and hard-of-hearing children throughout the USA. All children in the study had an identified sensorineural hearing loss which qualified them for special education services as defined by federal and state guidelines in their respective states of residence.

There is some possible overlap between the deaf and hard-of-hearing samples of the BTNRH epidemiological study (which included subjects only from Nebraska) and the data reported in this section (which include consecutive deaf and hard-of-hearing referrals from the national pool). In the BTNRH epidemiological study, there were 183 abused deaf and hard-of-hearing children within the 3001 abused sample, and 66 non-abused deaf and hard-of-hearing children in the 880 non-abused sample from Nebraska. In the current study of only deaf and hard-of-hearing children, there were 119 children within the four abused subgroups and 36 children within the non-abused control group from Nebraska.

Data collection and analysis

The medical records of the abused and non-abused deaf and hard-of-hearing children were reviewed to determine type, severity and duration of maltreatment and perpetrator characteristics. To establish the reliability of the data collection procedure, 55 records were selected randomly and reviewed by a research assistant who was not involved in the initial review of records. Inter-coder agreement was computed by use of Cohen's kappa coefficients for a subset of variables included in the study: type, severity and locus of maltreatment and perpetrator characteristics. The kappa coefficients for these variables ranged from 0.70 to 1.00, with an average of 0.90, suggesting high agreement between the coders.

Table 7.1 Abuse subgroups broken down by type of abuse

Subgroup	Sexual	Physical	Sexual/Physical	Emotional	Total
Abused	66	12	27	18	123
Abused & Perpetrator	33	8	17	0	58
Abused & Alcohol/ Chemically Dependent	5	1	1	0	7
Abused, Perp. & Alcohol/ Chemically Dependent	10	2	11	0	23
Total	114	23	56	18	211

Descriptive statistics, including frequency counts, percentages, and means and standard deviations, and Chi-squared tests of independence, were completed. Using a modified Bonferroni adjustment, the alpha level was set at 0.006 for the Chi-squared tests of independence. This was implemented in order to control for Type 1 errors because multiple Chi-squared tests were conducted.

Results

Type of maltreatment

The type of maltreatment endured by the children in the four abused subgroups is displayed in Table 7.1. There was not a significant relationship between the abuse subgroup and type of maltreatment endured ($\chi^2 = 20.07$; $p = 0.0175$). Sexual, as well as combined sexual and physical abuse, were the most prevalent types of maltreatment for each of the subgroups, followed by physical abuse, and emotional abuse. This finding is consistent with other research involving clinical, hospital and residential treatment centres for children and adults with disabilities in Canada (Sobsey and Doe, 1991), Australia (Turk and Brown, 1992), the UK (Westcott, 1991) and in the USA (Willging, Bower and Cotton, 1992). Among clinical samples, sexual abuse and a combination of sexual and physical abuse are the most prevalent forms of maltreatment. However, epidemiological data utilizing a Child Protective Service (CPS) nationally representative sample in the USA (Westat Inc., 1993) and a national hospital sample utilizing both social service and police child maltreatment registries (Sullivan and Knutson, 1998) found type of maltreatment among children with disabilities to mirror that found for non-disabled children, with neglect being the most prevalent, followed by physical abuse, sexual abuse and emotional or psychological abuse. In the current data, becoming a perpetrator of abuse and/or developing an alcohol or chemical dependency problem was not associated with any particular form of maltreatment.

Gender

There were no differences between boys and girls regarding type of maltreatment endured. Both boys and girls were victims, in descending order of frequency, of sexual abuse, a combination of sexual and physical abuse, and emotional abuse. Significantly more males than females were found in the perpetrator (APERP) and alcohol and/or chemically dependent (ACD) groups ($\chi^2 = 13.27$; $p < 0.004$). This suggests that deaf males are more likely than deaf females to become perpetrators of abuse and to develop alcohol and drug abuse-related problems. There were no gender differences between the abuse subgroups and the non-abused control groups. More males than females were found in both the abused and non-abused groups.

Table 7.2 Gender broken down by abuse subgroup

Subgroup	Male	Female
Abused	73	50
Abused & Perpetrator	46	12
Abused & Alcohol/Chemically Dependent	3	4
Abused, Perp. & Alcohol/Chemically Dependent	20	3
Non-abused Control	56	45

Ethnicity and multiple disabilities

The ethnicity of the entire sample of deaf and hard-of-hearing children was consistent with 1994 US Census data for Caucasians (74%), African Americans (12%), Hispanics (10%), Asian Americans (3%), and Native Americans (1%). There were no differences in ethnicity between the abused and non-abused control groups or among any of the abused groups. This is consistent with findings among non-disabled populations in which ethnicity has not emerged as a risk factor for maltreatment (Knutson and Schartz, 1994). Approximately one-third of both the non-abused control group and all abuse groups combined had multiple disabilities. There were no significant relationships between abuse status or abuse subgrouping and the presence of multiple disabilities. Thus, deaf and hard-of-hearing children with multiple disabilities are not at greater risk of being victims of maltreatment than peers without multiple disabilities.

Type of schooling

There was not a significant relationship between type of school placement and the four abuse subgroup categories ($\chi^2 = 14.24$; $p = 0.0271$). However, as indicated in Table 7.3, for each abuse subgroup, the majority of abused children attended residential schools. Previous research with a sample of children having a broad range of communication disorders (Sullivan et al., 1991), including children with speech and language disabilities, cleft lip and palate, learning disabilities, mental retardation and hearing impairment, found being male and attending a residential school were significantly related to being a victim of maltreatment. Although the type of schooling was not significantly related to becoming an abuse perpetrator, or alcohol or chemically dependent, among this sample of deaf and hard-of-hearing abused children, the majority of deaf and hard-of-hearing children in each abuse grouping attended residential schools. In addition, the majority of children in the non-abused control group (72%) attended mainstreamed or other non-residential placements. There was a significant difference in schooling type between the four abuse subgroups combined and the non-abused control group ($\chi^2 = 84.57$; $p < 0.001$) indicating that a residential placement is a major risk factor for experiencing sexual and/or physical abuse among deaf and hard-of-hearing children.

The deaf and hard-of-hearing abused subjects from Nebraska included a cohort of youngsters from a residential school who were referred specifically for psychotherapy. In order to determine if this cohort of residential subjects were responsible for the significance of residential placement as a risk factor between the abused and non-abused groups, Chi-squared analysis was completed without any Nebraska subjects. The results were also significant ($\chi^2 = 65.11$; $p < 0.001$), indicating that residential placement is a significant risk factor for the occurrence of maltreatment for deaf and hard-of-hearing children.

Site of abuse

Table 7.4 shows the relationship between location of abuse and abuse subgroups. The most prevalent site of abuse for each abuse subgroup was school, followed by home and a combination of home and school. For each of the abuse subgroups, the primary location at school where the abuse occurred was the dormitory. Abuse occurred in the dormitory in 62% of the abused group, 88% of the abused and perpetrator group, 100% of the abused and chemically dependent group, and 83% of the perpetrator and chemically dependent group. This is consistent with previous research which has indicated that much of the abuse in residential institutions occurs

Table 7.3 Schooling broken down by abuse subgroup

Subgroup	Mainstream	Residential	Other
Abused	35.3%	55.2%	9.5%
Abused & Perpetrator	17.9%	78.6%	3.6%
Abused & Alcohol/Chemically Dependent	14.3%	85.7%	0.0%
Abused, Perp. & Alcohol/Chemically Dependent	13.0%	82.6%	4.3%
Non-abused Control	72.0%	9.0%	19.0%

Table 7.4 Site of abuse broken down by abuse subgroup

Subgroup	Home	School	Home + School	Foster Home	Perp's Home	Other
Abused	30.1%	45.1%	9.7%	3.5%	3.5%	8.0%
Abused & Perpetrator	27.3%	41.8%	23.6%	0.0%	1.8%	5.5%
Abused & Alcohol/ Chemically Dependent	33.3%	50.0%	16.7%	0.0%	0.0%	0.0%
Abused, Perp, & Alcohol/ Chemically Dependent	21.7%	60.9%	17.4%	0.0%	0.0%	0.0%

Table 7.5 Location at school where abuse occurred

Subgroup	Class	Dorm	Other
Abused	5.8%	61.5%	32.7%
Abused & Perpetrator	4.2%	87.5%	8.3%
Abused & Alcohol/ Chemically Dependent	0.0%	100.0%	0.0%
Abused, Perp. & Alcohol/ Chemically Dependent	0.0%	82.4%	17.6%

Table 7.6 Severity of sexual abuse broken down by abuse subgroups

Subgroup	1	2	3	4
Abused	4.8%	27.7%	13.3%	54.2%
Abused & Perpetrator	9.5%	21.4%	14.3%	54.8%
Abused & Alcohol/Chemically Dependent	16.7%	0.0%	50.0%	33.3%
Abused, Perp, & Alcohol/Chemically Dependent	0.0%	0.0%	20.0%	80.0%

around caretaking activities of the residents (Sullivan and Scanlan, 1987; Siskind, 1986; Sobsey, 1994). Some abuse also occurred in foster placements (3.5%) as well as in the home of the perpetrator (5.3%). The Other category accounted for 33% of the abused group, 8% of the perpetrator group, and almost 18% of the abused and chemically dependent group. Sites of abuse within the Other category included non-dormitory sites within the school, such as the gym, showers in the gym, swimming pool, hallways, tunnels, and in buses, vans and taxicabs transporting the children to and from school. Table 7.5 delineates the site of abuse for the four abuse categories.

Severity of abuse

The severity of sexual and physical abuse was coded according to a four-point scale. For sexual abuse, the scale included:

1. Witnessing sexual abuse.
2. Fondling.
3. Oral and/or digital penetration.
4. Anal and vaginal intercourse.

Table 7.6 demonstrates that most deaf and hard-of-hearing children were victims of severe levels of abuse, attaining ratings of either 3 or 4. This is consistent with previous research which has indicated that children with disabilities tend to experience severe levels of sexual abuse (Sullivan et al., 1991; Sobsey, 1994; Sullivan and Knutson, 1998).

The severity of physical abuse coding scheme was as follows:

1. Potentially injurious to child.
2. Tissue-damaging event, including harmful restraint or control.
3. Serious injury requiring medical or dental services.
4. Fatality or life-threatening physical event.

For each of the abuse subgroups, the majority of deaf and hard-of-hearing children were harmfully restrained or controlled. Within the ABUSED group, some 36% of the children endured injuries requiring medical or dental services compared to almost 10% of the APERP and 8% of the APERCD groups. Only the APERP (4.5%) and APERCD (8.3%) groups suffered life-threatening physical events. Severity data of physical abuse for the sample are given in Table 7.7.

Duration of sexual and physical abuse was coded along the following continuum:

1. One episode.
2. Less than one year.
3. One to three years.
4. More than three years.

There was a significant difference in duration of sexual abuse across the four abuse subgroups ($\chi^2 = 25.06$; $p = 0.0029$). The majority of sexually abused children in the APERCD subgroup were victimized for more than three years, whereas the majority of children in the other three abuse subgroups were sexually victimized for three years or less (see Table 7.8). Thus, becoming a sexual abuse perpetrator and developing an alcohol or chemical dependency problem is associated with long durations of sexual abuse among deaf and hard-of-hearing children. For physical abuse, there was not a significant relationship between duration and abuse subgroup. However, Table 7.8 indicates that 62% of the ABUSED group, 77% of the APERP group, and 91% of the APERCD group endured physical abuse for one year or longer. Thus, there is a strong association between duration of physical abuse and becoming a perpetrator and/or alcohol or chemically dependent among deaf and hard-of-hearing youth.

Table 7.7 Severity of physical abuse broken down by abuse subgroups

Subgroup	1	2	3	4
Abused	9.7%	54.8%	35.5%	0.0%
Abused & Perpetrator	18.2%	68.2%	9.1%	4.5%
Abused & Alcohol/Chemically Dependent	0.0%	100.0%	0.0%	0.0%
Abused, Perp, & Alcohol/Chemically Dependent	0.0%	83.3%	8.3%	8.3%

Table 7.8 Duration of sexual and physical abuse

Subgroup	Sexual 1	2	3	4	Physical 1	2	3	4
Abused	17.2%	32.8%	35.9%	14.1%	12.5%	25.0%	33.3%	29.2%
Abused & Perpetrator	5.9%	38.2%	20.6%	35.3%	5.9%	17.6%	41.2%	35.3%
Abused & Alcohol/ Chemically Dependent	0.0%	66.7%	16.7%	16.7%	0.0%	100.0%	0.0%	0.0%
Abused, Perp, & Alcohol/ Chemically Dependent	0.0%	10.0%	35.0%	55.0%	0.0%	9.1%	27.3%	63.6%

Perpetrators

Perpetrator data for the abuse groupings for sexual and physical abuse are given in Tables 7.9 and 7.10, respectively. For sexual abuse, there are some differences between perpetrator identity and abuse subgroup. For all abuse subgroups, a high percentage of sexual abuse was perpetrated by older children or peers: ABUSE (49%), APERP (49%), ACD (50%) and APERCD (42%). Parents and step or foster parents accounted for 10% of the ABUSE, 5% of the APERP, 10% of the ACD, and none of the APERPCD groups. Houseparents in residential facilities accounted for 18% of the ABUSE, 24% of the APERP and 40% of both the ACD and APERCD groups. Males were most often the perpetrators of sexual abuse (M = 88.8%; F = 11.2%). Deaf and hard-of-hearing children are at higher risk of being sexually abused by houseparents, older students and peers than by their parents. These perpetrator risk factors are important concerns for residential placements.

For physical abuse, the majority of perpetrators were also male (M = 76.3%; F = 23.7%). The majority of perpetrators of the physical abuse were biological parents, step and foster parents, or houseparents for all abuse subgroups. Deaf and hard of hearing children are at highest risk of physical abuse by parent or parent substitutes. The physical abuse perpetrators are given in Table 7.10.

These data on a sample of clinically referred deaf and hard-of-hearing children suggest that residential placement is a major risk factor for child maltreatment for this population. Safety concerns for peers and older students as perpetrators of sexual abuse in residential schools emerge as well. These factors necessitate a consideration of institutional abuse and the dynamics of abuse within residential settings.

Child maltreatment in residential institutions

The problem of maltreatment of children in institutions is longstanding and has been reported for over two centuries. Sobsey (1994) provides the

Table 7.9 Sexual abuse perpetrator characteristics

Perpetrator	Abused	Abused/Perp.	Abused/Drug	Abused/Perp./Drug
Parent	7.1%	4.7%	10.0%	0.0%
Teacher	2.4%	0.9%	0.0%	0.0%
Houseparent	17.9%	24.3%	40.0%	40.0%
Older Child	22.6%	19.6%	50.0%	25.0%
Sibling	4.8%	7.5%	0.0%	0.0%
Peer	26.2%	29.0%	0.0%	17.5%
Relative	3.6%	4.7%	0.0%	2.5%
SF Parent	3.0%	0.0%	0.0%	0.0%
Other	12.5%	9.3%	0.0%	15.0%

Table 7.10 Physical abuse perpetrator characteristics

Perpetrator	Abused	Abused/Perp.	Abused/Drug	Abused/Perp./Drug
Parent	45.9%	44.1%	50.0%	42.9%
Teacher	4.9%	2.9%	0.0%	7.1%
Houseparent	9.8%	29.4%	0.0%	50.0%
Older Child	1.6%	5.9%	0.0%	0.0%
Sibling	3.3%	0.0%	0.0%	0.0%
Peer	4.9%	0.0%	0.0%	0.0%
Relative	0.0%	0.0%	0.0%	0.0%
SF Parent	14.8%	5.9%	50.0%	0.0%
Other	14.8%	11.8%	0.0%	0.0%

most recent review of abuse in institutions that serve individuals with disabilities. A great deal of attention was afforded the abuse of children in institutions in the mid-1960s with the publishing of *Christmas in Purgatory: A Photographic Essay on Mental Retardation* (Blatt and Kaplan, 1966) which chronicled photographically widespread abuse of children and adults in institutions for the mentally retarded. A few years later, Cole (1972) visited institutions in four states and reported horrific cases of maltreatment, including rape and sodomy of children by caregivers. These landmark works ultimately led to the 'deinstitutionalization' movement, the advent of mainstreaming, and standards of care to serve children in the 'least restrictive environment' rather than in institutions.

In the late 1960s and early 1970s there were numerous large-scale investigations of abuse of residents in institutions throughout the USA. The first exposé at Willowbrook in New York gained Rivera (1972) national attention and he wrote a book about his experiences in investigating the abuse allegations. Major investigations of maltreatment of residents in institutions occurred in Alabama, Maryland, Massachusetts, Nebraska,

New York, North Dakota, Pennsylvania and Tennessee. Reports of abuse of individuals with disabilities residing in institutions also occurred in the 1970s in England and Wales (Oswin, 1979) and Canada (Chase, 1976). There was widespread cognizance of the precarious position of institutions as a method of caring for children and youth, and institutions were fighting for their very existence (Whittaker and Trieschman, 1972; Taylor and Bodgan, 1980; Taylor, 1981). Many institutions closed as deinstitutionalization and mainstreaming became the methods of choice of serving children and youth. Attention and emphasis were directed toward concerns regarding the range of maltreatment endured by children and youth residing in institutions (Whittaker and Trieschman, 1972; Gil, 1979; Hanson, 1982) including:

- Neglect (Blatt and Kaplan, 1966; Cole, 1972; Rivera, 1972; Oswin, 1979; Schinke et al., 1981).
- Physical abuse (Cole, 1972; Chase, 1976; Harrell and Orem, 1980; Taylor, 1981; Gil, 1982; Hanson, 1982; Rindfleisch and Baros-Van Hill, 1982; Wexler, 1982).
- Sexual Abuse (Blatt and Kaplan, 1966; Cole 1972; Harrell and Orem, 1980; Tilelli, Turek and Jaffe, 1980; Schultz, 1981; Solomons, Abel and Epley, 1981; Corrigan, 1982; Gil, 1982; Hanson, 1982; Shore, 1982).

During this time, the populations of residential schools for the deaf in the USA decreased and the numbers of children served in day programmes within the public schools increased dramatically.

Abuse and deafness: brief chronology

From 1983 to 1987 there were multiple investigations into allegations of sexual and physical abuse in residential schools for the deaf throughout the USA and Canada. Abuse allegations emerged in schools for the deaf in Alabama, California, Florida, Iowa, Maine, Maryland, Michigan, Mississippi, Missouri, Nebraska, New York, South Dakota, Texas, Virginia, Washington, West Virginia, and Wisconsin. There was keen awareness on the part of administrators and staff at residential schools for the deaf of these investigations of child abuse, which were interpreted to be threats to close the schools (Sullivan, Vernon and Scanlan, 1987). In many cases, staff and administrators lost their jobs and this heightened concern and contributed to reactive rather than proactive responses to the situation.

In 1984, the first US National Conference on the Habilitation and Rehabilitation of Deaf Adolescents was held in Oklahoma and was attended by almost 200 people from throughout the USA. The topic of abuse of children in residential schools was addressed by Dr Henry Klopping, Superintendent of the California School for the Deaf. In his keynote presentation, Dr Klopping stated:

> In recent months, we have been exposed to a number of incidents involving abuse of deaf students attending several residential schools for the deaf. Charges of child abuse have led to three employees of one school being arrested for child molestation and at least one of these employees being convicted. A superintendent and dean of students in another school were recently arrested in front of TV reporters and newsmen and charged with felony child abuse for failure to report to police the sexual assault of one student upon another. In another case, a superintendent has been removed from his position for failure to report a child abuse incident. A superintendent of one residential school was fired because abuse had occurred in the school, although he was not aware of the specific abuses. Finally, another school suspended a dean of students for some inappropriate disciplinary measures which were being interpreted as child abuse. Although we do not have the complete facts on these cases, it appears that the failure to report suspected child abuse to appropriate authorities has led to the current problem that these administrators must face.

In December of 1984, the Center for Abused Children with Disabilities was established at the Boys Town National Research Hospital, in response to the large numbers of child abuse victims with disabilities, particularly deaf and hard-of-hearing children, being referred to the Center. In 1986, the Center hosted a national conference of experts on child abuse and neglect to address the issue of maltreatment among children with disabilities. This conference resulted in one of the first books published on the topic: ***Special Children – Special Risks: The Maltreatment of Children with Disabilities*** (Garbarino and Authier, 1987). An entire chapter was devoted to institutional abuse (Whittaker, 1987). Other articles addressed medical (Brookhouser, 1987), therapeutic (Sullivan and Scanlan, 1987), legal (Melton, 1987), educational (Garbarino and Authier, 1987) and media issues (McCall and Gregory, 1987).

In 1987, a presentation entitled 'Sexual Abuse of Deaf Youth' was made at the Convention of American Instructors for the Deaf (CAID) and Conference of Educational Administrators Serving the Deaf (CEASD). This is the national major conference for administrators and teachers from residential schools for the deaf throughout the USA and Canada. This presentation was later published (Sullivan, Vernon and Scanlan, 1987), and addressed the scope, nature and incidence of sexual abuse of deaf children and behavioural/emotional characteristics of sexually abused children and adolescents. These authors also addressed issues in the prevention, intervention and reporting of abuse, while specific resources that could be contacted for assistance, consultation or diagnostic/treatment services for suspected or identified victims of child sexual abuse were described. Preliminary prevalence data were presented on sexual abuse in residential schools for the deaf and a discussion of reporting problems in residential schools was also included in the article.

An article specifically addressing sexual abuse issues and risk factors among deaf children to be victims of maltreatment (Brookhouser et al., 1986) provided an overview of the incidence, demographic characteristics, risk factors and dynamics of sexual abuse within the deaf population, specifically discussing abuse in residential schools for the deaf.

In the UK, Kennedy (1989, 1990, 1992) has written exclusively about the abuse of deaf and hard-of-hearing children and established the Keep Deaf Children Safe Programme in London in 1987 which has served as a resource and advocacy centre on maltreatment issues for children who are deaf and hard of hearing.

Dynamics of abuse in institutions

Siskind (1986) enhanced understanding of the dynamics of institutional abuse in his article. He broadened the definition of child sexual abuse by including 'sexual abuse committed by a person under the age of 18 when that youngster is either significantly older than the victim or when the perpetrator is in a position of power or control over the child he or she is abusing'. He also identified several reasons for the under-reporting of child sexual abuse in institutions.

Given the frequent lack of physical evidence, sexual abuse is easier to hide for longer periods of time than is the case with physical abuse. Because sexual abuse tends to remain a secret, it is less likely that a sexually abusive residential worker or victimized child will seek help. Children are unlikely to report sexual abuse because of shame and fear surrounding their victimization. Children may be unable to discern abuse and may have confusion regarding:

- Their involvement in the seduction phase of the abuse.
- Their ambivalent feelings about sexual contact.
- The malicious versus affectionate intentions and contact with the abuser.

The helpless feeling of being victimized, with accompanying shame and guilt, may be experienced by adolescents as childish and they may, accordingly, hide, deny or retract disclosures of the incident. Finally, children may fear punishment and/or reprisals if they disclose the abuse. Siskind (1986) emphasizes that it is not as easy to hide abuse in an institution which has more people involved with and observing the children and their caregivers than does a family.

Most sexual abuse in institutions involves caregivers closest to the child in terms of daily contact and function. Parent surrogate and direct care roles require a certain amount of physical and affectionate contact during times when sexual stimulation might be more intense, such as at bedtime or at wake-up time. In contrast, there are fewer reports of abuse by professional teaching staff, possibly because these professionals spend less time in close proximity to the children they serve and the relationship of professionals to children is governed by clear expectations and guidelines.

There are some comparisons between institutional abuse and incest (Siskind, 1986). Institutional abuse can be conceptualized in terms of a familial model. Institutional living unit systems, like incestuous families, can also defend themselves vigorously by denying the abuse. Some abusive adult institutional caretakers may behave like incestuous parents and use power differentials and manipulation to coerce and seduce the children into sexual activity. Systemic issues must be evaluated in the case of institutional sexual abuse. If sexual abuse is repeated or thematic in an institution then clearly one needs to look at the institutional system. If patterns of sexual and non-sexual maltreatment can be traced beyond the occasional deviant staff member to the culture, values, economics and style of the institution itself then only a systemic solution can be realistically expected to resolve the abusive environment.

There has been a substantial Canadian contribution to the understanding of the dynamics of the maltreatment of children in institutions, ranging from the identification of administrative and management styles that foster abuse (Rindfleisch, 1984), the delineation of potential abuse indicators and guidelines for their investigation (Docherty, 1989), and the unique characteristics of institutional abuse and abusive subcultures within institutions (Sobsey, 1994). In a speech entitled 'Factors Which Influence the Severity of Adverse Events in Residential Facilities', in Montreal in September of 1984, Rindfleisch (one of the foremost experts on institutional child abuse of the time) addressed the International Congress on Child Abuse and Neglect and identified four administrative styles associated with patterns of institutional sexual abuse (Rindfleisch, 1984):

1. An autocratic senior administrator, protected by a strong political and administrative network, who discourages participation by staff and residents and inculcates a feeling of helplessness and powerlessness.
2. Stress is placed on the difficulty of handling the residents, with subtle or overt permission by administrative staff to control at any cost and thus, finally, to abuse.
3. Reliance is placed on an ideological model which tends to distance, dehumanize, and devalue relationships with residents.
4. An oppressor mentality that reflects, encourages or tolerates hostility toward females, children, or minorities exists.

In Toronto, Docherty and associates have published several manuscripts pertaining to the maltreatment of children in residential care, providing a description of indicators of abusive residential care facilities, a compendium of indicators that cut across all aspects of institutional life. A primary indicator is lack of frequent access to family and friends whereby children become disassociated from their homes and families if they do not have contact with family or visit them for long periods. Residential settings in which abuse occurs frequently are lax in informing children of their rights and in reinforcing those rights. The fact that some children may be incapable of making full use of their rights, even when fully informed, underscores the importance of having an advocacy system operating within the institution that is monitored by external involvement, including ethical review and an audit system. An on-site school is a potential additional risk factor for abuse because it affords the residential care programme an opportunity to keep children more isolated. Docherty emphasizes that programmes in which all components are fully enclosed within a single location need to be monitored more closely than one in which children have freer access to the community at large.

Excessive control over daily living functions, including eating, bathing, toileting, and conversation and communication, is inherently abusive. These controls reinforce a sense of powerlessness among residents and increase their vulnerability to abuse. Low wages for personnel working in the dormitories is another indicator. The low salary levels indicate the staff are poorly educated and trained for the positions they assume. Given this lack of training and education they are all too often unable to respond adequately to the needs of the children they supervise. The age difference between staff and children may be only four or five years, particularly if the school tends to hire former students as staff members. Young and unskilled staff rarely ask threatening questions or report abusive situations. Limited supervision of staff and long staff hours over extended periods of time also contribute to abuse within institutions.

In 1989, Docherty also produced guidelines for the investigation of abuse allegations in residential facilities. He cautioned that an organization responsible for placement, supervision, licensing, funding, monitoring or provision of the service in a specific case should not also be given investigating authority. He also recommended that guidelines be developed for investigating abuse in residential care settings that are based upon both an understanding of institutional dynamics and investigative practices. Individuals undertaking abuse investigations within residential placements should receive special training, and all children should be interviewed within their respective means of communication or interpreted by a person of their choosing in a safe location away from the institution.

Sobsey, Director of the Abuse and Disability Project at the University of Atlanta, has extensive experience in residential facilities, as an attendant at a residential facility for 10 years, and as a psychologist and researcher in the field. He has written the most comprehensive book to date on the abuse of people with disabilities (Sobsey, 1994) which has an entire chapter devoted to institutional abuse. Sobsey (1994) indicates that institutional abuse is distinguished by four factors which make it unique from other types of abuse. The first is the extreme power inequities between staff and residents, in which staff have control over most aspects of the lives of the residents (i.e. waking, sleeping, eating, toileting, exercising, bathing, communicating) and can obtain and maintain this control through the use of various tools, including compliance training, drugs, locks, restraints, institutional routines and condoned punishment interventions. Secondly, institutional abuse is collective in nature and there is often more than one offender and more than one victim. The third characteristic of institutional abuse is that it typically involves some kind of cover-up wherein the abuse is known within the institution, but is not reported to supervisors, and administrators attempt to control the problem internally by avoiding any action that could lead to public awareness of the problem. The fourth characteristic is the remarkable environmental similarity of institutions which often includes geographic isolation, large institutional settings in rural areas far from public transportation systems, sociocultural differences between the residents and the larger society, limited parental involvement, and limited resources in a highly isolated environment.

Certain administrative structures within institutions described by Sobsey (1994) make change and reform very difficult. These include non-enforcement, whereby administrators permit abuse and implicitly condone it, covert facilitation by taking actions which encourage abuse, and escalation which promotes the occurrence of abuse. Sobsey (1994) provides additional insights into the nature and effects of institutional abuse by describing the phenomena of dehumanization and detachment, clustering and abusive subcultures.

Children in institutional settings typically encounter some 50 – 80 caregivers (Rutter, 1989) given high staff turnover and caregiver burnout rates, making the development of healthy attachments with others virtually impossible. The mixing or clustering of highly naïve and vulnerable children with more sexually aggressive children is a recipe for abuse. Abusive subcultures exist within institutions wherein violence and sexual abuse is the norm. Residents of the institution are victims of that abusive subculture on a daily basis and are typically powerless to confront or control it.

Sobsey (1994) also describes several strategies for developing safer human service environments for people with disabilities, including sound organizational planning, thoughtful policies and procedures, careful staff recruitment, screening and training of staff, support programmes for staff, and environmental risk management strategies for staff and residents. This latter strategy encompasses the identification of potentially abusive occurrences within the residential facility and providing staff and residents with *in vivo* prevention training to address them. He is highly critical of administrators at residential facilities who make strong and sincere statements against abuse but are unwilling to confront it within their own institutions. In so doing, they take great care to be unaware of the existence of child maltreatment within the facility. Sobsey (1994) maintains that avoiding the discovery of abuse during an extended administrative career is analogous to spending 20 years in the desert without discovering sand: considerable effort is required. Of particular concern are administrators who claim they were unaware that abuse was occurring and who assist in its cover-up when allegations emerge. Antidotes to abusive residential environments include maltreatment prevention programmes for deaf and hard of hearing children and safety features which can be implemented within residential environments.

Existing prevention programmes for deaf and hard of hearing children

The '*No, go, tell*' sexual abuse prevention programme for deaf children was developed and disseminated by the Lexington Center at the Lexington School for the Deaf in New York (Trevelyn, 1988) and has been widely used by residential schools for the deaf as a prevention programme for sexual abuse in the USA and Canada. It was originally developed to provide self-protection training to young deaf and hard-of-hearing children and was extended to third to sixth graders and renamed '*Safe and Okay*'. A programme developed for deaf and hard-of-hearing students in Vancouver, British Columbia identified specific prevention training needs, including additional time for processing information, introduction of a standard vocabulary for discussing maltreatment issues, and the need to implement a variety of instructional media (Anderson, 1987). This programme has been used throughout Canada. In the UK, the Keep Deaf Children Safe (KDCS) programme (Kennedy, 1989) was developed and disseminated. A major weakness of these prevention programmes (developed specifically for deaf and hard-of-hearing children) is that there are no outcome data to evaluate their efficacy and, perhaps even more important, the prevention concepts taught are not derived from risk factors empirically identified through well-controlled epidemiological research.

Child-focused sexual abuse prevention efforts are not a viable method to implement with deaf and hard-of-hearing children because they place the onus of self-protection on the child and do not reflect the complex processes and outcomes inherent in the dynamics of sexual abuse within residential institutions or within the families of these children. Deaf and hard-of-hearing children require prevention programmes with modifications and content based upon both risk and protection factors appropriate for their disability. A child-centred approach is much too simple a solution for the complex problem of sexual maltreatment of deaf and hard-of-hearing children.

Prevention programmes which specifically target families of children with disabilities are predicated on the assumption that the stress of dealing with the child's disability, especially just after identification, increases the risk of maltreatment and that prevention efforts should consist of providing information and support to parents to decrease that risk (Friedrich and Boriskin, 1978; Bax, 1983; Gothad, Runyan and Hadler, 1985; Schirmer, 1986; Garbarino, 1987; Ammerman, Hersen and Lubetsky, 1988). However, other research suggests that the presence of a difficult to manage or disabled child within a family system does not, in itself, increase the risk of maltreatment (Schilling and Schinke, 1984; Adler, 1986; Benedict et al., 1990). Most research and commentary in the area of prevention efforts directed toward the family emphasize that complex interactions and contributions of risk factors must be considered in both content and evaluation of programmes (Kolko, 1988; Daro, Casey and Abrahams, 1990; Wurtele, Kast and Melzer, 1992; National Research Council, 1993). These include poverty, living conditions, substance abuse and the presence of adult role models within the family (Daro, Casey and Abrahams, 1990). The development level of the child with disabilities (Conte, Wolf and Smith, 1989; Miller-Perrin and Wurtele, 1988) and the interactive effects of the individual child and family characteristics (Kolko, 1988; Daro, Casey and Abrahams, 1990; National Research Council, 1993) have also been identified as important factors in prevention programme content and evaluation.

Child maltreatment prevention efforts directed towards various social institutions, including healthcare, judicial, social work and educational professionals, may be the prevention target of choice for children with disabilities. Prevention efforts directed towards training professionals to teach children how to protect themselves are not recommended for children with disabilities (Zirpoli, 1986; Brookhouser, 1987; Wurtele and Miller-Perrin, 1992; Sobsey, 1994). The onus for protection should not be placed upon the individual child. Rather, protection efforts should encompass the total ecological milieu with which the child interacts (National Research Council, 1993; Sobsey, 1994). Accordingly, professionals who have contact with children with disabilities should have training in the signs, symptoms and risk factors associated with maltreatment so that they can protect the children who cannot protect themselves (Nightingale and Walker, 1986; Kolko, 1988; Daro, Casey and Abrahams, 1990; Wurtele and Miller-Perrin, 1992).

Safety recommendations for residential environments

The 1987 article by Brookhouser specifically outlined and discussed risk factors for abuse of deaf children in residential schools, attitudes of staff, standards for out-of-home residential child care, institutional impediments to abuse/neglect reporting, administrative strategies for preventing and detecting maltreatment, and necessary components of health services in residential schools. The standards recommended by Brookhouser (1987) are a compilation of available recommendations based upon the out-of-home child care literature of the day (Whittaker, 1987) and contemporary recommendations for residential programmes for deaf children

(Phillips and Sullivan, 1985; Brookhouser et al., 1986; Sullivan, Vernon and Scanlan, 1987; Whittaker, 1987). These administrative strategies for preventing and detecting maltreatment specifically in residential schools for the deaf included:

1. **Policies and procedures**. Clearly stated policies and procedures regarding building safety, staff pre-employment screening, confidentiality of children's records, children's and families' rights, codes of conduct for staff regarding discipline and sexual conduct with children and youth, and requirements and procedures for reporting suspected maltreatment were recommended.
2. **Staff training**. The importance of staff training was heavily emphasized and defined as being systematic, comprehensive, and on-going to include child maltreatment and institutional abuse issues, stress management and the development of basic life skills for the children in their care. Within this training, staff must demonstrate competence in handling stressful situations with children without resorting to coercion or threats and be assured that consultation and assistance from supervisors will be available to them on an on-going basis. Avoiding a 'shift-mentality' (Phillips and Sullivan, 1985) wherein no one is ultimately responsible for the safety and progress of an individual child because *'I'm only responsible for what happens on my shift'* was strongly recommended.
3. **Direct observation and evaluation of staff performance**. In addition to thorough and on-going staff training, institutional policies should include provisions for on-going unannounced observation of staff by responsible supervisors of line staff who interact with children. Staff compensation, retention, promotion and certification within the system should be based upon satisfactory performance of objective rating criteria, known to staff and supervisors, on child care and work responsibilities.
4. **Open environment**. An open environment policy wherein family, visitors, social workers, inspectors, the media, etc. are given ready access to the facility and prompt responses to inquiries about programmes and practices within the residential school was recommended.
5. **Consumer evaluations: youth and general.** The consumers of the 'product' of residential youth care are: the youth in residence; their families; referral agencies; significant others associated with the youth (i.e. teachers, healthcare providers, therapists, coaches, etc.), and society in general. Information from these consumers should be gathered on a regular basis to garner their impressions of the quality of the programme to provide important additional information for improving the programme, to establish a line of communication for positive and negative feedback about staff practices and policies and

procedures, and to detect questionable practices. The children and youth themselves should also be queried about their impressions of the quality of care being provided for them.

6. **Youth abuse questions**. An exceptionally effective antidote to child maltreatment in institutions is an audit system in which the residents are specifically asked a series of questions dealing with abuse on a timely and regular basis by a non-employee of the school. This procedure was thoroughly explained (Brookhouser, 1987; Sullivan, Vernon and Scanlan, 1987) and specific questions were listed: (a) Has a staff member ever forced you to do anything that you did not want to do, touched your private body parts or asked you to take drugs? (b) Has any staff member ever threatened you or told you not to talk to a supervisor? (c) Have any other children hit you, threatened you, touched your private body parts or told you not to tell a supervisor?
7. **Staff practice inquiry process**. Institutional policies and procedures should provide for prompt and thorough internal and external investigations of allegations of abuse of children and youth in residence. Particular emphasis is placed upon having a structured procedure to be followed given allegations of abuse, and that the investigation be completed by both internal and external agents.
8. **External ethical review**. A programme ethics committee comprising parents, alumni, professionals and community representatives, should be established with regular meeting times. Some members should not have special knowledge or expertise in deafness-related issues. There is probably no better antidote to institutional abuse of children and youth than the presence of volunteers and concerned citizens asking 'naïve' questions about policies and procedures influencing the daily lives of children and youth.

Daly and Dowd (1992) extensively described the group care practice model implemented at Father Flanagan's Boys' Home. This model has applications for use within residential placements for deaf and hard-of-hearing children and youth. There are specific elements in residential child care programmes which foster effective and harm-free out-of-home care. These elements are predicated upon an underlying model or theme of care that is clearly visible and understood, which guides child care workers in their interactions with children and adolescents in care. The recommended caregiver to child ratio is 1:4 and individual living units or family homes should not exceed 10 children (Daly and Dowd, 1992). The key components of the child care model which seem to foster a harm-free residential environment are a focus on positive behaviour of the children and youth in care and extensive caregiver support, which includes adequate relief time, good on-going in-service training, and responsive and consistent supervision.

Conclusions

Residential schools are an integral component in the education of many deaf and hard-of-hearing children. For many of them, this is the only viable and appropriate educational placement, given their unique socio-cultural needs and the characteristics of their linguistic community. Residential schools for the deaf are the crucible of Deaf culture in which membership is defined by knowledge of sign language and Deaf cultural norms. American Sign Language (ASL) or BSL is acquired in young children primarily from the Deaf community within residential settings (Kyle and Pullen, 1988). Given that 90% of deaf children have hearing parents, the acculturation of deaf children into the Deaf community and culture tends to occur in residential schools. Thus, Deaf culture is transmitted from child to child in many cases, rather than from adult to child (Moores, 1987) and residential schools are the milieu in which this transmission occurs (Dolnick, 1993).

Unfortunately, maltreatment of Deaf and hard-of-hearing children is a risk factor that parents and caregivers must consider along with the positive cultural and linguistic benefits of residential placements. Accordingly, exceptional care and vigilance must be exercised to ensure the safety of Deaf and hard-of-hearing children in residential placements. This chapter has identified the maltreatment characteristics and dynamics of abuse within residential settings for Deaf and hard-of-hearing children. It has also described methods, policies and procedures for ensuring the safety of Deaf children in residential settings and provided a model protocol for interviewing Deaf and hard-of-hearing children and adults who are suspected victims of child maltreatment. However, with professional cognizance of these maltreatment risk factors and appropriate preventive procedures in place, residential schools can be safe placements for Deaf and hard-of-hearing children.

Therapeutic methods

In establishing a therapeutic programme for deaf and hard-of-hearing victims of sexual abuse at the Center for Abused Children with Disabilities, the available literature on therapeutic intervention with children was reviewed. Because psychotherapy research is largely silent on therapy with children with disabilities, knowledge of childhood deafness was applied to develop a sexual abuse therapy programme which delineated specific treatment goals and therapeutic methods to be used to assist the deaf and hard-of-hearing child in meeting these goals.

Therapeutic techniques

The specific therapeutic techniques used with sexually abused children with hearing impairments are eclectic in nature and thereby consistent with the current trends in child psychotherapy. Cognitive/behavioural techniques are very applicable to children who are deaf or hard-of-hearing. However, insight techniques are generally limited to those children and youth with sufficient affective vocabulary and language reasoning skills to benefit from them.

A structured set of psychotherapy goals has been established (Sullivan and Scanlan, 1987, 1990; Sullivan, 1993) and is implemented with the children at a level commensurate with their overall developmental status. Accordingly, children's cognitive, linguistic, psychosexual and emotional development are taken into consideration. These goals are both didactic and therapeutic in nature. Children who are deaf or hard-of-hearing are often not provided with basic human sexuality information. Therefore, human sexuality, sexual abuse issues, sexual preference issues, sexually transmitted diseases, dating skills and interpersonal relationships are emphasized with adolescent deaf and hard-of-hearing youth. Particular emphasis is placed on 'date rape' given its high incidence among college students who are deaf and hard-of-hearing in the USA. Younger children are taught body parts and social interaction skills with other children, both hearing and hearing-impaired. Self-protection skills are also addressed. Other goals include alleviating the guilt engendered by the sexual abuse, assisting children to regain the ability to trust peers and adults, helping them to express anger relating to the sexual abuse in appropriate and productive ways, and treating the secondary behavioural characteristics many children exhibit as a direct result of the abuse (i.e. aggression, withdrawal, somatic complaints, unrealistic fears and sexualized behaviour).

Communication issues

Therapists providing treatment to sexually abused deaf and hard-of-hearing children and youth must make sure the language used in therapy is appropriate for them. Communication abilities and preferences present distinct challenges to the therapist working with children and youth with hearing impairments. They are a heterogeneous group with a wide variety of linguistic and cognitive abilities, and communication skills are strongly influenced by environment and experiences — and particularly by the communication skills of family members with the deaf or hard of hearing child (Sullivan, 1995).

Therapists must take into consideration the client's specific communication abilities and preferred modalities (Sobsey, Mansell and Sullivan, 1995). To this end, the therapist must accept the client's communication abilities and understand the corresponding practical therapy implications. In particular, the therapist needs to know how the client with a hearing impairment typically communicates. Are there specific circumstances or contexts that affect the person's ability to communicate? Does this ability to communicate change in strange and unfamiliar environments or when the person is feeling angry, upset, depressed, withdrawn or anxious? How expressive is the client and how large are the client's receptive and expressive vocabularies? Does the client have other differences or challenges, such as vision and motor impairments, which may affect communication? Does the client use augmentative or alternative communication devices? Does the client typically use an interpreter? Does the client have consistent access to an interpreter whom he trusts and with whom he feels comfortable? What issues may using an interpreter in the therapy setting present? And, perhaps most critically, which sign language system is the client's preferred modality and how fluent is he within that particular system? Kennedy (1992) has an excellent review of communication systems with children with communication differences, which includes children who are deaf or hard-of-hearing. She provides an overview of available communication methods to use with deaf and hard-of-hearing children in assessment and therapeutic settings.

Deaf adolescents prefer counsellors fluent in sign language to those who use an interpreter or write notes to communicate (Freeman and Conoley, 1986; Haley and Dowd, 1988). The therapist should be well-versed in the use of sign language and communication alternatives which the deaf or hard-of-hearing child or adolescent typically uses in communicative discourse.

Family issues

Deaf and hard-of-hearing children are frequently victims of abuse and neglect perpetrated by family members. In these cases, therapeutic efforts need to be directed to the entire family. All too frequently, family members and other professionals want the child treated alone, sometimes within a residential setting, and returned to the family or school after treatment is completed. The current trends towards 'wrap-around' services, wherein the child receives treatment within an ecological context that involves both individuals and agencies with whom the child has frequent contact, is very applicable and appropriate for deaf and hard-of-hearing children and their families. This type of intervention is both therapeutic and didactic and requires that the family therapist participates within and co-ordinates community-based individualized services in pertinent life domains of both child and family.

Individualized services are based upon therapeutic needs and not a particular categorical intervention model. Life domains include areas of basic human needs that everyone experiences, including residential, family, social (friends and contact with other people), educational, vocational, medical, psychological/emotional, legal, safety, and cultural and ethnic needs.

A deaf or hard-of-hearing victim of neglect may require interventions across all of those life domains that involve medical evaluation of the neglect, and parent informational counselling and assistance regarding the educational, vocational, psychological/emotional, safety and cultural needs of children with hearing impairment. Victims of physical abuse will need parent training, anger control, behaviour modification and conflict resolution skills incorporated in the individualized therapy, with access to support systems for assistance in their respective life domains. Victims of sexual abuse require intensive intervention at the individual, family and ecological life domain levels to assist in reducing risk factors for sexual victimization to improve the outcomes of victims of sexual abuse, and to enhance compensatory and protective factors for children which may mitigate or buffer the deaf or hard-of-hearing child from the effects of sexual victimization.

Outcome research

The effectiveness of these therapeutic methods has been assessed in two separate studies with children referred to the Center for Abused Children with Disabilities for treatment because of sexual abuse.

The first study (Sullivan et al., 1992) was an outcome study using a sample of 72 sexually abused Deaf children and youth from a single residential school. An extensive police investigation had identified a large cohort of children and youth sexually abused within the residential school. An untreated comparison group emerged when about half of the parents of these children refused the offer of psychotherapy from the school. The sexual abuse investigation was highly publicized and many parents and school employees adamantly denied its occurrence and were therefore unsupportive toward the provision of therapy. Similar patterns of denial in school settings have been reported involving parents who refuse to believe their children's allegations of abuse (Summit and Kryso, 1978; Finkelhor et al., 1988). This untreated group of sexually abused Deaf children and youth were used as a control group for the study. Treated and untreated children were randomly assigned to pre- and post-test groups. Both groups evidenced high rates of behaviour problems prior to the initiation of therapy for the treatment group. Mean T-scores on the *Total Problems Scale of the Child Behaviour Checklist* (CBC) were above 70 for both the treatment and no-treatment groups. Among the girls, there were no significant differences between the treatment and no-treatment groups on the pre-test. Although boys tended to be more aggressive in the no-treatment group, the treatment group had significantly more behaviour problems. Children and youth receiving therapy had significantly lower scores on the CBC one year post-therapy than children not receiving therapy. There was a differential response to therapy on the basis of gender. Boys had significantly lower scores on the following CBC scales: Total, Internal, External, Somatic, Uncommunicative, Immature, Hostile, Delinquent, Aggressive and Hyperactive. There were no differences on the Schizoid and Obsessive scales. Girls receiving therapy had significantly lower scores on: Total, External, Depressed, Aggressive and Cruel. There were no differences on the Internal, Anxious, Schizoid, Immature, Somatic and Delinquent scales. These behaviours may be more resistive to intervention in deaf girls than boys.

The comparison no-treatment group was not a true random sample. However, it is most difficult to obtain such a comparison group given ethical constraints and the urgency of intervention for child sexual abuse victims. This type of comparison group, which naturally emerged because of parental refusal of treatment, might possibly be employed in future treatment outcome studies. Taking advantage of this fortuitous control group and completing any outcome study with a clinical sample is consistent with current trends in treatment outcome research (Peterson and Bell-Dolan, 1995). Innovative work utilizing new treatments with difficult populations is strongly encouraged in order to complete urgently needed clinical research. A cost–benefit analysis of methodological issues that can feasibly be addressed is suggested to create quality clinical research which may otherwise be discouraged by rigid methodological standards which may not yield clinically relevant results.

The Center has just completed gathering data on another psychotherapy outcome study with a wider range of children with disabilities who were victims of sexual abuse. In addition to children with hearing impairments, the subjects also included children with speech and language difficulties, learning disabilities, visual impairments, cleft lip and palate, health impairments and attention deficit disorder.

Initial data analyses, which combined children across age groups and treatment conditions, have been completed to assess an overall effect of therapy on some of the outcome measures. Such comparisons of pre-treatment and post-treatment scores indicate that statistically significant improvements were reported on several measures that have theoretical and practical importance. Based on systematic assessments of reports of deviant behaviour in the home (parental daily report), significant declines in the children's total behaviour problem score ($p < 0.05$) and the Children's Anxiety Questionnaire ($p < 0.025$) were obtained. Perhaps most importantly, the children evidenced significant change in several areas assessed with Wurtele's 'Index of Sexual Knowledge: Personal Safety and Prevention Skills'. All of these measures are completed by research assistants independent of the therapists and are administered individually to both parent and child. Thus, these preliminary data indicate that the therapies are having a positive influence on the behaviours of the treated children and are reducing their vulnerability to repeated sexual exploitation.

Conclusions

Deaf and hard-of-hearing children and youth are at increased risk of becoming victims of maltreatment, including neglect, physical abuse and sexual abuse (Sullivan and Knutson, 1998b). The primary perpetrators of the neglect and physical abuse are parents and other family members. They contribute to about half of the sexual abuse, with extrafamilial perpetrators (including care attendants, babysitters, van drivers, peers, older students, friends of siblings, clergy, teachers and houseparents) accounting for a significant portion of sexual abuse.

Deaf and hard-of-hearing children and youth and their families require psychotherapists with clinical competence and training in the psychology of deafness. In order to meet the need for therapeutic services, more accessible treatment programmes need to be developed. Psychotherapists with training and expertise in working with hearing children and their families cannot assume that they can also effectively serve children who are deaf or hard of hearing. As more treatment programmes for sexually abused deaf and hard-of-hearing children appear, the necessity of standards for service providers and certification will become more apparent.

In the interim, consumers of mental health services have a right to be informed of the competence and skill level of the providers of assessment and interventions to children and youth who are deaf and hard-of-hearing. In particular, they have a right to evaluate the communication skills of the prospective therapist and make a decision regarding their abilities to communicate with one another. A common error made by therapists unfamiliar with the psychodynamics of deafness is to become too controlling and didactic in the therapeutic process. Accordingly, providers need to implement therapeutic techniques which capitalize on clients' individual strengths and abilities and thereby empower them to resolve the trauma of the abuse and gain the courage and confidence to prevent future abusive experiences.

Macbeth: *Canst thou not minister to a mind diseased, pluck from the memory a rooted sorrow, raze out the troubles of the brain, and with some sweet oblivious antidote cleanse the stuffed bosom of that perilous stuff which weighs upon the heart?*

Doctor: *Therein the patient must minister to himself.*

(William Shakespeare)

References

Adler R (1986) Physical maltreatment of children. Australian and New Zealand Journal of Psychiatry 20: 404–412.

American Humane Association (1988) Highlights of Official Child Neglect and Abuse Reporting, 1986. Denver, CO: American Humane Association.

Ammerman RT (1991) The role of the child in physical abuse: a reappraisal. Violence and Victims 6: 87–101.

Ammerman RT, Hersen M, Lubetsky MJ (1988) Assessment and treatment of abuse and neglect in multihandicapped children and adolescents. International Journal of Rehabilitation 11: 313–314.

Ammerman RT, Van Hasselt VB, Hersen M (1988) Maltreatment of handicapped children: a critical review. Journal of Family Violence 3: 53–72.

Anderson J (1987) Educating deaf children about sexual abuse and their safety. Child Sexual Abuse Newsletter 13: 335–343.

Bax M (1983) Child abuse and cerebral palsy (editorial). Developmental Medicine and Child Neurology 25(2): 141–142.

Benedict M, White R, Wulff L, Hall B (1990) Reported maltreatment in children with multiple disabilities. Child Abuse and Neglect 14: 207–217.

Blatt B, Kaplan F (1966) Christmas in Purgatory: A Photographic Essay on Mental Retardation. Boston, MA: Allyn and Bacon.

Brookhouser PE (1987) Ensuring the safety of deaf children in residential schools. Otolaryngology–Head and Neck Surgery 97: 361–368.

Brookhouser PE, Sullivan PM, Scanlan JM, Garbarino J (1986) Identifying the sexually abused deaf child: the Otolaryngologist's role. Laryngoscope 96: 152–158.

Chase NF (1976) A Child is Being Beaten: Violence Against Children, An American Tragedy. New York: McGraw-Hill.

Cole L (1972) Our Children's Keepers: Inside America's Kid Prisons. New York: Grossman Publishers.

Conte JR, Wolf S, Smith T (1989) What sexual offenders tell us about prevention strategies. Child Abuse and Neglect 13: 293–301.

Corrigan JP (1982) Prevention and appropriate handling of maltreatment of children in residential facilities. In Washburne C, Hull JV, Rindfleisch N (eds) Multiregional Conference on Institutional Child Abuse and Neglect. Columbus, OH: Ohio State University School of Social Work, pp 1–14.

Daly DL, Dowd TP (1992) Characteristics of effective, harm-free environments for children in out-of-home care. Child Welfare 71: 487–496.

Daro D, Casey K, Abrahams N (1990) Reducing child abuse 20% by 1990: preliminary assessment. National Committee for Prevention of Child Abuse Working Paper, Number 843.

Docherty J (1989) Potential Abuse Indicators and Guidelines for Their Investigation. Unpublished manuscript.

Dolnick E (1993) Deafness and its culture. The Atlantic Monthly, September, 37–53.

Finkelhor D, Williams LM, Burns N, Kalinowski M (1988) Sexual abuse in daycare: a national study. Executive Study. University of New Hampshire: Family Research Laboratory.

Freeman ST, Conoley CW (1986) Training, experience and similarity as factors of influence in preferences of deaf students for counselors. Journal of Counseling Psychology 33: 164–169.

Friedrich WN, Boriskin JA (1978) Primary prevention of child abuse: focus on the special child. Hospital and Community Psychiatry 29: 248–256.

Frodi AM (1981) Contributions of infant characteristics to child abuse. American Journal of Mental Deficiency 85(4): 342–349.

Garbarino J (1987) What can the school do on behalf of the psychologically maltreated child and the community. School Psychology Review 16: 181–187.

Garbarino J, Authier KH (1987) The role of educators. In Garbarino J, Brookhouser PE, Authier KJ (eds) Special Children–Special Risks: The Maltreatment of Children with Disabilities. New York: Aldine de Gruyter, pp 69–82.

Garbarino J, Brookhouser PE, Authier KJ (1987) Special Children – Special risks: The Maltreatment of Children with Disabilities. New York: Aldine de Gruyter.

Gil E (1979) Handbook for Understanding and Preventing Abuse and Neglect of Children in Out-of-Home Care. San Francisco, CA: Child Abuse Council.

Gil E (1982) Institutional abuse of children in out-of-home care. In Hanson R (ed) Institutional Abuse of Children and Youth. New York: Haworth Press, pp 7–14.

Gothard TW, Runyan DK, Hadler JL (1985) The diagnosis and evaluation of child maltreatment. Journal of Emergency Medicine 3: 181–194.

Haley TJ, Dowd ET (1988) Response of deaf adolescents to differences in counselor method of communication and disability status. Journal of Counseling Psychology 35: 258–262.

Hanson R (ed) (1982) Institutional Abuse of Children and Youth. New York: Haworth Press.

Harrell SA, Orem RC (1980) Preventing Child Abuse and Neglect: A Guide for Staff in Residential Institutions. (Kirschner Associates, Inc., eds) Washington, DC: US Government Printing Office (Dept. 76).

Jaudes PK, Diamond LD (1985) The handicapped child and child abuse. Child Abuse and Neglect 9: 341–347.

Kennedy M (1989) The abuse of deaf children. Child Abuse Review Spr: 3–7.

Kennedy M (1990) The deaf child who is abused: is there a need for a dual specialist? Child Abuse Review 4: 3–6.

Kennedy M (1992) The case for interpreters – exploring communication with children who are deaf. Child Abuse Review 1: 191–193.

Knutson JF (1988) Physical abuse and sexual abuse of children. In Routh DK (ed) Handbook of Pediatric Psychology. New York: Guilford Press, pp 32–70.

Knutson JF, Schartz HA (1994) Evidence pertaining to physical abuse and neglect of children as parent–child relational diagnoses. In Widiger TA, Frances AJ, Pincus HA (eds) DSM-IV Sourcebook. Washington, DC: American Psychiatric Association.

Knutson JF, Sullivan PM (1993) Communicative disorders as a risk factor in abuse. Topics in Language Disorder 13: 1–14.

Kolko DJ (1988) Educational programs to promote awareness and prevention of child sexual victimization: a review and methodological critique. Clinical Psychology Review 8: 195–209.

Kyle JG, Pullen G (1988) Cultures in contact: Deaf and hearing people. Disability, Handicap and Society 3: 49–61.

McCall RB, Gregory TC (1987) Mass media issues. In Garbarino J, Brookhouser PE, Authier KJ (eds) Special Children – Special Risks: The Maltreatment of Children with Disabilities. New York: Aldine de Gruyter, pp. 211–230.

Melton GB (1987) Special legal problems in protection of handicapped children from parental maltreatment. In Garbarino J, Brookhouser PE, Authier KJ (eds) Special Children – Special Risks: The Maltreatment of Children with Disabilities. New York: Aldine de Gruyter, pp 179–193.

Miller-Perrin CL, Wurtele SK (1988) The child sexual abuse prevention movement: a critical analysis of primary and secondary approaches. Clinical Psychology Review 8: 313–329.

Moores DF (1987) Educating the Deaf: Psychology, Principles and Practices. Boston, MA: Houghton Mifflin.

Morgan SR (1987) Abuse and Neglect of Handicapped Children. Boston, MA: Little, Brown and Co.

National Research Council (1993) Understanding Child Abuse and Neglect, first edition. Washington, DC: National Academy Press.

Nebraska Department of Education (1992). Rule 51: regulations and standards for special education programs, 1–84.

Nightingale NN, Walker EF (1986) Identification and reporting of child maltreatment by Head Start personnel: attitudes and experiences. Child Abuse and Neglect: the International Journal 10: 191–199.

Oswin M (1979) The neglect of children in long-stay hospitals. Child Abuse and Neglect 3: 89–92.

Peterson L, Bell-Dolan D (1995) Treatment outcome research in child psychology: realistic coping with the 'Ten Commandments of Methodology'. Journal of Clinical Child Psychology 24: 149–162.

Phillips EL, Sullivan PM (1985) The Boys Town Teaching Family Model: Applications to residential programs for hearing impaired children and youth. In Anderson GB, Watson D (eds) The Habilitation and Rehabilitation of Deaf Adolescents. Little Rock, Arkansas: University of Arkansas Rehabilitation Research and Training Center on Deafness and Hearing Impairment, pp 286–303.

Porter S, Yuille JC, Bent A (1994) A comparison of the eyewitness accounts of deaf and hearing children. Child Abuse and Neglect 19: 51–61.

Rindfleisch NA (1984) Identification, Management and Prevention of Child Abuse and

Neglect in Residential Facilities. Columbus, OH: Ohio State University Research Foundation.
Rindfleisch N, Baros-Van Hill J (1982) Direct care worker's attitudes toward use of physical force with children. In Hanson R (ed) Institutional Abuse of Children and Youth. New York, Haworth Press, pp 115–125.
Rivera G (1972) Willowbrook: A Report on How It Is and Why It Doesn't Have to Be That Way. New York: Vintage Books.
Rutter M (1989) Intergenerational continuities and discontinuities in serious parenting difficulties. In Cichetti D, Carlson V (eds) Child Maltreatment: Theory and Research on the Causes and Consequences of Child Abuse and Neglect. Cambridge: Cambridge University Press, pp 317–348.
Sangrund A, Gaines RW, Green AH (1974) Child abuse and mental retardation. A problem of cause and effect. American Journal of Mental Deficiency 7 : 327–330.
Saywitz K, Geiselman RE, Bornstein G (1992) Effects of cognitive interviewing and practice on children's recall performance. Journal of Applied Psychology 77: 744–756.
Schilling RF, Schinke SP (1984) Maltreatment and mental retardation. In Bern JM (ed) Perspectives and Progress in Mental Retardation 1. Baltimore: University Park Press, pp 11–20.
Schilling RF, Kirkham MD, Schinke SP (1986) Do child correction services neglect developmentally disabled children? Education and Training of the Mentally Retarded 21: 21–26.
Schinke SP, Blythe BB, Schilling RF, Barth R (1981) Neglect of mentally retarded persons. Education and Training of the Mentally Retarded 16: 299–303.
Schirmer BR (1986) Child Abuse and Neglect: Prevalence, Programs and Prevention with the Hearing Impaired. Paper presented at the 70th Annual Meting of the American Educational Research Association, San Francisco, CA (ERIC Document Reproduction Service No. ED 270-954), April.
Schlesinger H, Meadow K (1972) Sound and Sign: Child Deafness and Mental Health. Berkeley, CA: University of California Press.
Schultz GL (1981) Sexual contact between staff and residents. In Shore DA, Gochros HL (eds) Sexual Problems of Adolescents in Institutions. Springfield, IL: Charles C Thomas, pp 90–103.
Shore DA (1982) Sexual abuse and sexual education in child care institutions. In Conte JR, Shore DA (eds) Social Work and Child Sexual Abuse. New York: Haworth Press, pp 171–184.
Siskind AB (1986) Issues in institutional child sexual abuse: the abused, the abuser, and the system. Residential Treatment for Children and Youth 4: 9–30.
Sobsey D (1994) Violence and Abuse in the Lives of People with Disabilities: The End of Silent Acceptance. Baltimore, MD: Paul H. Brookes.
Sobsey D, Doe T (1991) Patterns of sexual abuse and assault. Journal of Sexuality and Disability 9: 243–259.
Sobsey D, Varnhagen C (1988) Sexual Abuse, Assault, and Exploitation of People With Disabilities. Ottawa, Ontario: Health and Welfare Canada.
Sobsey D, Mansel S, Sullivan PM (1995) Therapy Accommodations for Sexually Abused People with Developmental Disabilities. Poster session presented at the annual meeting of the American Psychological Association. New York, NY: August.
Solomons F, Abel CM, Epley SA (1981) Community development approach to the prevention of institutional and societal child maltreatment. Child Abuse and Neglect 5: 135–140.
Solomons G (1979) Child abuse and developmental disabilities. Developmental Medicine and Child Neurology 21: 101–105.
Starr RH, Dietrich KN, Fischoff J, Ceresnie F, Zweier D (1984) Contribution of handicapping conditions to child abuse. Topics of Early Childhood Special Education 4: 55–69.
Sullivan PM (1993) Sexual abuse therapy for special children. Journal of Child Sexual Abuse 2: 117–125.
Sullivan PM (1995) Assessment and Treatment Issues with Maltreated Children with

Disabilities. Paper at the annual meeting of the American Psychological Association. New York, NY: August.

Sullivan PM, Knutson JF (1998a) Maltreatment and behavioral characteristics of youth who are deaf and hard of hearing. Sexuality and Disability 16(4): 295–319.

Sullivan PM, Knutson JF (1998b) The association between child maltreatment and disabilities in a hospital based epidemiological study. Child Abuse and Neglect 22(4): 271–288.

Sullivan PM, Scanlan JM (1987) Therapeutic issues. In Garbarino, J, Brookhouser PE, Authier KJ (eds) Special Children – Special Risks: The Maltreatment of Children with Disabilities. New York: Aldine de Gruyter, pp 127–159.

Sullivan PM, Scanlan JM (1990) Psychotherapy with handicapped sexually abused children. Developmental Disabilities Bulletin 18: 21–34.

Sullivan PM, Scanlan JM, Knutson JF, Brookhouser PE, Schulte LE (1992) The effects of psychotherapy on behavior problems of sexually abused deaf children. Journal of Child Abuse and Neglect 16: 297–307.

Sullivan PM, Vernon M, Scanlan J (1987) Sexual abuse of deaf youth. American Annals of the Deaf: 132(4): 256–262.

Sullivan PM, Brookhouser PE, Scanlan JM, Knutson JF, Schulte LE (1991) Patterns of physical and sexual abuse of communicatively handicapped childen. Annals of Otology, Rhinology and Laryngology 200: 188–194.

Summit R, Kryso J (1978) Sexual abuse of children: a clinical spectrum. American Journal of Orthopsychiatry 48: 237–251.

Taylor RB (1981) Discarded children. In Taylor RB (ed) The Kid Business: How it Exploits the Children it Should Help. Boston, MA: Houghton Mifflin, pp 38–66.

Taylor RB, Bogdan R (1980) Defending illusions: The institution's struggle or survival. Human Organization 39: 209–218.

Tilelli JA, Turek D, Jaffe AC (1980) Sexual abuse of children: clinical findings and implications for management. New England Journal of Medicine 302: 319–323.

Trevelyn J (1988) When it's difficult to say no. Nursing Times 84: 16–17.

Turk V, Brown H (1992) Sexual Abuse of Adults with Learning Disabilities. Paper presented at the Conference of the International Association for Scientific Study of Mental Deficiency Conference, Brisbane (August 5–7).

Westat Inc. (1993) A Report on the Maltreatment of Children with Disabilities. Washington, DC: National Center on Child Abuse and Neglect.

Westcott H (1991) The abuse of disabled children: a review of the literature. Child Care, Health and Development 17: 243–258.

Wexler DB (1982) Seclusion and restraint: lessons from psychiatry and psychology. International Journal of Law and Psychiatry 5: 185–294.

Whittaker JK, Trieschman AE (eds) (1972) Children Away from Home: A Sourcebook of Residential Treatment. Hawthorne, NY: Aldine de Gruyter.

Whittaker JK (1987) The role of residential institutions. In Garbarino J, Brookhouser PE, Authier KJ (eds) Special Children – Special Risks: Maltreatment of Children with Disabilities. New York: Aldine de Gruyter, pp 83–100.

Willging JP, Bower CM, Cotton RT (1992) Physical abuse of children: a retrospective review and an otolaryngology perspective. Archives of Otolaryngology – Head and Neck Surgery 118: 584–590.

Wurtele SK, Miller-Perrin CL (1992) Preventing Child Sexual Abuse: Sharing the Responsibility. Lincoln: University of Nebraska Press.

Wurtele SK, Kast LC, Melzer AM (1992) Sexual abuse prevention education for young children: a comparison of teachers and parents as instructors. Child Abuse and Neglect 16: 865–876.

Yuille J (1988) The systematic assessment of children's testimony. Canadian Psychology 29: 247–262.

Zirpoli TJ (1986) Child abuse and children with handicaps. Remedial and Special Education (RASE) 7: 39–48.

Chapter 8
Psychological Assessments

LYNN BLENNERHASSETT

> An unlearned carpenter of my acquaintance once said in my hearing: 'There is very little difference between one man and another; but what little there is, is very important.' This distinction seems to me to go to the root of the matter.
>
> (William James, 1842–1910)

Introduction

In what ways is a given individual like all others? In what ways is that individual like members of only certain subgroups? And in what ways is that individual unique among all others? Questions posed by early functional psychologists paved the way for differential psychology and the subsequent development of mental tests — norm-referenced tests that enabled assessment of an individual's unique and shared abilities. Individual psychological assessment was rooted in intelligence testing of schoolchildren (Binet and Simon, 1905). Assessments now are carried out in a variety of settings — educational, medical, legal or clinic-based — and form part of a broader multidisciplinary approach. Psychological assessment is a comprehensive process using a variety of techniques, evaluating multiple areas of functioning and serving a variety of purposes (Table 8.1).

Professional ethics guide assessment practices and examiner qualifications (American Psychological Association, 1985, 1986, 1992; National Association of School Psychologists, 1992).

Although these professional codes of conduct do not address services to the deaf specifically, adherence to them is required with any client population. What follows is a discussion of assessment practices with the deaf, including assessment of intelligence, achievement, personality and social-emotional functioning. The reliability and validity of various

Table 8.1 Assessment components

Techniques	Areas of functioning	Purposes
Case history	Intelligence	Screening
Observation	Social–emotional	Diagnostic
Interview	Personality	Prescriptive
Standardized tests	Adaptive behaviour	Rehabilitative
Informal testing	Vocational aptitude	Progress evaluation
	Achievement	

techniques are examined, along with issues related to qualification of examiners. The discussion will be organized around ethical principles of psychologists, the professional codes of conduct that guide assessment practices for all clients, hearing or deaf.

Qualifications of psychologists to deaf people

Among the many competencies outlined in professional codes of conduct are four that appear particularly relevant for psychologists who conduct assessments of deaf clients.

Recognizing the strengths and limitations in one's training and experience

Awareness of one's personal or professional limitations is key to ensuring competent, professional delivery of service to deaf clients. Limitations may be based on training, experience, or personal differences such as language and culture.

In 1982, the Council on Education of the Deaf adopted and approved for distribution *Standards for the Certification of Specialized Professional Personnel in the Education of the Hearing Impaired*. Training and communication competencies for psychologists working with hearing-impaired students included:

- Academic preparation (master's degree or higher from an NCATE or APA accredited psychology programme or department of psychology in an accredited university).
- Satisfaction of existing state certification/licensure requirements for the practice of psychology.
- Communication competency, defined as the ability 'to communicate with deaf individuals and have competency in use of both oral and manual communication skills'. (Standard 10, p. 6)

The first two areas acknowledge that psychologists to deaf people should first meet all existing standards put forth by their professional organizations and accreditation bodies. As Edna Levine (1981) once quoted a deaf colleague: 'The deaf deserve no less!' (p. 228). Yet Levine's (1974) classic survey of psychologists to deaf people found that of the 93% who held postgraduate degrees, only 10% were doctorates. Spragins, Karchmer and Schieldroth (1981) found only a slightly higher percentage of doctorates (16.3%) among the school psychologists they surveyed, with 79.5% credentialled at the master's, master's-plus, or dual-master's level.

The third area, communication competency, addresses linguistic requirements unique to those who would provide psychological services to deaf people. Improvement in sign language skills is an acknowledged need within the profession (Gibbins, 1989). Research suggests that sign communication competency has improved somewhat since Levine (1974) first reported that 50% of practitioners could not understand or communicate with their deaf clients. For example, McQuaid and Alovisetti (1981) found that two-thirds of the school psychologists in their sample had some sign communication training. And Spragins, Karchmer and Schieldroth (1981) found increased sign communication competency among psychologists who work full-time with deaf people. Still, standards for communication competency are needed to guide psychological services to deaf people.

The Council on Education of the Deaf recommends a minimum of two courses in sign communication (excepting deaf graduates of colleges or universities using *Total Communication*). But even at universities using sign communication, deaf and hearing trainees need to evaluate their competency (Table 8.2), respecting that some deaf clients will require a psychologist fluent in American Sign Language (ASL), others in sign-supported speech, still others in auditory–oral or cued speech.

The National Association of State Directors of Special Education (NASDSE) also endorsed communication competency in their recent issuance of standards for school psychologists who serve deaf students. Their recommendations included — but were not limited to — the requirement that school psychologists be competent in 'communicating with deaf and hard-of-hearing students in their primary language or preferred communication mode or using an interpreter or transliterator according to the student's communication mode' (Roed and Sass-Lehrer, in press).

But communication competence alone is not sufficient to assure appropriate psychological service to deaf people. Broader cultural awareness is required. NASDSE requires that psychologists understand the sociological and psychological aspects of deafness, the linguistic and cultural factors related to deafness, and the implications of such factors,

Table 8.2 Communication policy, Gallaudet University School Psychology Programme

It is the ethical responsibility of school psychologists to:

- Recognize that effective communication between child and psychologist is of the highest priority.
- Recognize the diversity of languages and communication modes used by deaf, hard-of-hearing and hearing children.
- Evaluate their own communication skills and the communication needs of each child with whom they work.
- Develop self-understanding and acceptance of the fact that, given the diversity of languages and communication modes used by deaf and hard-of-hearing children, not all psychologists will have the communication skills to work with every deaf, hard-of-hearing or hearing child.

Source: Gallaudet University School Psychology Handbook (1994–1995), p. 46.

particularly upon assessments. Similarly, Levine proposed knowledge-imperatives for psychologists to deaf people (Table 8.3). Ethics dictate that psychologists acquire the requisite knowledge-imperatives and communication competencies to serve deaf clients.

Using only those techniques that are within one's area of training or expertise

Sattler's (1992) multiple assessment approach describes four techniques used by psychologists when evaluating clients: norm referenced testing, informal testing, observations, and interviews. Although psychologists are trained in all, each poses additional challenges when applied to deaf people.

In norm-referenced testing, standardized tests are used to obtain a score that compares the client's performance to that of some normative group. Intelligence tests, for example, are norm-referenced techniques used to assess whether a client's performance is 'average' (or above, or below) compared to established norms. If the norms were established using a non-representative sample then the risk of discriminatory assessment increases. The use of norm-referenced tests with deaf clients is problematic because most commercially available tests do not include deaf subjects within their normative sample. Psychologists need specialized training in selecting, administering and interpreting norm-referenced tests with deaf clients. Even with informal testing techniques, special training is required, especially when psychologists attempt to develop test items or pursue questioning. Knowledge of linguistic and cultural aspects of deafness is necessary to ensure non-discriminatory assessment.

Interview techniques present special challenges related to communication and rapport (Table 8.4). Levine (1981), reporting on the Spartanburg Conference (the national conference on The Preparation of Psychological Service Providers to the Deaf), reiterated that psychologists must be able 'to express and receive messages in whatever communicative modes and concept levels are habitually used by deaf subjects' (p. 226). Until such skills are obtained, the use of interpreters is not ruled out, but caution is advised.

Table 8.3 Levine's knowledge-imperatives for psychologists to the deaf

- To 'know' the deaf in terms of heterogeneity, culture, community and persons.
- To know the impact of deafness on family and child.
- To know the diverse educational practices to which the deaf are exposed, for these represent major influences in their fashioning, adjustments and problems.
- To know the educational reform movements and their rationale, because educational reforms represent the best preventive mental health moves undertaken on behalf of the deaf.
- Above all, to know … how to 'think deaf' and 'talk deaf' when such is required.

Source: Levine (1981) pp. 226–227.

Table 8.4 Potential problems in the psychologist–client relationship arising from use of interpreters during the assessment process

Rapport issues

- possible inhibiting effect of conveying confidential, sensitive or evaluative information through a third party
- use of interpreters introduces possible dependency issues, which may encourage feelings of resentment, guilt, etc.

Interaction issues

- use of interpreters results in decreased eye-contact between the psychologist and client, which may inhibit conversational exchanges or turn-taking between the psychologist and client
- interpreted messages risk loss of information conveyed non-verbally by the psychologist (e.g. through natural gestures, facial expressions, body axis and posture, etc.) which may distort messages between psychologist and client
- altering the timing or pace of the interaction to facilitate interpreter services may result in distorted, edited or abbreviated communication between psychologist and client
- seating requirements for interpreters may interfere with presentation of test materials, standardized instructions and item demonstration
- inappropriate light sources (e.g. light from behind the interpreter, psychologist or client) may interfere with receiving visual messages

Translation issues

- assessment protocol typically requires standardized instructions; interpreted or transliterated messages may introduce semantic, syntactic, or morphological variations which alter meaning within the psychologist's text
- assessment protocol requires verbatim transcriptions of client responses; interpreted or transliterated messages may introduce semantic, syntactic or morphological differences which alter meaning within the client's response
- some features of sign (e.g. directionality, handshape, etc.) may inadvertently reveal answers to test questions or clues not conveyed in spoken text

Rapport may suffer significantly if the art and skill of sign interpretation is not fully understood. Furthermore, the client's trust and confidence in the psychologist may be jeopardized if interpreted communication is used.

Consulting with or referring to appropriate specialists

Interpreters are not the only deafness specialists with whom psychologists might consult. Ethical practice requires that psychologists seek whatever consultation, supervision or referral is needed to serve their client. The consultative/referral network might include audiologists, medical/health providers, speech and language specialists, deaf educators/vocational personnel, community support systems, advocacy groups and the like. (See Cherow, Matkin and Trybus (1985) for a comprehensive listing of resources.) Psychologists have an ethical responsibility to recognize, respect and utilize appropriate resources in providing assessment services to deaf clients.

A multidisciplinary model of assessment, or what Cherow (1985) termed interactive interdisciplinary teaming, provides a holistic frame within which psychological assessments occur. Interdisciplinary teaming helps to bridge the gap between initial referral and subsequent treatment (or intervention) plans. Even highly trained psychologists may have difficulty diagnosing and treating dysfunctional behaviour within the context of deafness. This is especially true for psychologists who work in isolation, relying upon a single-discipline perspective. The ethics of consulting and referring to appropriate specialists not only protect the welfare of the client but serve also to protect the psychologist from error and burnout.

Seeking additional training, experience or supervision

Ethics require that psychologists continually seek additional training, experience and supervision to improve service to their clients. Indeed, research shows that psychologists to deaf people acknowledge their need for additional training in assessment, sign communication, delivery of psychological services, and knowledge about deafness and the needs of deaf people (Levine, 1974; McQuaid and Alovisetti, 1981; Spragins, Karchmer and Schieldroth, 1981; Gibbins, 1989). Since few specialized training programmes exist*, practitioners often rely on regional conferences, national meetings, and summer courses or workshops to meet their continuing education needs (Gibbins, 1989).

Specific assessment practices with deaf people

Psychological assessment and psychological testing are not synonymous. Testing is only one part of a comprehensive assessment process. The process is guided by ethical principles and codes of conduct, three of which pose significant challenges for psychologists to deaf people. Each is discussed below.

Multiple sources of data are needed to provide a comprehensive, valid picture of the client. Ethics require that psychological tests not be used as the sole basis of assessment. Although standardized tests provide important information about an individual's functioning and ability levels, Kaufman (1990) reminds us that 'the focus of the assessment is the Person being assessed, not the test' (p. 24) and that 'the goal of any examiner is to be better than the tests he or she uses' (p. 25). Towards this goal, psychologists practise both the 'art' and 'science' of assessment. That is, the assessment process has both subjective and objective components. Matarazzo (1990) describes the psychologist as:

*Gallaudet University offers training for school psychologists (Master's plus Specialist level) and clinical psychologists (Doctoral level). The Rochester Institute of Technology has a school psychology and deafness programme for practising school psychologists seeking additional training.

> ... an artisan familiar with the accumulated findings of his or her young science, who each instance uses tests, techniques, and a strategy that, whereas also identifying possible deficits, maximizes the chances of discovering each client's full ability and true potential (p. 1000).

The art of psychological assessment requires the ability to integrate case history, interviews, observations and test results, all in an effort to derive the most comprehensive, valid picture of the individual.

Case history, interviews and observation techniques with deaf people

There are few guides for conducting case histories, interviews, or observations of deaf clients. For case histories, Levine's (1981) *Inventory Guide for Case History Information on Deaf Children and Adults* provides the most comprehensive system of integrating information (Table 8.5). Although some of the information may be obtained from files or tests, most is gathered informally by interview or observation. Again, it should be stressed that conducting interviews with deaf clients requires considerable communication competence and knowledge about deafness, particularly about cultural differences in interpersonal communication. Skill is

Table 8.5 Categories in Levine's case history guide for deaf clients

Category	Exemplary inclusions
Identifying data	name, birthdate, ethnic/religious affiliation, history of family deafness, onset of deafness
Developmental history	pre-natal and birth events, developmental milestones
Family background	family line, size, home language, socio-economic and cultural background, physical/health background
Medical/health status	chronology of physical and mental dysfunctions, history of treatments, medications, reactions
Auditory history	degree/configuration of hearing loss, age diagnosed, aided measures and auditory training, speech and language training, intrafamily reactions
Educational background	infancy/pre-school programme, chronology of education programmes, scholastic achievement, educational goals
Psychosocial profile	childhood reaction patterns, parent and sibling relationships, recreational interests and activities
Vocational	interests, aptitude, training, goals, adjustment
Social participation	clubs, interests, friendship circles, social roles
Self-concept	attitudes towards deafness, deaf culture, hearing society, self-assessment of assets and liabilities

Source: Levine (1981).

required of both the psychologist and client when communicating across languages (English or ASL) and when using various modes of communication (speech, speechreading, signs, written language) (Stewart, 1981; Stokoe and Battison, 1981).

Three deafness-specific scales may prove useful in conducting structured or unstructured interviews. The Bronfenbrenner Hearing Attitude Scale (Levine, 1981) elicits the client's response to loss of hearing. This scale is made up of 100 items with which the client 'agrees' or 'disagrees'. Because it was developed for hard-of-hearing adults, some items may be inappropriate for profoundly deaf clients. Meadow-Orlans' Impact of Childhood Hearing Loss on the Family Questionnaire is a 24-item questionnaire for parents designed to assess the family's reaction to having a deaf child. Parents are asked questions that cluster into three scales: Stress, Communication and Professionals. In addition to revealing parental attitudes, each scale may be scored to reflect the degree to which the family is adjusting. Interviews with teachers might be guided by the Meadow–Kendall Social–Emotional Assessment Inventory for Deaf and Hearing Impaired Students. In addition to revealing teacher perceptions of students' social adjustment, scores are derived which assess the child's self-concept and emotional adjustment compared to other deaf children.

Psychological tests used with deaf people

A list of psychological tests most frequently used with deaf people can be compiled from surveys conducted over the past 20 years (Table 8.6). Unfortunately, most of these tests were not developed specifically for use with deaf people. Braden (1994) provides a comprehensive review of the assessment of intelligence in deaf people. Inappropriate items and over-reliance on verbal language necessitate significant modifications in administration, scoring, and interpretation when used with deaf people (Spragins, Blennerhassett and Mullen, 1993).

Practitioners frequently select only performance-based or non-verbal sections of psychological tests when assessing deaf clients. Although this is a reasonable strategy when faced with the need to eliminate bias due to verbal items, it is problematic for a number of reasons (Gibbins, 1992). Firstly, many 'performance-based' tests are assumed incorrectly to be 'non-verbal', when actually they require extensive English instructions. For instance, the *Wechsler Performance Scales* appear non-verbal because client responses are 'performance-based' (pointing, arranging cards and blocks, etc.); however, the instructions are heavily verbal and clients with limited receptive language may not completely understand the tasks. Secondly, the alternative use of test items presented in print (e.g. *MMPI-II, Piers–Harris Children's Self-Concept Scale*) may well exceed the client's reading ability. Thirdly, any altering or elimination of items is a violation of

Table 8.6 Psychological tests most frequency used with the deaf

Tests of intelligence/cognitive functioning
- Wechsler Performance Scales (WISC–R, WAIS–R, WISC–III)
- KABC Non-verbal Scale
- CID Preschool Performance Scale
- Hiskey–Nebraska Test of Learning Aptitude
- Raven's Progressive Matrices
- Leiter International Performance Scale
- Columbia Mental Maturity Scale

Social–emotional/personality measures
- Meadow–Kendall Social–Emotional Assessment Inventory for Deaf and Hearing Impaired Students
- Projective drawings
- Piers–Harris Children's Self-concept Scale
- Bender Gestalt Test
- School Behavior Checklist
- Thematic Apperception Test
- Children's Apperception Test
- Walker Problem Behavior Checklist
- Tennessee Self-Concept Scale
- Minnesota Multiphasic Personality Inventory — II
- Rorschach

Achievement
- Stanford Achievement Test — Hearing Impaired
- Peabody Individual Achievement Test
- Test of Early Reading Ability — Deaf or Hard of Hearing
- Woodcock Reading Mastery Tests
- Woodcock–Johnson Psychoeducational Battery
- Wide Range Achievement Test — Revised
- Keymath
- Sequential Assessment of Mathematics Inventories
- California Achievement Test
- Brigance Diagnostic Inventory of Basic Skills
- KABC Achievement Tests

Adaptive behaviour
- Vineland Adaptive Behavior Scale
- AAMD Adaptive Behavior Scale
- Scales of Independent Behavior
- Vineland Social Maturity Scale

Sources: Levine, 1974; Gibbins, 1989; McQuaid and Alovisetto, 1981; Spragins, Blennerhassett and Mullen, 1993.

that test's standardization. Scores obtained under non-standard administration may not be reliable or valid.

Psychological tests must be reliable and valid for the purpose for which they are used

Ethics require that psychological tests meet standards of reliability and validity. Test manuals provide data supporting the reliability and validity of their tests. These data are derived from research conducted on the standardization (or norm) sample during test development. Since most psychological tests were not standardized using deaf subjects, their reliable and valid use with this client population is open to question. What follows is a discussion of the reliability and validity of psychological tests most frequently used with deaf people, including tests that have been standardized on deaf people and those that have not.

Tests standardized for use with deaf people

Of the 35 psychological tests listed in Table 8.6, only seven were standardized for use with deaf people. Three are tests of intelligence, three are emotional–behavioural scales, and one provides measures of academic achievement. What follows is a discussion of the reliability and validity of these, and other, tests standardized for use with deaf people.

Tests of intelligence/cognitive functioning

Few non-verbal cognitive tests were developed specifically for deaf people. One such instrument, the *Hiskey–Nebraska Test of Learning Aptitude*, was standardized on a sample of 1077 deaf residential school students between the ages of 2;6 and 17;5. From 12 subtests, a median mental age and a learning quotient (derived by ratio IQ formula) is obtained for deaf children. The manual reports strong split-half reliability (r = 0.947) and concurrent validity (r = 0.89). However, criterion-related validity was found to vary as a function of grade: the learning quotient predicts reading achievement at lower grades (2nd, 3rd, and 4th) and upper grades (9th–12th), but not at 5th and 8th grade levels.

The *Snijders–Oomen Non-verbal Intelligence Scale* (SON) provides two levels of assessment, one standardized on Dutch deaf children between the ages of 2;6 and 7;0, the other extending upward to 17 years of age. Although not cited as one of the tests most frequently used, the SON has been reviewed favourably for its reliability (r = 0.91–0.93) in the assessment of deaf children (Detterman, 1985; Keith, 1985). English translations of both levels are available.

Specific to preschool assessment, the *Central Institute for the Deaf (CID) Preschool Performance Scale*, was standardized on a sample of 521 hearing-impaired children between the ages of 2;0 and 5;6. The manual reports moderate test–retest reliability (r = 0.71) and concurrent validity (r = 0.485). The *Smith–Johnson Non-verbal Performance Scale* also was developed specifically for use with deaf pre-school children, although it does not rank among the tests used most frequently. Its lack of popularity may be due to questionable reliability (r = 0.27–0.81) and to the limited age range assessed (2- to 4-years).

The popular *WISC-R Performance Scale*, although not developed specifically for deaf people, has been the focus of subsequent standardization procedures (Anderson and Sisco, 1977; Ray, 1979). Scores derived from over 1200 residential deaf students provide norms for comparing a student's performance against that of same-age deaf peers. Students between the ages of 6 and 16 are covered by the WISC-R deaf norms. Deaf norms are not available for the upper age scale, the WAIS-R, nor are they available for the revised WISC-III.

Tests of social–emotional and adaptive behaviour

In the area of social–emotional assessment, the *Meadow–Kendall Social–Emotional Assessment Inventory for Deaf and Hearing Impaired Students* provides both school-age and pre-school scales. The school-age scales were standardized on a sample of approximately 2000 students in residential and day programmes for deaf children. The manual reports adequate interscorer reliability (r = 0.58–0.93) and concurrent validity (r = 0.54–0.70). The preschool scales were standardized on a sample of 857 hearing-impaired students between the ages of 2;0 and 5;6. Variable interrater reliability (r = 0.75–0.95) and validity (r = 0.34–0.70) coefficients were reported within the scales. The only other social/adaptive measure with deaf norms is found in the expanded form of the *Vineland Adaptive Behavior Scales*. Although deaf subjects were not included among the 3000 individuals in the original standardization sample, 300 deaf residential students became part of a supplemental norm project. The manual reports appropriate split-half reliability (r = 0.84–0.97) and moderate criterion-related validity (r = 0.47) of these adaptive behaviour scales for the deaf sample.

Achievement tests

The *Stanford Achievement Test — 8th Edition* (SAT-8) provides the most extensive standardization of achievement tests for deaf students. This battery contains group-administered tests of reading, spelling, mathematics, science, and social studies, available in eight difficulty levels. The SAT-8 used with deaf students includes the same items and questions that are administered to hearing students, but special screening tests in reading and mathematics are used to determine which of the eight difficulty levels should be administered. The screening tests and special norms for deaf students (e.g. percentile rankings by age, grade equivalent score, score distributions at each age level) are available through the Center for Assessment and Demographic Studies (CADS, 1989, 1991). A guide is also available for interpreting the performance of deaf students (Holt, Traxler and Allen, 1992).

For an individually administered assessment of reading achievement, the *Test of Early Reading Ability — Deaf or Hard of Hearing* recently became available. Standardized on a sample of 1146 hearing-impaired students, this test measures knowledge of the alphabet and its functions, awareness of the conventions of print, and ability to construct meaning from print. Adequate test–retest reliability (r = 0.90) and criterion-related validity (r = 0.77–0.78) were reported in the manual.

Statistical properties of other tests used with deaf people

Because most of the tests listed in Table 8.6 have not been standardized on deaf people, their manuals do not include statistical data for this population. Therefore, psychologists depend upon subsequently published studies to determine the validity of each test for use with deaf clients. Criterion-related validity studies fall into two categories: *concurrent (or diagnostic) validity* (i.e. the degree to which scores on one test correlate with scores on other tests that purport to measure the same ability) and *predictive (or prognostic) validity* (i.e. the degree to which scores on one test, such as IQ, correlate with scores on other tests that measure a different but relevant criterion, such as achievement). What follows is a review of criterion-related validity studies of psychological tests used with deaf people.

Tests of intelligence/cognitive functioning

Table 8.7 presents a summary of concurrent validity studies of cognitive tests used with deaf people. As evidenced, concurrent validity has been established for the use of several non-verbal intelligence tests, including the Wechsler Performance Scales, KABC Non-verbal Scale, *Hiskey–Nebraska Test of Learning Aptitude*, *Raven's Progressive Matrices* and the Leiter International Performance Scale. (Interested readers are referred to Braden (1992, 1994) for a synthesis on research related to intellectual assessment of deaf people.)

Studies of predictive validity using achievement tests with deaf people reveal a less consistent picture. This is illustrated by research summarized in Table 8.8. Scores on the Stanford Achievement Test have been found to correlate with IQ scores derived from the Wechsler Performance Scales, KABC Non-verbal Scale, and Hiskey–Nebraska Test of Learning Aptitude. Similarly, WRAT-R Spelling, KABC Reading, and MAT Reading scores of deaf students correlated with non-verbal intelligence. But predictive validity involving the Woodcock Reading Mastery Test and WRAT-R Reading achievement was not consistently established.

The Wechsler Verbal Scales present an interesting dilemma for psychologists to deaf people. Best practice recommends that the Verbal Scales be omitted when assessing intelligence of deaf people. This is because low Verbal Scale IQ may be due to linguistic delays or differences rather than intellectual delays (Vernon and Brown, 1964; Vernon, 1968). Indeed, research supports the lack of concurrent validity between the Verbal and Performance scales with this population. Deaf subjects with average or

Table 8.7 Concurrent validity studies: cognitive tests used with the deaf

Study	Non-verbal or performance measures	r
Blennerhassett, Gibbins and Kachman (1994)	WISC-III PIQ and WISC-R PIQ (deaf norms)	0.90**
	WISC-III PIQ and WISC-R PIQ (hearing norms)	0.90**
Porter and Kirby (1986)	WISC-R PIQ and KABC Non-verbal (pantomime/gesture administration)	0.675**
	WISC-R PIQ and KABC Non-verbal (ASL administration)	0.635**
Ulissi, Brice and Gibbins (1989)	WISC-R PIQ and KABC Sequential	0.670**
	WISC-R PIQ and KABC Simultaneous	0.845**
	WISC-R PIQ and KABC Non-verbal	0.859**
Phelps and Branyan (1988)	WISC-R PIQ and HNTLA	0.661**
	WISC-R PIQ and KABC Non-verbal	0.729**
	WISC-R PIQ and LIPS	0.739**
Phelps and Branyan (1990)	WISC-R PIQ and KABC Non-verbal	0.731**
Ulissi and Gibbins (1984)	WISC-R PIQ and LIPS	0.822*
Paal, Skinner and Reddig (1988)	WAIS-R PIQ and HNTLA	0.75*
Blennerhassett, Strohmeier and Hibbett (1994)	RPM and WISC-R PIQ (deaf norms)	0.598**
	RPM and WISC-R PIQ (hearing norms)	0.616**
Spragins (1991)	CID PIQ and Battelle	–0.02

*p <0.01
**p <0.001.
Adapted from Blennerhassett, Strohmeier and Hibbett (1994).

above-average performance IQs score significantly lower on verbal IQ measures (Goetzinger et al., 1966; Hine, 1970; Geers and Moog, 1989; Moores and Sweet, 1990; Rush et al., 1991; Maller and Braden, 1993).

Although the Wechsler Verbal Scales are not recommended as a measure of 'intelligence' for deaf clients, their related use in assessment of deaf people warrants attention. Gibbins (1989) found that 60% of psychologists to deaf people sometimes use these Verbal Scales for ' ... purposes other than assessing cognitive ability' (p. 98). And as a measure of 'verbal comprehension and expression', the criterion-related validity of the Verbal Scales with deaf students has been investigated. Moores and Sweet (1990) found strong, positive correlations between WAIS-R Verbal Scale scores and literacy measures (r = 0.62–0.70 for both reading and writing achievement). This was true for deaf students of deaf parents as well as deaf students of hearing parents. In a parallel study of auditory–oral deaf adolescents, Geers and Moog (1989) confirmed the criterion-related validity of WAIS-R Verbal Scale scores in predicting literacy skills. More

Table 8.8 Predictive validity studies: cognitive and achievement measures with the deaf

Study	Cognitive test	Achievement measure	r
Maller and Braden (1993)	WISC-III PIQ	SAT-HI Reading	0.46*
	WISC-III PIQ	SAT-HI Language	0.54*
	WISC-III PIQ	SAT-HI Math	0.63*
Blennerhassett, Gibbins and Kachman (1994)	WISC-III PIQ	SAT-HI Reading Comprehension	0.77**
	WISC-III PIQ	SAT-HI Language	0.82**
	WISC-III PIQ	SAT-HI Math	0.83**
Kelly and Braden (1990)	WISC-R PIQ	SAT-HI Reading Comprehension	0.32**
	WISC-R PIQ	SAT-HI Spelling	0.24**
Ulissi, Brice and Gibbins (1989)	WISC-R PIQ	SAT-HI Combined Reading	0.588**
	KABC Non-verbal	SAT-HI Combined Reading	0.706**
Paal, Skinner and Reddig (1988)	WAIS-R PIQ	SAT-HI Reading Comprehension	0.73*
	HNTLA	SAT-HI Reading Comprehension	0.53*
Phelps and Branyan (1990)	WISC-R PIQ	WRAT-R Reading	0.317
	WISC-R PIQ	WRAT-R Spelling	0.494**
	WISC-R PIQ	KABC Reading/Decoding	0.652**
	WISC-R PIQ	KABC Reading/Understanding	0.593**
	KABC Non-verbal	WRAT-R Reading	0.513**
	KABC Non-verbal	WRAT-R Spelling	0.517**
	KABC Non-verbal	KABC Reading/Decoding	0.647**
	KABC Non-verbal	KABC Reading/Understanding	0.570**
Porter and Kirby (1986)	KABC Non-verbal	MAT Reading Comprehension (pantomime/gesture administration)	0.539*
	KABC Non-verbal	MAT Reading Comprehension (ASL administration)	0.463*
Watson et al. (1986)	WISC-R/WAIS-R PIQ	Woodcock Reading Mastery (Grade Level)	0.12–0.53

*p <0.01
**p <0.001
Adapted from Blennerhassett, Strohmeier and Hibbett (1994).

recently, Maller and Braden (1993) found WISC-III Verbal IQ to be highly correlated with SAT-HI total reading (0.80), total language (0.85), and total math (0.83). In all three studies, Wechsler Verbal Scale scores of deaf students were found to be better predictors of achievement than were Performance Scale scores.

Slate and Fawcett (1995) retrospectively reviewed the educational assessments of 47 deaf and hard-of-hearing children who used either spoken language only or Total Communication. The mean age of the children at their initial assessment, using the WISC-R, was 9;9, and 12;9 at their second assessment using the WISC-III. Forty-three of the children underwent both assessments.

Performance IQ on the WISC-R was significantly correlated with Performance IQ on the WISC-III. However, the mean Performance IQ on the WISC-III (88.0) was three points lower than the mean Performance IQ using the WISC-R (91.0). Performance IQ on the WISC-III correlated moderately with the three WRAT-R subscales (Reading, Spelling and Arithmetic), most significantly with the Arithmetic subscale. Slate and Fawcett (1995) undertook a factor analysis of the Performance subtests. This factor analysis provided partial support for the notion of two main factors with the Performance subscale, Perceptual Organization and Processing Speed. Interestingly, the mean Performance IQ of children using Total Communication was 10 points higher than the Performance IQ of children using spoken language only.

Social–emotional, personality and adaptive measures

The reliability and criterion-related validity of social–emotional and adaptive measures is less well-established. Although support has been documented for the ***Meadow–Kendall Social–Emotional Assessment Inventory*** (Bransky, 1990; Kluwin, Blennerhassett and Sweet, 1990) and the ***Vineland Adaptive Behavior Scale*** (Altepeter, Moscato and Cummings, 1985; Bransky, 1990), other measures have been reviewed less favourably. For instance, the ***Bender Gestalt Test for Young Children*** was found to yield a number of false positive emotional indicators for deaf children, even though the mental maturity score appeared to be a valid developmental index (Johnston, 1975). And although the concurrent validity of human figure drawings was supported by Johnson (1989) and Cates (1991), predictive validity was not confirmed.

Deaf adaptations of personality measures have met with difficulties related to reliability, validity and administration (Gibbins, 1992). For instance, a deaf adaptation of the ***Tennessee Self-Concept Scale*** was attempted, but found to be only moderately reliable, and no validity data were provided (Gibson-Harman and Austin, 1985). Deaf norms were attempted for Form E of the ***Sixteen Personality Factor Questionnaire***, but reliability data were very low (Trybus, 1973; Jensema, 1975, 1976). An ASL videotape version of Form E was also initiated, but a strong relationship was not found between videotape and pencil–paper forms (Dwyer and Wincenciak, 1977). Despite these weaknesses, Bannowsky (1983) supports the use of Form E in vocational rehabilitation assessment with deaf clients. An ASL videotape version of the *Minnesota Multiphasic Personality Inventory* (MMPI) is now available in the *Brauer Gallaudet MMPI-168* (Brauer, 1989), but Riley-Glassman (1989) found that, like its written English version, it over-identified control subjects as 'disturbed'.

The use of projective techniques is even more difficult as these require considerable communication fluency on the part of both psychologist and client. The *Rorschach* is recommended only for deaf clients with above-average intellectual and communicative abilities (Vernon and Brown, 1964) and only with psychologists fluent in the client's mode of communication (Sachs, 1976; Schwartz, 1989). But the problematic nature of scoring ASL signs on English-based protocols remains unresolved. Currently, Gibbins (personal communication, March 16, 1994) is investigating inter-rater reliability of *Rorschach* scores when client responses are transliterated from ASL to English by use of Exner's Comprehensive System of Rorschach scoring (Exner, 1986). In a companion study, Santistevan (personal communication, March 16, 1994) is researching the effect of using direct ASL responses upon the Exner system of *Rorschach* scoring.

Ethical practice requires that psychologists recognize and report whenever adjustments in test administration violate procedures established during test standardization. They must also recognize and report whenever the reliability or validity of instruments is lacking, suspect or altered. These codes of conduct are critically important when assessing special populations. The 'state of the art' in assessment of deaf people is such that psychologists may find themselves lacking appropriate tests of intelligence, social–emotional, adaptive or educational achievement for deaf clients. Psychologists may be forced to use or adapt tests of unestablished reliability and validity with deaf people, and to derive scores based on inappropriate norms. Under such conditions, psychologists have an ethical responsibility to report any and all reservations about the tests used, the scores obtained, and the interpretation of findings.

Psychologists refrain from using outdated or obsolete tests and techniques

Ethics dictate that psychologists refrain from using tests or test data that are outdated or obsolete. This standard poses a special challenge to psychologists to deaf people, since many of the tests standardized for deaf people are now decades old and contain out-of-date norms upon which scores are derived. For instance, deaf norms on the *Hiskey–Nebraska Test of Learning Aptitude* were established nearly 30 years ago and norms for the *Leiter International Performance Scale* date back to 1948. The *CID Preschool Performance Scale*, although published in 1983, contains normative data that were derived 20 years prior to publication. And norms for the *Smith–Johnson Non-verbal Performance Scale*, gathered back in 1960, render it obsolete as well.

Even the (relatively) recent WISC-R Performance Scale, upon which deaf norms and deafness-based research were subsequently compiled, is now rendered obsolete by the revised WISC-III Performance Scale. Practitioners are well advised to use the updated edition — even though deaf norms have yet to be established for the WISC-III — for at least three reasons. Firstly, most of the WISC-III revisions occurred within the Performance Scale, the scale typically used with deaf people. As a result, most of the differences in scores between the WISC-R and WISC-III appear within the Performance Scale. Using the old WISC-R may inflate IQ by about 5 points (Wechsler, 1991; Weiss, 1991). Secondly, the revised WISC-III Performance Scale includes a new subtest and new factor index, Processing Speed, which represents a significant change in measurement not enabled by the former WISC-R. Finally, the deaf norms (Anderson and Sisco, 1977) to which psychologists would refer when defending use of the old WISC-R, may not be all that appropriate for most deaf students. Not only are those norms now nearly 20 years old, but they were derived solely from students in residential and day schools for deaf people. Current demographic data indicate that most deaf students now are educated in mainstream settings rather than residential or day schools (Allen and Karchmer, 1990).

Ethical, responsible, assessment practice is not always easy with special populations, especially when advances in test development exceed the deafness research base upon which psychologists depend. Psychologists to deaf people, like all psychologists, must make use of the most recently developed professional tools while pursuing research on their most effective application with deaf clients.

Closing comments

In this chapter, the psychological assessment of deaf people was examined within the context of ethical standards and codes of conduct that guide all psychologists in the art and science of assessment. The discussion focused on ethics related to the competency of psychologists who wish to work with deaf people, particularly the communication competencies and knowledge-imperatives related to deafness. Ethical standards for conducting multifactored, research-based assessments were also discussed, with particular attention to reliability and validity of psychological tests most frequently used with deaf people. As with all clients, psychologists to deaf people practise the art and science of assessment with these goals in mind: to discover the unique and shared abilities of their client, to interpret these within the social-cultural context relevant to that client, and to enable recommendations supportive of the client's growth across all psychological domains.

References

Allen TE, Karchmer MA (1990) Communication in classrooms for deaf students: student, teacher, and program characteristics. In Bornstein H (ed) Manual Communication: Implications for Education. Washington, DC: Gallaudet University Press, pp 45–66.

Altepeter T, Moscato E, Cummings J (1985) Comparison of scores of hearing-impaired children on the Vineland Adaptive Behavior Scale and the Vineland Social maturity Scale. Psychological Reports 59: 535–639.

American Psychological Association (1985) Standards for Educational and Psychological Tests. Washington, DC: APA.

American Psychological Association (1986) Guidelines for Computer-Based Test Interpretations. Washington, DC: APA.

American Psychological Association (1992). Ethical Principles of Psychologists and Code of Conduct. Washington, DC: APA.

Anderson RJ, Sisco FH (1977) Standardization of the WISC-R Performance Scale for Deaf Children. Washington, DC: Gallaudet University Center for Assessment and Demographic Studies.

Bannowsky A (1983) Issues in assessing vocationally relevant personality factors of prelingually deaf adults utilizing the 16PF-E. Journal of Rehabilitation of the Deaf 17: 21–24.

Binet A, Simon H (1905) New methods for the diagnosis of the intellectual level of subnormals. L'annêe Psychologique 11: 191–244.

Blennerhassett L, Gibbins S, Kachman W (1994) Criterion related validity of the WISC-III for deaf residential students. Unpublished raw data.

Blennerhassett L, Strohmeier SJ, Hibbett C (1994) Criterion-related validity of Ravens' Progressive Matrices. American Annals of the Deaf 139: 104–110.

Braden JP (1992) Intellectual assessment of deaf and hard of hearing people: a quantitative and qualitative research synthesis. School Psychology Review 21: 82–94.

Braden JP (1994) Deafness, Deprivation and IQ. London and New York: Plenum Press.

Bransky B (1990) The discriminative validity of selected instruments in identifying well-adjusted and poorly adjusted hearing-impaired students. Doctoral dissertation, University of Kansas, Lawrence.

Brauer B (1989) A translation of the MMPI into sign language for use with deaf individuals: an assessment of translation accuracy. Unpublished manuscript, Gallaudet University, Washington, DC.

Cates J (1991) Comparison of human figure drawings by hearing and hearing-impaired children. Volta Review 93: 31–39.

Center for Assessment and Demographic Studies (1989) Administering the 8th Edition Stanford Achievement Test to Hearing Impaired Students. Washington, DC: Gallaudet Research Institute.

Center for Assessment and Demographic Studies (1991) Stanford Achievement Test 8th Edition Form J: Hearing impaired norms booklet. Washington, DC: Gallaudet Research Institute.

Cherow E (1985) Through the looking glass. In Cherow E, Matkin N, Trybus R (eds) Hearing Impaired Children and Youth with Developmental Disabilities: An Interdisciplinary Foundation for Service. Washington, DC: Gallaudet University Press, pp 3–15.

Cherow E, Matkin N, Trybus R (eds) (1985) Hearing Impaired Children and Youth with Developmental Disabilities: An Interdisciplinary Foundation for Service.

Washington, DC: Gallaudet University Press.

Council on Education of the Deaf (1982) Standards for the Certification of Specialized Professional Personnel in the Education of the Hearing Impaired. Tucson, AZ: CED.

Detterman DK (1985) Review of Snijders–Ooman Non-verbal Intelligence Scale for Young Children. In Mitchell JV, Jr (ed) The Ninth Mental Measurements Yearbook. University of Nebraska Press, pp 1406–1407

Dwyer C, Wincenciak S (1977) A pilot investigation of three factors of the 16PF-Form E comparing the standard written form with an Ameslan videotape revision. Journal of Rehabilitation of the Deaf 10: 17–23.

Exner J (1986) The Rorschach, A Comprehensive System. Volume 1: Basic Foundations (second edition). New York: John Wiley.

Gallaudet University School Psychology Handbook (1994) Communication Policy. Washington, DC: Gallaudet University.

Geers A, Moog J (1989) Factors predictive of the development of literacy in profoundly hearing-impaired adolescents. Volta Review 91: 69–86.

Gibbins S (1989) The provision of school psychological assessment services for the hearing-impaired. Volta Review 91: 95–103.

Gibbins S (1992) Personality assessment of deaf children: the dismal state of the art. Paper presented at the National Association of School Psychologists. Nashville, Tennessee, March.

Gibson-Harman K, Austin G (1985) A revised form of the Tennessee Self-Concept Scale for use with deaf and hard of hearing persons. American Annals of the Deaf 130: 218–225.

Goetzinger EP, Ortiz JD, Bellerose B, Buchan LG (1966) A study of the SO Rorschach with deaf and hearing adolescents. American Annals of the Deaf 111: 510–522.

Hine WD (1970) The abilities of partially hearing children. British Journal of Educational Psychology 40: 171–178.

Holt JA, Traxler CB, Allen TE (1992). Interpreting the Scores: a User's Guide to the 8th Edition Stanford Achievement Test for Educators of Deaf and Hard of Hearing Students. Washington, DC: Gallaudet University Center for Demographic Studies.

Jensema C (1975) Reliability of the 16PF Form E for hearing impaired college students. Journal of Rehabilitation of the Deaf 8: 14–28.

Jensema C (1976) A statistical investigation of the 16PF, Form E as applied to hearing impaired college students. Journal of Rehabilitation of the Deaf 9: 21–29.

Johnson G (1989) Emotional indicators in the human figure drawings of hearing-impaired children: a small sample validation study. American Annals of the Deaf 134: 205–208.

Johnston K (1975) The relationship between emotional indicator scores on the Bender Gestalt Test and teacher ratings on a behavior scale with young hearing impaired children. Doctoral dissertation, University of Utah.

Kaufman AS (1990) Assessing adolescent and adult intelligence. Boston, MA: Allyn & Bacon.

Keith TZ (1985) Review of Snijders–Oomen Non-verbal Intelligence Scale for Young Children. In Mitchell JV, Jr (ed) The Ninth Mental Measurements Yearbook. University of Nebraska Press, pp 1407–1408.

Kelly MD, Braden JP (1990) Criterion-related validity of the WISC-R Performance Scale with the Stanford Achievement Test–Hearing Impaired Edition. Journal of School Psychology 28: 147–151.

Kluwin T, Blennerhassett L, Sweet C (1990) The revision of an instrument to measure the capacity of hearing-impaired adolescents to cope. Volta Review 92: 283–291.

Levine ES (1974) Psychological tests and practices with the deaf: a survey of the state of the art. Volta Review 76: 298–319.

Levine ES (1981) The Psychology of Early Deafness. New York: Columbia University Press.

McQuaid MF, Alovisetti M (1981) School psychological services for hearing-impaired children in the New York and New England Area. American Annals of the Deaf 126: 37–42.

Maller SJ, Braden JP (1993) The construct and criterion related validity of the WISC-III with deaf adolescents. Journal of Psychoeducational Assessment, WISC-III Monograph, 105–113.

Matarazzo J (1990) Psychological assessment versus psychological testing: validation from Binet to the school, clinic, and courtroom. American Psychologist 45: 999–1017.

Moores, DF, Sweet, C (1990) Factors predictive of school achievement. In Moores D, Meadow-Orlans K (eds) Educational and Developmental Aspects of Deafness. Washington, DC: Gallaudet University Press, pp 154–201.

National Association of School Psychologists (1992) Professional Conduct Manual Silver Spring, MA: NASP Publications.

Paal N, Skinner S, Reddig C (1988) The relationship of nonverbal intelligence measures to academic achievement among deaf adolescents. Journal of Rehabilitation of the Deaf 21: 8–11.

Phelps L, Branyan BJ (1988) Correlations among the Hiskey, K-ABC Nonverbal Scale, Leiter, and WISC-R Performance Scale with public school deaf children. Journal of Psychoeducational Assessment 6: 354–358.

Phelps L, Branyan BJ (1990) Academic achievement and nonverbal intelligence in public school hearing-impaired children. Psychology in the Schools 27: 210–217.

Porter LJ, Kirby EA (1986) Effects of two instructional sets on the validity of the Kaufman Assessment Battery for Children-Nonverbal Scale with a group of severely hearing impaired children. Psychology in the Schools 23: 37–43.

Ray S (1979) An Adaptation of the WISC-R for the Deaf. Northridge, CA: Steven Ray Publications.

Riley-Glassman N (1989) Discriminating clinic from control groups of deaf adults using a short form of the Minnesota Multiphasic Personality Inventory. Doctoral dissertation. Tucson, AZ: University of Arizona.

Roed K, Sass-Lehrer (in press) Deaf Education Initiative: Program Guidelines for Students who are Deaf or Hard of Hearing. Alexandria, VA: National Association of State Directors of Special Education.

Rush P, Blennerhassett L, Epstein K, Alexander D (1991) WAIS-R Verbal and Performance profiles of deaf adolescents referred for atypical learning styles. In Martin D (ed) Advances in Cognition, Education, and Deafness. Washington, DC: Gallaudet University Press, pp 82–87.

Sachs B (1976) Some views of a deaf Rorschacher on the personality of deaf individuals. Hearing Rehabilitation Quarterly 2: 13–14.

Sattler JM (1992) Assessment of Children. (Revised and updated third edition.) San Diego, CA: Jerome M Sattler.

Schwartz N (1989) Effects of alternate modes of administration on Rorschach performance of deaf adults. Doctoral dissertation Fuller Theological Seminary, School of Psychology.

Slate JR, Fawcett J (1995) Validity of the WISC-III for Deaf and Hard of Hearing Persons. American Annals of the Deaf 140: 250–254.

Spragins AB (1991) Preschool Deaf Children: Cognitive Assessment with the CID and Battelle. Paper presented at the National Association of School Psychologists Dallas, TX: March.

Spragins AB, Blennerhassett L, Mullen Y (1993) Review of Five Types of Assessment Instruments used with Deaf and Hard of Hearing Students. Washington DC: Gallaudet University.

Spragins AB, Karchmer M, Schieldroth AN (1981) Profile of psychological service providers to hearing-impaired students. American Annals of the Deaf 126: 94–105.

Stewart LG (1981) Counseling the deaf client In Stein LK, Mindel ED, Jabaley T (eds) Deafness and Mental Health. New York: Grune & Stratton, pp 133–159.

Stokoe WC, Battison RM (1981) Sign language, mental health, and satisfactory interaction. In Stein LK, Mindel ED, Jabaley T (eds) Deafness and Mental Health. New York: Grune & Stratton, pp 179–194.

Trybus R (1973) Personality assessment of entering hearing impaired college students using the 16PF-Form E. Journal of Rehabilitation of the Deaf 6: 34–40.

Ulissi SM, Brice PJ, Gibbins S (1989) Use of the Kaufman Assessment Battery for Children with the hearing impaired. American Annals of the Deaf 134: 283–287.

Ulissi SM, Gibbins S (1984) Use of the Leiter International Performance Scale and the Wechsler Intelligence Scale for Children — Revised with hearing-impaired children. Diagnostique 9: 142–153.

Vernon M (1968) Fifty years of research on the intelligence of deaf and hard-of-hearing children. Journal of Rehabilitation of the Deaf 1: 1–12.

Vernon M, Brown DW (1964) A guide to psychological tests and testing procedures in the evaluation of deaf and hard-of hearing children. Journal of Speech and Hearing Disorders 29: 414–423.

Watson B, Goldgar D, Kroese J, Lotz W (1986) Nonverbal intelligence and academic achievement in the hearing-impaired. Volta Review 88: 151–158.

Wechsler D (1991) Manual for the Wechsler Intelligence Scale for Children — Third Edition. New York: Psychological Corporation.

Weiss LG (1991) WISC-III: The revision of the WISC-R. Assessment News 1: 1–9.

Chapter 9
Forensic Psychiatry and Deaf People

PETER HINDLEY, NICK KITSON AND VALERIE LEACH

Introduction

Forensic psychiatry literally means those aspects of psychiatric practice that pertain to the law. It would be impossible for us to review forensic psychiatry with deaf adults, children and families in relation to the different legal systems of the world. We have chosen to discuss English law, hoping that our discussion of the principles will be of relevance to other national laws. Chapter 7 reviews child protection procedures in the USA.

Forensic psychiatry with adults will inevitably have different emphases and concerns from forensic psychiatry with children and families. As far as adults are concerned the following areas are covered here: assessment of responsibility, involuntary treatment and the Mental Health Act (1983); court proceedings (the experiences of interpreters and Deaf people) and fitness to plead; the propensity of Deaf people to offend and the types of offences committed; the disposal of mentally disordered Deaf offenders; and the experiences of Deaf prisoners. With respect to children and families we shall cover laws concerned with child care and protection, the legal responsibilities of local authorities, and juvenile offenders. Reference is made to two major pieces of legislation, the Mental Health Act 1983 and the Children Act 1989 but our reviews are focused on how these laws relate to Deaf people. Readers needing more detailed accounts are directed to authoritative guides such as White, Carr and Lowe (1990) which provides the full Children Act and a detailed commentary on the legislation. Hoggett (1984) gives a full account of mental health law with respect to adults.

As will be seen, the literature pertaining to forensic psychiatry and Deaf people is patchy and so, perhaps more than in any other area, we have drawn on our personal experiences to provide examples.

Deaf adults

Deaf adults, like deaf children, tend to be overprotected by the criminal justice system. It is not uncommon for Deaf offenders to be 'let off' or merely cautioned out of pity for their Deafness or avoidance of the burdensome procedures necessary to give a Deaf person full access to the system, such as interpreters. In a similar fashion to other situations of overprotection, rejection lurks covertly. Some Deaf offenders are 'let off' for offences of increasing seriousness, until finally they commit grievous bodily harm, murder, rape or arson, and are imprisoned or incarcerated in mental institutions for very long periods. From our experience, it is our view that it is in the interests of Deaf offenders, with respect to their mental health and general quality of life, that they follow the usual course of the law, provided that it is conducted in a Deaf-appropriate manner.

Adults are generally considered responsible for their actions, unlike children. Although the views of children are being given increasing importance (see below), they are balanced by the views of parental figures and involved professionals. In contrast, with adults the starting point is that the person has the freedom to choose and the responsibility for the consequences of those choices. The practice of forensic mental health work centres on the diagnosis and treatment of conditions that negate responsibility. A significant aim of treatment is to return the patient to the state of someone who is responsible for their actions. This is not to suggest that those responsible for their actions behave responsibly or within the law. In the latter case forensic mental health services might attempt to help offenders, though responsible for their actions, to modify their behaviour to avoid conflict with the law where this is their wish and there is a reasonable possibility of a successful outcome.

Assessment of responsibility, involuntary treatment and the Mental Health Act 1983

Monteiro and McNeeney (1992) note that the ancient Greeks denied deaf infants the right to live, the Romans chained deaf people for the entertainment of the public, and that even in America, Deaf people were declared legally incompetent until the 1940s. Deaf people in most countries have historically been regarded as legally incompetent and formally 'protected' by the courts. They have, by these measures, been treated as not responsible for their actions, or worse.

The assessment of people's responsibility for their actions is not only necessary when they have offended. Some people need care due to an inability to manage their financial affairs. Others need care or treatment of the mental disorder that has limited the responsibility for their actions. Although most patients being treated by mental health services attend and receive medication of their own free will, some will need compulsory treatment. The British Deaf Association (BDA) ensured provision for deaf people in the Mental Health Act 1983. 'Approved Social Workers', social workers with special training, whose duty it is to apply for individual patients to be detained, are required under Section 13 of the Act to interview patients 'in a suitable manner'. The then Government Department of Health and Social Security's Memorandum on the Act (Department of Health, 1987) explained that this means 'taking into account any hearing or linguistic difficulties the patient may have'. The BDA (1984) goes further to recommend that social workers working with deaf people should be 'Approved' under the act; failing that, social workers working with deaf people should work with the Approved Social Worker, and failing that, attempts to gain the help of social workers with deaf people should be recorded and they should be involved as soon as possible afterwards. The BDA adds that the training of Mental Health Act Approved Social Workers should include information on access to social workers with deaf people. The Department of Health (England) and Welsh Office (1993) Code of Practice to the Mental Health Act confirms many of the BDA's earlier recommendations and is generally an example of good practice. In paragraph 2.11 it clarifies the Approved Social Worker's (ASW) duty to interview deaf patients in a 'suitable manner', stating:

- Where the patient and ASW cannot understand each other's language sufficiently, wherever practicable recourse should be made to a trained interpreter who understands the terminology and conduct of a psychiatric interview and if possible the patient's cultural background.
- Where another ASW with an understanding of the patient's language is available, consideration should be given to requesting this ASW to carry out the assessment, or to assist the ASW assigned to the assessment.
- Where the patient has difficulty either in hearing or speaking, wherever practicable an ASW with appropriate communication skills should carry out the assessment, or assist the ASW initially assigned to the case. Alternatively the ASW should seek the assistance of a trained interpreter.

There is no such legal obligation on the doctors concerned to interview deaf patients in a suitable manner, despite the likelihood of doctors needing to interview patients about highly complex and often bizarre personal experiences. Doctors, along with ASWs, are told that they should consider not only the statutory criteria but also, amongst other things, the risk of making assumptions based on an individual's social and cultural background and the possibility of misunderstandings which may be caused by medical/health conditions, including deafness, when judging whether compulsory admission is appropriate (para. 2.6). In our view, doctors, and any other mental health professionals involved in assessments under the Mental Health Act, should be required to interview patients in a 'suitable manner'.

The Code of Practice implies support for our view, without stating it clearly. In paragraph 1.4 it states that:

> 'individuals should be as fully involved as practicable . . . in the formulation and delivery of their care and treatment, and that, where linguistic and sensory difficulties impede such involvement reasonable steps should be taken to attempt to overcome them.'

and more clearly states (para. 2.19):

> . . . proper medical examination requires: direct personal examination of the patient's mental state, excluding any possible preconceptions based on the patient's . . . social and cultural background . . . where the patient and doctor cannot understand each other's language the doctor should, wherever practicable, have recourse to a trained interpreter, who understands the terminology and conduct of a psychiatric interview (and if possible the patient's cultural background).

Harry (1986) cautions that interviews conducted through a sign language interpreter may inhibit the interaction and therefore both diagnosis and therapy.

The BDA document (1984) comments that social workers with deaf people will know of the specialist psychiatric services for deaf people. We would go further and suggest that all deaf patients detained under any mental health law should have their detention and treatment reviewed by a specialist psychiatrist for deaf people as soon as is practicable.

> A Mental Health Review Tribunal psychiatrist, appointed to ensure the patient's appeal is properly heard, attributed the detained Deaf patient's interest in graphic gory movies to be indicative of psychopathy, a diagnosis likely to lead to the patient's appeal being denied. In the author's view the patient's behaviour was adequately explained by the patient's deprivation of words and love of action. The patient's dangerousness was historically related to impulsive beha-viour in response to frustration and in no way related to psychopathic tendencies.

Denmark (1985) notes that Deaf people are prone to over- and under-diagnosis. It is as important that specialist mental health workers for deaf people are involved in their release as in their detention.

Psychiatrists are the principal diagnosticians in most mental health work, and psychiatrists for deaf people should be involved where practicable. Deaf mental health services not uncommonly reveal deaf patients whose mental illness has been significantly neglected, to their risk and detriment, in addition to any risk to society.

> A deaf patient had been admitted to an inpatient unit for deaf people with florid psychosis of many years' standing and a history of walking down the middle of the road and taking overdoses. Despite the neglect of care having been at last noticed, there was continued resistance to admission by persons responsible for health care.

The difficulties in diagnosing mental illness in deaf people are described in Chapter 4. It is all the more important to make correct assessments where a deaf patient's liberty might be removed or his protection, or that of the public, from serious harm is concerned. In cases of learning disability, termed 'Mental Impairment' in the Mental Health Act 1983, particular caution in diagnosis is required (see Chapter 5) Some deaf patients may be inappropriately diagnosed as 'mentally impaired', though some will function as 'mentally impaired' until given an adequate learning environment in a deaf world, such as deaf mental health services. In WHO terms (see Chapter 1) the patients are handicapped, but to such a degree that the Mental Health Act 1983 definition of 'mental impairment' may be correct.

The disorders of mental health that affect people's responsibility are generally the psychoses (see Chapter 4). Organic psychoses, such as forms of dementia, will have a long-term effect—mostly on ability to manage one's own affairs. Here, various powers are required by carers to ensure adequate care. It is fundamental to the law and its operation that in situations of care the least restrictive options on freedom, and the options least disabling of the patient's responsibility, should be pursued. Which laws and practices achieve this is always debatable, balancing freedom, responsibility and adequate care within national cultures. In the UK, for those in receipt of state-funded income only, the choice of an 'appointee' is their least restrictive option. On the other hand, for those with significant financial resources, the added safeguards of the Court of Protection are required. In the latter case, in addition to the legal proceedings, the deaf person will need a medical assessment, but there is no legal requirement for the medical practitioner to use sign language or an interpreter.

The Commission of Enquiry into Human Aids to Communication (1992) recommends that human aid communicators should not function where impartiality can be questioned, yet 'Second Opinion Approved Doctors' from the Mental Health Act Commission regularly use mental health staff involved in detaining patients as communicators, or interpreters employed by the mental health services. Similarly, mental health review tribunals expect detaining mental health services to employ the interpreters for reviews of detention. As well as being against the recommendations of the Commission of Enquiry, it is against those of HM Government. Despite one author's attempt to challenge these practices with the Mental Health Act Commission (MHAC) and HM Government's Minister for the Disabled, they continue, although there have been very notable improvements in the MHAC's own direct practice.

When assessing whether patients should be detained in hospital against their will, the Mental Health Act 1983 Memorandum on Parts I–VI, VII and X of the Act (Department of Health, 1987) states that the Approved Social Worker must be satisfied that detention in a hospital is the most appropriate way of providing the care and medical treatment that the patient needs. Approved Social Workers are expected to consider options other than hospital. The authors assert that the Approved Social Workers cannot satisfy themselves over hospital detention unless they have considered the services of specialist deaf mental health services, including their hospital and community provision. There will be situations where compulsory detention is only appropriate, where it is to a specific Deaf Mental Health Service, and situations where the community provision of a Deaf Mental Health Service is the only effective alternative to detention.

Crime

Deaf people's access to the protection and control provided by the criminal justice system should be equal. For this they and hearing people involved will require aids to communication in the hearing worlds of the police and the courts. The Code of Practice for the Police and Criminal Evidence Act 1984 (HMSO, 1991) provides some examples of good practice, ensuring that interpreters are made available for all relevant police actions. Once in court, misunderstandings of the role of the interpreter can be a problem (see Chapter 13).

> Attending court as an expert witness for a Deaf offender patient suffering a paranoid psychosis, one of the authors was asked by the judge, via the defence counsel, to interpret the court proceedings, despite not being a registered interpreter and being a witness for the defence. Refusal was met with a further request to interpret, and an explanation for refusal. Refusal was repeated with an explanation. Fortunately the booked interpreter eventually arrived after a prolonged delay and the outcome was satisfactory.

Interpreter issues in court have recently been the subject of much debate within Deaf and legal worlds, following an observed interpreter error leading to an expensive retrial in a murder case. A trial for alleged rape was postponed because only one interpreter was available. The interpreter withdrew from the task, with the support of the BDA and the Royal National Institute for Deaf People (RNID), to the reported fury of the judge (British Deaf News, October 1995). A separate trial for alleged rape was postponed due to possible interpreter error (British Deaf News, November 1995). As a result of these unfortunate incidents, it is to be hoped that the legal officers have a better understanding of the issues, unlike the judge in the first trial for alleged rape, who is reported to have threatened the BDA and RNID with withdrawal of state funding (British Deaf News, October 1995).

There is still institutional discrimination against deaf people in UK courts. Though institutional discrimination generally does not apply to witnesses, victims or offenders, the deaf population is not allowed to serve on juries due to their need for interpreters. There is an element of discrimination against alleged deaf offenders in the UK in that interpreters can be called as witnesses. In the USA the involvement of interpreters, even in counselling, is regarded as as privileged as the counselling sessions themselves. In the USA interpreters cannot be ordered by a court to disclose or act as witnesses to the information gained in a counselling session (Roe and Roe, 1991).

Fitness to Plead

Monteiro and McNeeney (1992) remind us that the concept of being 'unfit to plead' was established in 1836 from the case of an accused 'deaf mute', Pritchard. The criteria for fitness to plead include:

- Being aware of the nature of the charge.
- Appreciating the difference between 'guilty' and 'not guilty'.
- Being able to challenge a juror.
- Being able to examine a witness and being able to instruct legal counsel.

In the UK, until the Criminal Procedure (Insanity and Unfitness to Plead) Act of 1991, it had great significance. A person found unfit to plead was detained under the equivalent of Section 37/41 of the Mental Health Act 1983. That means an indefinite 'sentence' to detention in a mental institution, until the Home Secretary, a senior government minister, sees fit to release, which is usually then only on strict conditions, 'conditional discharge'. The effect was often that alleged offenders were detained for much longer than if they had been tried in the ordinary way and given a finite sentence or gained parole. The 1991 Act allows the courts a sensible range of disposals, from very restrictive to absolute discharge.

For deaf offenders, the involvement of specialist deaf mental health workers in providing recommendations to the courts is essential to appropriate disposal. The criteria for fitness to plead, if interpreted rigidly, would exclude many of us. The authors are in the practice of stating that the client is 'fit to plead provided . . .' and stating the required behaviour of the court to enable the client to take full part in the court proceedings. The most obvious proviso is the presence of suitably qualified and experienced interpreters, but courts are not always well versed in the use of sign language interpreters and guidance might also be included.

Propensity to offending behaviour

There is no direct evidence that deaf people are any more likely to offend than the general population. The high incidence of behaviour disorder in deaf children and in deaf psychiatric populations might indicate a higher incidence of offending. The paucity of statistics is in part due to lack of routine recording of deafness in convicted criminals in the UK or USA.

In a retrospective mental health service case note study, Denmark (1985) found that over one-fifth of patients referred to a deaf mental health service in the north of England had behavioural problems and maladjustment, and Hamblin and Kitson (1992) found 25% of patients had a history of criminal offences, including crimes against property 10%, sexual offences 8% and assault 8%. Thirteen per cent of inpatients, at a time when 35% of patients were offered admission, had had more than one violent incident per month. There are high levels of past and present offending behaviour in deaf versus hearing mental health patients. This cannot necessarily be extrapolated to the whole deaf community. A study of violent behaviour amongst patients of a psychiatric hospital in 1987 (Lim, Tobin and Falkowski, 1991) included the London specialist Deaf Unit. The Deaf Unit (N = 34) produced the highest number of incidents per patient (4.9) compared to rehabilitation wards (3.5) and locked intensive care wards (2.5). Characteristics of violent compared with non-violent deaf inpatients were analysed.

Male patients were more involved in violent incidents, but not significantly so, and this sex distribution reflected the average inpatient deaf population. Within the deaf population, 75% of violent patients were below the age of 39 compared to 50% of the non-deaf violent inpatients, though this did reflect the average age of the deaf inpatient population. It is of note that in this study, apart from a diagnosis of schizophrenia, deaf, Afro-Caribbean and Asian patients predominated in the frequently violent group. This points to the possibility or likelihood that language and cultural mismatches between staff and patients played a significant part in offences.

Despite the Deaf Unit being specific to that culture, its staff at the time were all hearing (see Chapter 12). A similar survey in the same service today would be likely to produce very different results. Lim, Tobin and Falkowski (1991) found no more violence generally nor a greater likelihood to be involved in serious violence amongst the Afro-Caribbean and Asian patients in contrast with deaf patients who, like patients with schizophrenia and those in rehabilitation wards, were more violent generally. Both the Deaf Unit and rehabilitation wards had longer stays, which may have been the cause and/or effect of violence.

Offences

Information from deaf mental health patient populations suggests a higher incidence of violent crime, though there is no support for this from less biased populations. Klaber and Falek (1963), in a study of 51 Deaf offenders, found a high incidence of sex offences (37%). The figure, when adjusted for what would now be considered criminal, though significantly reduced, remains high (18%). The high incidence of sexual offences is from only a small sample, including one case of indecent exposure, three of molesting females and five of paedophilia. These figures cannot reliably be extrapolated to the deaf population at large, but are in accord with clinical experience. In our view and experience, any increased incidence of sexual offences is highly likely to be related to a lack of sexual education (Tripp and Kahn, 1986) and the inappropriate sexual experiences more common amongst deaf people (see Chapter 7). Klaber and Falek (1963) found the same incidence of hearing versus deaf parents amongst the offending as the non-offending deaf population, but found a higher incidence of at least one deaf sibling (25%) amongst the offending population.

Disposal

Assessments are not only required to provide information on responsibility, they are also vital for appropriate sentencing. Gore and Critchfield (1992) describe the fate of a deaf girl, who was sexually abused by her alcoholic stepfather with the support of her alcoholic mother. Her promiscuous behaviour resulted in expulsion from residential school and return to the abuse at home. Her disturbance was noticed by a signing minister of religion, resulting in a referral to a psychiatrist who prescribed tranquillizers. At the age of 25 the young woman attacked her stepfather, was arrested and placed in a psychiatric hospital for 18 months, where she was treated with antipsychotic drugs without effect on her apparent hallucinations. She was hospitalized several times in the next 12 years. Finally, she was hospitalized, but released within 10 days. The next day the young woman shot her stepfather three times, killing him. She was found not guilty by reason of insanity and placed in a forensic psychiatric unit for two years followed by an intensive care unit. At last she was placed in a psychiatric unit with other deaf patients and shared her story of abuse and, though still needing antipsychotic medication, was successfully rehabilitated out of hospital to independent living and work. Had she been first assessed by a mental health service for deaf people a much better outcome would have been likely.

In the author's opinion deaf people charged with or convicted of offences, who are subject to any suspicion of mental disorder should receive an assessment by a specialist psychiatrist for deaf people. In England and Wales, if necessary, they can be remanded in hospital under the Mental Health Act 1983 for assessment under Section 35 or treatment under Section 36. Unlike compulsory admissions under the Mental Health Act for non-offenders, where there is specific guidance for social workers and doctors on interviewing deaf patients in an appropriate manner, there is no such specific guidance for medical recommendations to courts. In practice it has not been uncommon for deaf offenders to be diverted to the mental health system without the expertise of any specialist care professional for deaf people. With the increased availability in the UK of psychiatrists for deaf people, solicitors defending deaf patients would be unlikely to allow this practice to continue, though in law there is nothing formal to prevent it.

In assessing risk for the appropriate disposal of mentally disordered criminal offenders, the most significant predictor of future behaviour is past behaviour, including detail of potentially causative preceding events, immediate precipitants, physical and social environment and the patient's mental state in which the behaviour occurred. In other words, the circumstances of the crime should be taken into account. For deaf people a lack of availability of communication, and circumstances which enable the offender to have power and take responsibility over outcomes, are often crucial. Hamblin and Kitson (1992) noted that of the 16% of patients with a diagnosis of unsocialized conduct disorder, many had the phenomena of personality disorder, yet proved to be responsive to treatment. Basilier (1964) and subsequent psychiatrists for deaf people emphasize this better prognosis and this has significance for court disposal of deaf offenders. At present, in the UK, courts that wish to make a hospital disposal of a deaf mentally disordered offender have only the choice of Rampton Maximum Secure Hospital or the open wards of the three specialist Deaf Mental Health Services for their deaf offenders. Unlike the services available to hearing mentally disordered offenders, there are no medium or minimum secure units nor local intensive care wards for deaf people. Although the open wards of the three national Deaf Mental Health Services provide a 24-hour deaf environment, deaf maximum secure hospital patients have access to each other and deaf staff only during their day programmes, generally being nursed on separate wards.

Prisoners

Deaf prisoners have an exceptionally hard time.

> One of the authors recalls a deaf prisoner being called by the hospital wing officer to attend an appointment. The prisoner had his back to the officer, who shouted with increasing officiousness. It took a fellow prisoner to eventually notice the situation and attract the deaf prisoner's attention. The officer's expression and gesture unintentionally made the deaf prisoner aware of his plight, while the officer berated him. Many deaf prisoners complain of teasing, bullying or being used by fellow inmates. Worse, others accept it unconsciously as their lot to serve their hearing fellows for protection. It appears likely they will continue to be the dupes in crime on release.

In an unpublished survey commissioned by the Home Office (Home Office, 1987), Fiskin, a prison officer with signing skills and an interest in deafness, notes that receiving prison officers will be likely to make recourse to writing in ignorance of the poor literacy of some deaf people. The receiving prison medical officer will be in a similar position, yet is expected to judge a prisoner's mental state, especially suicidal risk, in addition to physical health. It appears that deaf people are commonly assigned to the hospital wing merely because they are deaf. Two out of four of Fiskin's subjects were so placed just because they were deaf. Fiskin asks how deaf prisoners can learn the detailed routine of prison and prison culture. They cannot hear the instructions of the officers, or advice and gossip from fellow prisoners. Deaf prisoners are uncommon but not a rarity. Fiskin describes five prisoners in four years at Lincoln Prison.

A Home Office survey (1987) found at least 45 deaf people in prison, just under 0.1% of the prison population that day, indicating the probability of deaf people being in prison is at least equal to the hearing population. The 45 prisoners were spread between 26 different prisons. Fourteen were assessed as requiring psychiatric treatment, but how valid were their assessments? Fiskin reports that the US Department of Justice, Federal Bureau of Prisons could find only two prisoners with hearing restrictions, despite Jensema (1990) finding the incidence of hearing impairment much higher in penal institutions in the USA. The Correctional Service of Canada, in contrast to other countries surveyed by Fiskin, has guidelines and relatively good services.

Fiskin points out that deaf prisoners suffer 'double imprisonment'. They are left alone with their thoughts, out of contact with fluent communication, yet usually not provided with text technology for televisions, telephones and video. Either their sentences should be reduced, or access to compensatory technology needs to be provided to achieve equity. Fiskin suggests that frustration often leads to breaches of discipline, which are rarely handled with an interpreter and lead to loss of remission. He recommends deaf awareness and sign language training for prison staff; sign language videos of rights, rules and 'handbook' type information; use of interpreters for reception and medical screening; a record of interpreters, staff with signing ability, approved deaf visitors and contact numbers; and appropriate text technology. More significantly, he recommends that deaf prisoners are carefully screened taking into consideration family visits and availability.

Fiskin further recommends that thought be given to regional units for deaf prisoners, for similar reasons to the need for regional mental health units (see Chapter 19). It is our experience that deaf prisoners, like deaf mental health patients, have often lost contact with their families and friends and would prefer to reside with other deaf people, even if they are distant from their home. The rehabilitation possibilities of a small prison deaf community should be balanced against the possibility of more trouble with deaf people ganging together against the regime. Clearly, thought should be given to ensuring adequate signing staff for prison security as well as rehabilitation. Regional centres could employ deaf prison officers for such units, following the successful example of mental health units. Bastikar (1995) urges deaf people to become prison visitors.

Deaf child and family psychiatry and the law

Child and family psychiatry interfaces with the law in the UK in four main areas. Firstly, in relation to parental responsibility and the quality of care that parents provide for their children. This extends to child protection and the risks of abuse and neglect that children face, both within their families and with non-family members and strangers. In a variety of circumstances concerns about the quality of parental care will lead to alternative carers being necessary — foster parents, children's homes or adoptive parents.

Secondly, the effects on children of marital breakdown within the family and the role that child and family psychiatry can play in determining the best interests of the child. Thirdly, with respect to the responsibilities that local authorities have for children with disabilities. Finally, in relation to the antisocial and criminal behaviour of children and young people.

Child care law in England and Wales

Child care law in England and Wales has recently undergone major changes. In the past, laws relating to public concerns — child protection, parenting breakdown, reception into care, etc. — were contained in separate statutes from those relating to private concerns, such as determination of where children should reside when marriages break up, and disputes over levels of contact with the non-resident parent. Under the Children Act 1989 both of these areas of law were brought together, along with laws describing the responsibilities of local authorities for children with disabilities, school attendance, residential placements for children and, to some extent, financial provision for children. In addition, the Children Act 1989 brought together the same powers to make orders in all courts, where in the past different courts had held different powers. The Act describes the powers and responsibilities of the courts in these areas and outlines a number of fundamental principles that should be used to determine decisions and actions relating to children and families. Finally, the Children Act shifts the balance of power away from statutory authorities and towards parents in a significant departure from previous legislation. What follows is a brief and highly selective summary of the legislation, in particular in relation to deaf children.

The Children Act 1989 and deaf families

General principles

Part I of the Act outlines the general principles of the Act.

The welfare principle

Section 1(1) of the Children Act states that when a court determines any question in relation to the upbringing of a child or administration of the child's property 'the child's welfare shall be the court's paramount consideration'. For deaf children, the court is likely to have to depend on other people to help it to determine what is in the child's best interest — be they interpreters, social workers or psychiatrists. Equally, deaf parents will find themselves talking to the court through an interpreter rather than directly.

In order to determine the child's welfare, the Act introduced a Welfare Checklist (Section 1(3)) which outlines the areas that the court should consider in determining the child's welfare:

a. The ascertainable wishes and feelings of the child concerned (considered in the light of his age and understanding);

Given the highly variable language environments in which deaf children find themselves, and the consequent effects on all aspects of psychological development, this area may need careful consideration. Non-signing clinicians, working with an interpreter, must ensure that they employ an interpreter with experience in working with children. They should be prepared to use a wide range of communication methods, including drawing, role-play and writing, to gain the deaf child's views. In these circumstances involving a deaf person as a responsible adult can give the deaf child and clinician an important sense of being understood. Careful double-checking with the interpreter is vital.

> Whilst interviewing a family with an interpreter, a deaf teenager made passing reference to abuse in her family of origin. The interpreter did not process the full meaning of the child's statement but the child confirmed it when the interviewer asked her directly.

b. his physical, emotional and educational needs;

For deaf children these needs are likely to be more complex than for hearing children. Physical needs will include full audiological assessment and support, and help for the family to develop appropriate communication skills. The child's emotional needs would include the extent to which the family has been able to accept the child as a deaf child. Educational needs would include early access to education services to facilitate language development. The family is likely to need continuing support to maintain and further develop their language skills, particularly with deaf children.

c. the likely effect on him of any change in his circumstances;

In order to assess the likely effect of change it is vital that the child has as full an understanding as possible, given his or her developmental stage. Given that many deaf children are excluded from family discourse, the deaf child may need additional input to understand fully what is happening within their families. For some hearing children of deaf parents the reverse may be true. Where such children have become parentified, not so for all such children, they may feel responsible and to blame for changes occurring within the family.

d. his age, sex, background and any characteristics of his which the court considers relevant;

Deaf children are at greater risk of additional physical and intellectual impairments. For the children of deaf parents, consideration needs to be given to cultural differences between deaf and hearing communities. There are occasions when these come into conflict.

> Jason a 6-year-old deaf boy of mixed race parentage was accommodated by his local authority at his mother's request. She subsequently severed all contact and the local authority sought an adoptive placement. Jason communicated in BSL and yet the adoption panel decided that he needed to be placed with a Black family rather than a family who could sign.

e. any harm which he has suffered or is at risk of suffering;

f. how capable each of his parents, and any other person in relation to whom the court considers the question to be relevant, is of meeting his needs;

It is difficult to see how deafness alone, either in child or parents, could account for difficulties in meeting the child's needs. Rather, difficulty in recognizing the deaf child's needs is more likely to be part of a more general difficulty.

> Two deaf children of hearing parents were made subject to care orders following disclosure of sexual abuse by the father. Whilst this allegation was not legally proven, their marked language and social delay was as a result of the combined effects of parental neglect and deafness. Transfer to permanent foster carers led to significant developmental gains for both children.

g. the range of powers available to the court under the Act in the proceedings in question.

In addition, the Act lays down the principle that a court should use the powers available to it under the Act only when it is satisfied that the making of an order will be better for the child than making no order

(S1(5)). Parties applying for an order must convince the court that the making of the order will improve the welfare of the child.

This principle reflects the philosophy of the Act that courts should respect the integrity and independence of families. The Act also introduces the concept of Parental Responsibility (S2). Under the Act, parental responsibility means 'all the rights, duties, powers, responsibilities and authority which by law a parent of a child has in relation to a child and his property'. (S3(1)). This broad definition was chosen deliberately in order to avoid the problems that might arise from a more prescriptive list of parental responsibilities. Parental responsibility is automatically granted to mothers and married fathers. Unmarried fathers must apply to the courts in order to be granted parental responsibility, or reach an agreement with the mother of the child.

Family proceedings

Part II of the Act relates to the court's powers in relation to family proceedings, primarily issues relating to children arising from disputes between parents which do not involve the local authority.

Under previous legislation, courts could make custody orders—who cared for the child—and access orders—whom the child could see. The Act replaces these orders with four orders under S8 of the Act: Residence orders; Contact orders; Prohibited Steps orders; and Specific Issue orders.

Residence orders determine where the child will live whilst allowing each parent to retain parental responsibility, subject to any conditions attached to the Residence order. Contact orders determine with whom and how often a child will have contact with their parent(s).

Prohibited Steps orders allow the court to proscribe certain actions in relation to the exercise of parental responsibility, such as removing the child from the UK.

Specific Issue orders relate to specific matters such as education and medical treatment.

Responsibilities of local authorities

Part III of the Act describes the responsibilities of local authorities. The fundamental principle contained in the Act is that local authorities have a responsibility to support family life and, as far as possible, to prevent children 'in need' having to be received into care. Deaf children are specifically defined as being in need by virtue of S17(11) of the Act. The duties of local authorities are to identify children 'in need'. They are to establish a register of disabled children in their area [Sch. 2, para. 1: S17(2)] and to provide services to disabled children that will minimize the effect of their disabilities and give them the opportunity to lead lives that are as normal as possible (Sch. 2 para. 6).

In the case of deaf children these responsibilities can clearly be interpreted to mean that the local authority should ensure that all newly diagnosed deaf children should have access to deaf communication workers who can help hearing parents to develop communication strategies and acquire signing skills in order to ensure that their child develops to their maximum potential. Equally, this provision of the Act could be interpreted as meaning that local authorities have a responsibility throughout a Deaf child's childhood to help parents maintain and develop their signing skills through direct provision of services for them.

Local authorities are given a general duty to promote the upbringing of children by their parents and to make provision to enable this to happen. They are also expected to take steps to prevent the abuse and neglect of children in their area. Provision of social workers with deaf people, working directly with children and families and able to communicate directly with deaf children and deaf parents, would seem an essential preventive component of this responsibility (see Chapter 16). Given the prevalence of childhood deafness and abuse it would seem sensible that local authorities collaborate in identifying specialist deaf child abuse workers and specialist interpreters who could undertake investigative work with deaf children who may have been abused (Kennedy, 1992).

Included within these recommendations is provision by the local authority to assist people who are living in the same house as a perpetrator to find safe accommodation, thus preventing children from having to be removed from their family if abuse is occurring or is suspected. They are expected to encourage children not to commit criminal offences and are to avoid the need to use secure accommodation. Local authorities are required to make provision for day care of children in need aged under 5, and to ensure that their provision of day care and foster care takes into account different racial groups.

The Act radically alters previous concepts of voluntary care, replacing them with accommodation. The parents of children who are accommodated by the local authority retain parental responsibility for their child, whereas in the past they passed their responsibility to the local authority, but this allows whoever is caring for the child to do whatever is 'reasonable' whilst the child is in their care. This includes medical consents.

George was a 15-year-old deaf boy who communicated in both BSL and spoken English. He had a long history of physically aggressive behaviour, mainly in relation to his sister and deaf peers and teaching staff, although occasionally directed towards his parents. He was permanently excluded from his residential school after threatening another pupil with a knife. He was not interviewed by the police. On his return home his parents felt unable to care for him and asked the local authority to accommodate him. George was placed in a local authority children's home with 24-hour interpreting support. Further episodes of violence occurred and he was finally arrested for being in possession of a gun. He was cautioned by police. Following this his unlawful behaviour diminished and he returned home. Throughout this period his parents had worked closely with the local authority sharing information and decision-making.

Care and supervision orders

Applications for care orders can be made only by local authorities or persons authorized by the Secretary of State, such as the National Society for the Prevention of Cruelty to Children (NSPCC). Courts at all levels — magistrates' courts (called 'family proceedings courts'), county court and the High Court — can now make care orders. Care orders cannot be made unless there is an application before the court, but courts may make interim care orders (see below) and ask local authorities to investigate a child's circumstances. When considering whether to grant a care order the court must be satisfied that two criteria have been satisfied:

- The child concerned is suffering significant harm or is likely to suffer significant harm.
- The harm or likelihood of harm is attributable to (i) the care given to the child, or likely to be given to him if the order were not made, not being what it would be reasonable to expect a parent to give him; or (ii) the child's being beyond parental control.

These are known as the 'threshold criteria'.

The court must also apply the welfare checklist and not make an order unless it considers that making an order would be better for the child than not doing so. Before making any order the court must consider the local authority's plans for the child and plans for any contact between the child and his parents. All the parties must have the opportunity to see these plans, known as 'care plans'.

Once a care order has been granted, it supersedes any other order that has been granted — residence order, supervision order, etc. — and the local authority acquires parental responsibility. Parent(s) do not lose their responsibility but the local authority can determine the extent to which they can meet it. The local authority cannot apply for freeing for adoption or appoint a guardian. A care order lasts until the child is 18 years old, or a residence order is made, or the care order is discharged.

John was the hearing 3-year-old son of a deaf mother, Diana. Diana had made frequent threats to harm herself and had threatened to poison John. She had severe episodes of anger during which she damaged property and threatened social work staff. She had been referred to psychiatric services for the deaf but discharged herself from treatment. Diana's upbringing had been disrupted by marital violence and the sudden death of her father. John was made subject to an interim care order and psychiatric reports requested. Assessment showed that John's mother could not see the effects of her behaviour on John and she could see no reason to change. He was at risk of suffering significant physical and psychological harm if he returned to his mother's care. John was made subject to a full care order and placed for adoption. The cause of Diana's difficulties were partly the consequences of her deafness but equally a reflection of a disturbed family life. Her parenting difficulties were more closely related to her upbringing than to her deafness.

Supervision orders can be granted only if the same criteria that apply to care orders are fulfilled. A supervision order places a child under the supervision of a local authority or probation officer. Supervision orders last for one year and can be renewed for up to three years.

Interim arrangements

Once an application for a care order has been made there is normally a period of time during which the local authority, parent(s) and guardian *ad litem* will prepare reports and if necessary instruct experts. During this time the court has four main options in the powers that it can use:

- To make no order.
- A residence order.
- An interim care order.
- An interim supervision order.

The court will also give directions as to what further investigations it considers need to be carried out, for example a psychiatric report or medical report. Interim care orders last for as long as the court specifies, up to eight weeks for the first order and up to four weeks for each subsequent order.

Contact with children in care and freeing for adoption

Under the Act the court has powers to determine who, where and how much contact a person has with a child in care. Children themselves or a local authority can also apply to prevent contact between children and specific people. The same principles that apply to care orders are used to determine the granting of contact orders, except that the threshold criteria do not apply and an order can be made if the court considers it to be in the children's best interest to do so.

Joanne was a 10-year-old deaf girl whose allegations of sexual abuse at age 5 had been found to be unproven, but who was received into care because of neglect. As her confidence with her foster carers grew she began to express increasing distress before and after fortnightly contact with her natural parents. Contact was reduced to monthly but her parents sought a contact order restoring it to fortnightly. The local authority sought an assessment by the Deaf Child and Family Team. At assessment Joanne made it clear that her father had consistently and frequently abused her. She expressed a profound dislike and fear of her father, but a wish to continue seeing her mother on an infrequent

> basis. The team's report supported Joanne's request for cessation of contact with her father but continuing but infrequent contact with her mother. A contact order providing six-monthly supervised contact with the family was made, with the stipulation that Joanne should decide with which family members she had contact.

Orders freeing a child for adoption, and adoption orders themselves, are still sought under the Adoption Act 1976. The court may need to consider an application for contact by the birth parent(s) under the Children Act at the same time as the adoption application.

Child protection

The Act includes three powers that may be used when concerns about a child's safety and well-being arise. In circumstances where parents refuse to allow local authorities to assess the risk of a child being harmed, the authority or other authorized persons (such as the NSPCC) can apply for a Child Assessment Order (S43). If granted, assessments, most commonly medical or social work, must be carried out within seven days. This has very rarely been upheld in practice. For social work to be undertaken with deaf children, considerable thought needs to be given to the communication needs of the child. Kennedy (1992) has made a strong case for the creation of dual-specialist posts — social workers with experience and training in working with Deaf people and in child protection. She has also been instrumental in establishing training courses for BSL interpreters in this field in the UK.

If the local authority or other people, such as health workers, are concerned that a child is at risk of suffering significant harm and is in need of safety they can apply for an Emergency Protection Order lasting eight days; this allows them to remove the child from the parents' care and confers limited parental responsibility on the local authority for eight days (S43/44). Finally, if a police constable is concerned that a child is likely to suffer significant harm he can take the child into police protection (S47/48).

Assessment of parenting with deaf families

Children need parents who can meet their primary needs for care, safety and affection. Parents need to be able to respond to their developing child's changing needs. In this sense, assessing parenting in deaf families is no different from assessing parenting in hearing families, except that the children or the parents or both are likely to use a different language from the clinician. In this respect the signing skills of professionals in the Deaf Child and Family Team offer a unique perspective, allowing deaf and hearing professionals to interview children and parents directly, without the need for an interpreter, and so allowing direct observation and engagement with the deaf individual.

However, deafness within the family brings an extra set of considerations that need to be borne in mind. For both deaf parents of hearing children (D:H) and hearing parents of deaf children (H:D) these concentrate on an awareness of the communication needs of deaf people, but the consequences for these two kinds of families are often different. The main factors for D:H and H:D families are described, recognizing that all families are different and that what we describe should be taken only as features of these families when they are seen as part of a clinical population; that is, they do not characterize all families containing deaf people.

D:H families

When assessing deaf parents two main factors need to be considered. Firstly, the impact of early onset deafness on the deaf person's social and psychological development. For some deaf people early deprivation of language and distortions of social environments may lead to two varying outcomes. For some, the repeated experience of failure leads to disempowerment and passivity. For others, poor impulse control and egocentricity (see Chapters 3 and 5) may be understood as compensations for the experience of disempowerment. Limited social experience, when combined with other family risk factors, may lead to parents who have difficulty in recognizing their children's needs and so putting them at risk either through neglect or through direct physical or emotional harm. This is often compounded by limited communication between parents and children and an over-reliance by the parents on the children to act as interpreters. For older hearing children this early parentification may lead to them protecting their parents when outside agencies intervene.

Susie, a profoundly deaf mother of two hearing sons, first came into contact with social services when her eldest son, Mark, presented with human bite marks at school. Both sons had appeared neglected from time to time and showed academic underachievement. Initial enquiries by social services were hampered by Mark's reluctance to describe life at home. Slowly a picture emerged of Susie's multiple relationships with abusive men, who at times physically, emotionally and sexually abused her sons. Educational and social support, followed by family therapy aimed at empowering Susie, was attempted but Susie failed to engage and change. Both sons were made subject to care orders but frequent contact was maintained because of the children's warm relationships with their mother.

H:D families

For H:D families, communication differences within the family can be used as a means of exerting and abusing power in the opposite way. Kennedy (1992) has argued that denying deaf children access to sign language amounts to emotional abuse and acts as the context for physical and sexual abuse. Certainly Gregory (1995) and Schlesinger and Meadow (1972) found that hearing parents of deaf children were more likely to use physical punishment rather than verbal punishment and explanation if their children misbehaved. When there is no deliberate intent to cause suffering by denying access to sign language, we cannot see that this, however misguided, amounts to abuse.

Sandy, the hearing mother of a deaf son and hearing daughter complained to social services of her son's behaviour. At assessment she presented as a cold and emotionally disengaged person, who used highly punitive language towards her children. At interview both children complained of excessively harsh physical punishment — beatings with belts and other objects. Sandy made no attempt to deny this, saying the children deserved it, but became intensely angry when the Team proposed notifying Social Services because of their concerns for the children's safety.

Writing court reports

A court report represents the findings of the assessment, the opinion and the recommendations of the clinician. It should start by identifying the author of the report and his or her professional qualifications and relevant professional experience. This introductory section should identify the individual who commissioned the report, the children or family assessed and the purpose of the assessment. Before outlining the findings of the assessment, the report should identify the documents which relate to the assessment and the people interviewed as part of the assessment, including when they were interviewed. A brief chronology of events leading up to the involvement of statutory services is also useful.

Following the chronology it is helpful to summarize the findings of previous assessments and interventions. The report should then go on to outline the findings of the assessment, confining itself to factual information and eschewing opinions as far as possible. This section should not be a verbatim account of the assessment but should identify sources of information, who said it and when, and where necessary, provide direct quotes and direct observations of behaviour. The report should provide a balance of the family's or child's history and present-day functioning. No assessment can be complete without integrating past and present.

The final section of the report should summarize the important aspects of the case by integrating it into a welfare checklist and then provide a clear opinion about the child's and family's difficulties and the prognosis. Possible interventions should be described and their advantages and disadvantages clearly outlined. On this basis the clinician can then make his or her recommendations to the court.

Juvenile delinquency and antisocial behaviour

'Juvenile delinquency' is not a psychiatric diagnosis but a socio-legal term, a juvenile delinquent being defined as a young person who has been prosecuted and found guilty of an offence that would be classified as a crime if committed by an adult (Sheldrick, 1994). Many young people commit delinquent acts, often minor ones, but few are ever prosecuted. There is, to our knowledge, only one study of delinquency in deaf young people (Harry and Dietz, 1985) and none of the large studies of juvenile delinquency make reference to deaf youth in their populations of young people (e.g. West and Farrington, 1977). Farrington (1995) summarizes the factors that are known to put boys and young men at risk of committing such acts but these all relate to hearing youth. We can give case examples of young deaf people committing antisocial acts, the response of the criminal justice and other social systems and possible treatment options.

Using information from the Cambridge Delinquency Study, Farrington (1995) has identified six risk factors which by themselves and in combination, at ages 8–10 years, predict a significant risk of later delinquency in hearing young people up to 32 years of age. No deaf children were involved in the study. The factors are:

1. Antisocial child behaviour, including troublesomeness at school, dishonesty and aggressiveness.
2. Hyperactivity–impulsivity–attention deficit, including poor concentration, restlessness, daring and psychomotor impulsivity.
3. Low intelligence and poor school attainment.
4. Parental criminality, including convicted parents, delinquent older siblings and siblings with behaviour problems.
5. Family poverty, including low family income, large family size and poor housing.
6. Poor parental child-rearing behaviour, including harsh and authoritarian discipline, poor supervision, parental conflict and separation from parents.

Patterson and his colleagues (Patterson, 1982) studied parenting styles in greater depth. Using direct observation they found parents of aggressive and conduct-disordered children to be more punitive, issue more commands, attend to deviant behaviour, issue more threats but at the same time fail to follow these through. Patterson and other workers have developed intervention strategies aimed at changing parenting (see Webster Stratton, 1991, for a comprehensive review) to prevent the development of delinquent behaviour.

In the study by Farrington and West (Farrington, 1995) protective factors at ages 8–10 were social isolation and lack of contact with a delinquent peer group. In early adulthood two factors have been shown to help juvenile delinquents avoid further offending — stable employment and a lasting sexual relationship (Sheldrick, 1994).

Antisocial behaviour and deaf youth

Investigating antisocial behaviour in deaf youth poses a number of difficulties for the criminal justice system. Firstly, the psychosocial development of deaf children varies and this can lead to uncertainties as to whether a deaf young person charged with an offence knew that he or she was committing an offence.

> A deaf young man who had experienced multiple traumatic experiences and had encountered sign language for the first time at 12 years, was charged with indecent assault. At interview the young man showed no awareness that he had committed an offence. The alleged victim was unable to give a consistent account of the assault and charges were dropped.

Secondly, the presence of deafness may lead the police to regard the deaf young person as handicapped and so not deserving of punishment.

> A 13-year-old boy was repeatedly arrested by the police for shoplifting. Despite his parents' wishes he was neither cautioned nor charged.

Finally, a deaf youth accused of committing an offence presents logistical problems to the police and courts — can interpreters be found, will they be sufficiently skilled to deal with the criminal justice system and work with children.

> A deaf youth charged with committing a serious sexual offence was interviewed by police with a colleague with signing skills acting as interpreter. The boy's solicitor challenged the interpreter's independence and the charges were dropped.

These accounts include a number of deaf young men who have been accused of committing sexual offences. Given that the rate of sexual abuse is probably higher amongst deaf children (see Chapter 7) the number of Deaf sexual offenders is also likely to be higher. At present no therapeutic services exist in the UK to assist these young people.

For many hearing youths who are convicted of criminal offences, diversion from custody via the child care agencies or Youth Justice programmes is the treatment of choice.

> We know of one young man who displayed a range of antisocial behaviours, including seriously aggressive behaviour, who was accepted on a Youth Justice programme with interpreter support provided by his local social services. He

was successfully diverted from offending and at 16 was referred to a residential training centre for Deaf youth with behaviour problems (RNID Court Grange).

Conclusions

It is our opinion that it is in the interests of deaf children and deaf adults that the law treat them as it treats hearing children and adults. In order to do so the criminal justice system will have to adapt to their specific communication needs and make special arrangements to ensure that deaf people have full access to decision-making. At the same time, it appears vital that a person's deafness is not used as an excuse either to deny them access to information or to protect them from the consequences of their actions. This does not always appear to happen at the moment. Both over-protection, by police and courts, and rejection, by failure to provide interpreters and appropriately qualified and experienced mental health workers, appear commonplace.

For deaf people who require compulsory treatment, it would seem eminently sensible that the excellent guidance offered to social workers in the use of the MHA should also apply to psychiatrists. Equally, deaf mental health workers should play an important part in determining the disposal of deaf mentally disordered offenders. It is perhaps not our responsibility to offer advice to the courts and other parts of the criminal justice system. However, it does appear that some members of the judiciary have little knowledge or understanding of the needs of deaf people, whilst others display much greater awareness. There may be a role for training in working with sign language interpreters and deaf awareness. The position of deaf offenders in prison is far more intractable but we believe that serious consideration should be given to Deaf Units within the prison system. The experience of deaf mental health services in the effects of providing an appropriate communication environment on violent behaviour, suggests that such arrangements could have a significant effect on deaf offenders.

Similar problems of communication and over-protection arise with children and families, but vary enormously according to location. In areas with social work departments for deaf people who work with deaf children, a child's chances of good access to legal proceedings are much greater. Equally, social workers in these areas are far likelier to be able to make use of Children Act provisions which enable them to provide early language intervention and so 'minimise the effect on disabled children within their area of their disabilities.' (Sch. 2 para. 6). For both deaf adults and deaf children there appear to be distinct advantages in gaining access to services with professionals who can communicate directly with them but, as with deaf adults, services for deaf juvenile offenders are extremely limited. There appears to be a considerable gap in services that might divert these young people from offending and so halt a progression through to the adult criminal justice system.

References

Basilier T (1964) Surdophrenia. The psychic consequences of congenital or early acquired deafness. Acta Psychiatrica Scandinavica 180: 362–372.

Bastikar R (1995) Sign On: Talking Point: Deaf people in prison. Channel 4 Television.

British Deaf News (1995) 'Furious judge threatens'. October, p 5.

British Deaf News (1995) 'Another trial of Deaf defendant collapses' November, p 5.

The Commission of Enquiry into Human Aids to Communication (1992) 'Communication is Your Responsibility'. Panel of Four, 25 Cockspur Street, London SW1Y 5BN.

Denmark J (1985) A study of 250 patients referred to a department of psychiatry for the deaf. British Journal of Psychiatry 146: 282–286.

Department of Health (1987) Mental Health Act 1983: Memorandum on Parts I to VI, VIII and X. London: HMSO.

Department of Health and Welsh Office (1993) Code of Practice: Mental Health Act 1983. London: HMSO.

Farrington DP (1995) The Twelfth Jack Tizard Lecture. The development of offending and antisocial behaviour from childhood: key findings from the Cambridge Study in Delinquent Development. Journal of Clinical Psychology and Psychiatry 36: 929–965.

Gore TA, Critchfield AB (1992) The development of a state-wide mental health system for deaf and hard of hearing persons. Journal of the American Deafness and Rehabilitation Association 26: Fall.

Gregory S (1995) Deaf Children and Their Families. Cambridge: Cambridge University Press.

Hamblin L, Kitson N (1992) Springfield supra-regional deaf unit: a retrospective case note survey. Abstracts, Royal College of Psychiatrists Annual Meeting p 73.

Harry B (1986) Interview, diagnostic and legal aspects in the forensic psychiatric assessments of deaf persons. Bulletin of the American Academy of Psychiatry Law 14: 147–162.

Harry B, Dietz PE (1985) 'Offenders in a silent world:hearing impairment and deafness in relation to criminality, incompetence and insanity.' Bulletin of the American Academy of Psychiatry and Law, 13: 85–96.

Hoggett B (1984) Mental Health Law, (second edition) London: Sweet & Maxwell.

Home Office (1987) Survey of Deaf or Hearing Impaired Inmates. Directorate of Health Care (unpublished).

Home Office (1991) Police and Criminal Evidence Act 1984 (s. 66): Code of Practice. London: HMSO.

Jensema CK (1990) 'Hearing loss within a jail population.' Journal of the American Deafness and Rehabilitation Association 24: 49–58.

Kennedy M (1992) Not the only way to communicate: a challenge to voice in child protection work. Child Abuse Review 3: 169–177.

Klaber MM, Falek A (1963) Delinquency and crime. In Rainer J, Altshuler M, Kallmann F, Deming E (eds) Family and Mental Health Problems in a Deaf Population. Department of Medical Genetics, New York State Psychiatric Institute, Columbia University, pp 141–151.

Lim L, Tobin M, Falkowski W (1991) The characteristics of patients who display violent behaviour in a psychiatric hospital. British Journal of Clinical and Social Psychiatry 8: 12–18.

Monteiro BT, McNeeney T (1992) Forensic aspects of deafness, Proceedings, second international congress, European Society of mental Health and Deafness. La Bastide, Avenue Vauban, 8, b-5000, Namur, Belgium, pp 235–238.

Patterson GR (1982) Coercive Family Process. Eugene, OR: Castalia.

Roe DL, Roe CE (1991) The third party: using interpreters for the deaf in counselling situations. Journal of Mental Health Counselling 13: 91–105.

Schlesinger H, Meadow K (1972) Sound and Sign. Berkeley, CA: University of California Press.

Sheldrick C (1994) Treatment of Delinquents. In Rutter M Hersov, Taylor E (eds) Modern Approaches to Child and Adolescent Psychiatry (third edition). Oxford: Blackwell Scientific.

Tripp AW, Kahn JV (1986) Comparison of the sexual knowledge of hearing impaired and hearing adults. Journal of the Rehabilitation of the Deaf 19: 3–4, 15–18.

Webster-Stratton C (1991) Strategies for helping families with conduct disordered children. Journal of Child Psychology and Psychiatry 32: 1047–1062.

West DJ, Farrington WP (1977) The Delinquent Way of Life. London: Heinemann.

White R, Carr P, Lowe N (1990) A Guide to the Children Act 1989. London: Butterworths.

Chapter 10
Addictive Behaviour and Deafness

SALLY AUSTEN AND KEN CHECINSKI

Addictive behaviour

In the last 40 years the definition of addictive behaviour has changed dramatically, reflecting a more holistic approach to diagnosis and treatment, a less judgemental perception, and an awareness of the commonality across addictive behaviours. Well into the 1960s 'addiction' was described only in terms of physical dependence. More recently, Orford (1985) described a person with an addictive behaviour as having an 'excessive appetite' for that activity and initiated the search for a definition which would be equally applicable to behaviours such as gambling, over-eating and drug use. Donovan and Marlatt (1988) responded to the challenge and defined addiction as:

> ... a complex, progressive behaviour pattern having biological, psychological and behavioural components. This pattern differs from others by the individual's overwhelmingly pathological involvement in or attachment to it, subjective compulsion to continue it, and reduced ability to exert control over it. An addictive behaviour pattern continues despite its negative impact on the physical, psychological and social functioning of the individual.

Drug use

In this chapter the focus is mainly on the field of drug use. However, many of the issues raised will be relevant to all addictive behaviours.

The World Health Organization defines 'a drug' as 'any substance that, when taken into any living organism, may modify one or more of its functions'. 'Drug abuse' is defined as 'persistent or sporadic excessive use of a drug inconsistent with or unrelated to, accepted medical practice'.

We shall try to avoid the terms 'drug abuse' or 'misuse' in favour of 'drug use' or 'drug-taking' as the former are determined by the judgemental attitudes of others and may relate more to legal/social factors than to harm caused to the individual. To imbue doctors with such omnipotence or to use medical practice as a measure when hundreds of thousands of people in the UK have (iatrogenic) addictions caused by badly prescribed tranquillizers and pain killers is illogical. Furthermore, medical opinion is not best-placed to comment on other addictive behaviours such as gambling or overwork. Again, a more holistic approach to definition is needed.

Whether a person is considered by society to have abused a drug may depend on whether the drug is legal or illegal, which may change over time. In the 1920s alcohol was illegal in some parts of the USA, whereas morphine and heroin were legal in the UK in the late nineteenth century. Whilst legislation, in part, exists to protect citizens, the profits made from the taxation of legal drugs such as alcohol and tobacco may interfere with objective decision-making. Some say that if alcohol had been invented in the 1990s it would have been outlawed instantly, such is the severity of its association with physical, psychological, social and legal problems.

People use drugs for two reasons:

- To increase their subjective experience of pleasure.
- To decrease their subjective experience of displeasure.

Drugs used may come in one of four categories:

- Legal drugs, e.g. alcohol.
- Illegal drugs, e.g. heroin.
- Prescribed drugs, e.g. barbiturates.
- Over-the-counter (OTC) drugs, e.g. solvents.

MacDonald and Patterson (1991) subdivide drug use into three levels of use:

- **Experimental** - using a drug 1-6 times then not using that drug again.
- **Recreational/social** - as an enjoyable pastime (as alcohol use is to many people).
- **Chronic** - use of the drug daily, often in isolation from others. With some drugs this leads to psychological and physical dependence, the use of the substance is seen as a solution to more fundamental problems and may be symptomatic of much more severe difficulties.

Dixon (1982) studied solvent use by young people in North London during 1981-1982 and found 33% to be experimental users, 57% to be recreational/social users, and only 10% to be chronic users.

Main classes of substances

Substances can be classified by the three different types of effect they have on the central nervous system:

- Stimulants.
- Depressants.
- Hallucinogens.

Stimulants

Stimulants or 'uppers' stimulate the central nervous system (CNS). They create an elevated mood (high, excited, bubbly). They can cause decreased sleep, dilated pupils, increased libido (especially cocaine), increased vital functions such as heartbeat, and decreased appetite. The effect on appetite is sometimes used medically in diets, but appetite increases on withdrawal of the drug. During withdrawal all these effects are reversed, for example, elevated mood changes to low mood, fatigue and headache. In some cases withdrawal causes a rebound depression so severe that the user commits suicide. Examples of stimulants are:

- **Cocaine** - often called 'Charlie', 'C' or 'Coke'. It can be sniffed, swallowed or injected. 'Crack' is a highly purified (free-based) cocaine which can be smoked. It can damage the nasal septum when sniffed.
- **Amphetamine** - often called 'speed', 'whizz' or 'billy', it is relatively cheap and widely used in the UK. It can be taken orally or intravenously. It tastes foul so people try all sorts of ways to get it down without tasting it, such as wrapping it in layers of paper before swallowing. It attacks the enamel of the teeth and the gums, making brushing the teeth painful. Regular users may stop brushing their teeth as a result and disfigurement and decay occurs. Amphetamine psychosis can occur, though this usually resolves on discontinuation of the amphetamine.
- **Amyl nitrate** - this comes in an ampoule which is sniffed. Medically it is used for angina and poor circulation as it relaxes artery walls. It is sometimes used by people having anal sex, as an anal relaxant.
- **Ecstasy** - Ecstasy works half like a stimulant and half like an hallucinogen. Legal until the 1960s, and used in some therapies because of its properties of making people want to communicate and be nice to each other, it is now a class A illegal drug. It is used mostly by young people at parties and 'Raves' to increase friendliness and the ability to dance for hours. Whilst some deaths result directly from lethal effects of the drug, most deaths following ecstasy use are due to dehydration or heart attacks caused by prolonged activity.
- **Nicotine** - nicotine in tobacco can be smoked in cigarettes, pipes and cigars, taken as snuff or chewed. All methods of administration permit the absorption of significant amounts of nicotine into the blood stream. In addition, smoking leads to tar-like substances entering and damaging the respiratory system. The effects of nicotine are subtle and

intoxication does not occur. Nicotine appears to act as a mood regulator and, in non-smokers, may enhance performance of psychomotor tasks. Within 24 hours of stopping smoking tobacco a number of withdrawal effects may occur, including mood changes, palpitations, irritability, restlessness and difficulty concentrating. Sleep is frequently disturbed and there is strong psychological craving. Mood changes resolve over four weeks or so, but there is increased hunger and appetite for at least three months.

- **Caffeine** - in the form of tea and coffee, drinking chocolate and soft drinks, caffeine is unconsciously used by millions of people to give them a 'lift', to increase activity or improve concentration. Withdrawal can result in headaches.
- **Anabolic steroids** - increasingly used by people who pay excessive attention to outstanding physical appearance, body builders and sports people. Taken by mouth and (increasingly) intravenously, these drugs can alter hormone balance, resulting in personality changes.

Depressants

Depressant or 'downers' sedate the Central Nervous System (CNS). A euphoria is experienced where the user feels removed from the situation and unaffected by surroundings. These kill pain and lower the metabolic rate, for example, gastric motility (leading to constipation), and promote sleep. They have an anticonvulsant property. During withdrawal all these properties are reversed, therefore there is a risk of convulsions which can be lethal.

Withdrawal fits are discrete: they do not continue after the withdrawal. However, if a person has experienced a withdrawal fit before it will be more likely to happen again. Examples of depressants are:

- **Alcohol** - alcohol is the most commonly used of the depressants. Although it is legal it is not necessarily safe. Consumed to experience euphoria, alcohol is in some way associated with 10% of deaths of those aged under 25 years; results in 40 000 deaths per annum in the UK; is associated with one-third of all road traffic accidents and 25% of admissions to male medical wards (Royal College of Physicians, 1987). In New York in 1972 alcohol was associated with 50% of road traffic accidents (Betros, 1974). Offences of vandalism or violence are commonly related to alcohol consumption and industry loses millions of pounds per year through working days lost because of alcohol. The majority of the aforementioned consequences require neither gross intoxication nor chemical dependence. Chronic excessive use can cause brain damage, liver damage and intra-uterine damage to the developing child. It is also associated with other gastrointestinal disorders and probably with a number of cancers (co-occurrence with tobacco smoking is important). Physical dependence can lead to alcoholic withdrawal, initial anxiety and agitation, progressing through paranoid ideas to delirium tremens which includes vivid visual hallucinations and convulsions. Alcohol use may be associated with acute thiamine deficiency leading to Wernicke's encephalopathy.

- **Opiates** - the original drug, opium, was refined to make morphine in the 1870s, then further refined to create heroin (diamorphine). Other opiates include codeine (or DF118), which is a commonly prescribed painkiller, and methadone, an orally administered heroin substitute used in drug maintenance or reduction programmes. They contain histamines which make the back of joints (knees, elbows) itch.
- **Barbiturates** - between 1920 and 1950 barbiturates were used as sleeping tablets. However, they are very dangerous in overdose so were discontinued. They are still used in the treatment of epilepsy. Taken by mouth, intravenously or intramuscularly, there is a cross-tolerance with alcohol.
- **Benzodiazepines** - the minor tranquillizers, as they are called, come in 'two forms': the *anxiolytics* such as valium and ativan, and the *hypnotics* such as temazepam. They are commonly prescribed for minor affective problems and, despite the knowledge that long-term use can lead to dependence, over a quarter of a million people in the UK have taken tranquillizers for seven years or more (Release, 1982).
- **Major tranquillizers** - used in the treatment of psychotic disorders and taken either orally or by slow-acting depot injection, these are not commonly abused as the effects are unpleasant.
- **Cannabis** - cannabis is mainly a depressant but also has some stimulant and hallucinogen properties. It is commonly used in the UK as part of youth culture and although a class B drug, those in possession of it for personal use are often not prosecuted. Dealers are still treated firmly.
- **Volatile substances** - this has been a problem area in the UK since 1970. Glue, solvents, petrol lighter fuel and the propellants from aerosols are inhaled. Their use is mainly a problem in school-age males. These substances are toxic to the body and can cause damage to the internal organs, anaemia, neurological damage and heart arrhythmia. Until approximately 1990 glue sniffing was the biggest problem; since then use of gases and aerosols has become more common. Most deaths and injuries, however, do not occur from the drug itself but from the environmental dangers, i.e. young boys may suffocate while using a plastic bag to sniff glue or may inhabit unsafe places such as canals and railway embankments while trying to hide their escapades. Others die when, intoxicated, they fall, knock themselves out and then asphyxiate on their own vomit (Rathod, 1992).
- **Minor analgesic** - asprin and paracetamol are in the depressant class and taken with cola or beer can give a minor euphoria.

Hallucinogens

Hallucinogens alter perceptions of reality, causing an altered state of consciousness or 'trip'. The senses are often heightened and hallucinations affecting space and colour along with auditory or tactile effects may occur. Occasionally there is a delusional lack of insight (e.g. a person tries to fly). Hallucinogens are taken in microdot form, meaning a tiny quantity of the substance on a piece of blotting paper is taken orally. Their effects last between 3 and 12 hours in general, but the drug can be stored in fat cells and then be discharged up to two years later, causing a 'flashback'. Whilst not physically addictive or damaging, the psychological damage can be vast. A 'bad trip' includes low mood, frightening psychotic experiences and an overriding sense of despair. Fears experienced while 'tripping' can induce phobias which may have numerous psychological triggers. Some examples of hallucinogens are:

- **Lysergic acid diethylamide (LSD)** - commonly known as 'acid'. Usually taken orally in microdot form or 'tabs' this drug has been popular as a recreational drug since the 1960s when altered states of consciousness were first examined in a public arena. It is still commonly used in youth and dance cultures.
- **Angel Dust or PCP** - this drug, phencyclide, can be taken transcutaneously so it may even be absorbed through the skin.
- **Ecstasy** - Half stimulant and half hallucinogen, this drug is used mainly by the youth and dance cultures (see Stimulants).
- **Magic Mushrooms** - 'Magic Mushrooms' refer to certain fungi, algae and lichen which contain the drug psilocybin.

Epidemiology of drug and alcohol problems in the general population

It is notoriously difficult to estimate the problems of drug and alcohol addiction in the general population because of major problems in finding people who admit to drug use, particularly of illegal substances. Different definitions make research difficult, e.g. addiction, dependence, abuse, misuse, problematic use. Addiction is stigmatized and in some cases illegal so it would be fair to assume there is a dramatic under-recording of drug and alcohol consumption.

Bearing in mind the problems with case definition indicated above, the Office of Population Census and Statistics (1988) estimated that 8% of men and 2% of women over the age of 16 admitted to drinking at a level that posed 'risk' or is 'unsafe'. The Royal College of Psychiatrists (1986) estimated that at least 300 000 people in the UK were 'alcohol-dependent'. In western Europe and Scandinavia the lifetime risk of suffering from serious problem drinking ('alcoholism') is estimated at 3-5% for men and 0.1-1% for women (Goodwill, 1989). Life-time risks are reported to be up to 20% for men and 10% for women in the USA (Schuckit, 1989) which leads to a suspicion that more inclusive definitions of 'problem drinking' were used in the USA research. Other research by McCornell (1986) estimated that 5% of Americans 'cannot voluntarily control their drinking'.

One source of information about patterns of drug addiction in England and Wales is the Home Office Index. Whenever a person with an addiction to certain opioids (including diamorphine and heroin) or cocaine is seen, medical practitioners are obliged to submit confidential data to the Home Office in London. Although this information provides a substantial under-estimate of the drug problem, it does supply data on trends of drug use. Recent figures are:

- 1977 3600 users
- 1980 5100
- 1983 10 200
- 1986 14 800
- 1988 19 200
- 1991 24 000

Epidemiology of drug and alcohol problems in the deaf population

Estimates of the incidence of drug and alcohol problems in the deaf population vary greatly. Steitler (1984) estimated that more than one million deaf Americans need 'substance abuse counselling' and that between one-quarter and one-third of all deaf Americans with mental health problems have problematic drug or alcohol use. Comparison between deaf and hearing populations range from a lower incidence (Adler, 1983) to a higher risk (Steitler, 1984). Block (1965) stated that there were three possible scenarios associated with the relative alcohol use by deaf people compared to hearing people.

The first hypothesis would be that the deaf would drink more to cope with additional stresses in their life caused by being deaf (i.e. self-medicate). Secondly, it could be hypothesized that by learning to adjust and deal with problems from a very early age, before alcohol was available, deaf people have found alternative coping methods to alcohol, resulting in reduced prevalence. The third hypothesis, that the two groups would drink the same amount comes from the view that the problems of existence which influence one's alcohol use are much more complex than audiology alone: relationships, money, jobs, media influences and so on. Most research, however, suggests that deaf people have at least the same risk of developing problems with their drug and alcohol use as hearing people (Johnson and Lock, 1978; Issacs, Buckley and Martin, 1979). Thus, in the USA, McCrone (1982) estimates that in the deaf population there 'may be 73 000 deaf alcoholics, 8500 deaf heroin users, 14 700 deaf cocaine users, and 110 000 deaf people who use marijuana on a regular basis'. Issacs, Buckley and Martin (1979) predict that the number of drug and alcohol users will rise among the deaf population as it has in the general population.

Issacs, Buckley and Martin (1979) in the USA, commenting on research into the use of alcohol by deaf people, said 'It is a sobering fact that we know more about a few thousand Lepch of the Himalayas than we do about the estimated 13 million hearing-impaired persons in our country'.

Researching drug and alcohol use in a deaf population

Research in this area is a fairly modern phenomenon. The first published acknowledgment of a Deaf person's need for drug or alcohol treatment was an Alcoholics Anonymous (AA) newsletter article by a recovering deaf alcoholic (BJ, 1968).

Research in the tightknit Deaf community may be limited by difficulties gaining their trust, suggest Issacs, Buckley and Martin (1979), in whose sample only 39 out of a possible 120 of their deaf subjects consented to being interviewed about their alcohol consumption. Watson, Boros and Zrimec (1979), in America, said that accurate statistics are unavailable as 'Deaf alcoholics are generally unreached, untreated and uncounted throughout the nation'. If deaf people are loath to attend treatment facilities or take part in research, or they do not know that either exists, the result will be unrepresentative and inaccurate statistics.

Accurate statistics are required to secure funding (Moses and Rendon, 1992). Hence, an impasse is quickly reached where, without funding, services will not be provided, and without services the statistics required to secure funding cannot be collected. The BDA (1995) claims that while social workers and educators deny the scale of the problem there will be no cause to mobilize the funding necessary for educational resources or outreach work.

Methodologically, variations in definitions of deafness may cause as much trouble as the definition of the particular type of drug use being researched. In the UK there is no comprehensive register of deaf people so random sampling is difficult: many a skewed population has been identified by choosing particular Deaf clubs, residential schools or social work case lists. Issacs, Buckley and Martin (1979) stated that by using such sampling techniques only those people who identify themselves as part of the Deaf community will be sampled. Given the severe problems of access to training for Deaf people, resulting in few individuals being qualified in research, it will commonly be the case that hearing researchers will be studying deaf people (Baker-Shenk and Kyle, 1990). This may result in deaf people feeling patronized and bring response rates down. For those deaf people whose preferred or first language is sign language then the hearing researchers' lack of ability in sign may restrict accurate information exchange. Similarly, written questionnaires may not be valid or response rates may be extremely low in a population whose adult average reading age is approximately 8.75 years (Conrad, 1979). Baker-Shenk and Kyle (1990) purport that failure to deal with such difficulties will undermine the validity of supposedly objective results.

Services for deaf drug and alcohol users

Given that the first public acknowledgment of a deaf person with an alcohol problem occurred only in 1968 it is not entirely surprising that there is a dearth of appropriate services for those Deaf people who are having problems with their drug or alcohol use. The Hearing Society of San Franscico was the first to address this problem in the mid-1970s by designing a service to aid deaf people in accessing generic alcohol treatment services and providing interpreters to residential treatment centres and police stations (Gorey, 1979).

Between 1975 and 1980 a few states in the USA established isolated treatment services, either residential or outpatient. Some provided services specifically for deaf people and some provided either integration with, or access to, hearing services. It was not until the American Deafness and Rehabilitation Association (ADARA) held its annual meeting in Texas in 1978 that the sharing of ideas began. Alcohol Intervention for the Deaf (AID) in Ohio subsequently sponsored special national conferences on deafness and drug use and promoted the sharing of information, evaluation of services and the accumulation and transmitting of findings. Further impetus was added in the USA during 1990 when Gallaudet University hosted the 'National Conference of Substance Abuse in the Deaf Community'.

Watson, Boros and Zrimec (1979) reported their belief that deaf drug users are unreached, untreated and uncounted. They said that the majority of services were designed for hearing people, where the counsellors have no knowledge of the psychosocial aspects of deafness and cannot use sign language. Boros (1981) suggests that this results in deaf people being neither diagnosed nor treated, whilst Hetherington (1979) reports that deaf people are 'bounced' from agency to agency getting help for everything except the alcohol (or drug) problems. He also claims that professionals in hearing services will not accept responsibility for the provision of services to this group. Boros (1979) claims that, similarly, Deaf experts shy away from working with this group as they do not have the alcohol expertise. Watson, Boros and Zrimec (1979) conclude that 'The deaf alcoholic faces a bleak situation'.

There is no consensus as to whether services should be designed to be integrated with hearing services, or independent and for only deaf people. Issacs, Buckley and Martin (1979) feel that alcohol and drugs should be handled by the general population, regardless of the audiological status of the user. They suggested that Deaf services would be concerned with issues of deafness and added that the deaf were not all in the same geographical region, so accessing Deaf-only services would not be easy. Glow (1989) reported that Deaf services should be mainstreamed so as to uphold the right of deaf people to equal access to services.

Ferrell and George (1984) describe interventions in Tucson where the Arizona State School for the Deaf and Blind had released high school students from classes to attend captioned films about 'Substance Abuse' and arranged talks with local police and teenage alcoholics. A committee was formed in 1982 comprising members of the Tucson Community Outreach Program for the Deaf (COPD) and the Association for Drug Abuse and Alcoholism Prevention and Treatment Inc (ADAPT); this committee decided to focus its attention on educating the professionals in deafness about alcohol, rather than educating the alcohol professionals about deafness. Ferrell and George (1984) conclude that Watson, Boros and Zrimec (1979) were unduly pessimistic and that the future for the deaf alcohol abuser (in Tucson at least) is not so bleak.

McCrone (1982) recommends that agencies adopt a philosophy of valuing all people, including deaf citizens who communicate manually, and suggests various means of increasing a Deaf user's access to a hearing drug service. These included the provision of a textphone (a telephone which enables deaf people to type to each other over a phone line), the use of certified sign language interpreters and education of staff in sign language. Boros (1981) adds that translation of written material into a simplified form to cope with the lower average reading age of deaf people is beneficial, as is a slightly longer admission to allow for the repetition of educational information which may be totally new to the deaf client. Adler (1983) added that as many deaf people have been neglected or patronized by their families, and later by professionals, it may take a great deal of time to build their trust.

Boros (1981) reported that in Cleveland, USA, where the AID project prepared alcohol agencies to treat deaf clients, integrating their clients into hospital programmes did not prove problematic, but finding 'half-way houses' and after-care facilities willing to accept deaf clients was very difficult. Facilities were unwilling to fund interpreters, and the support mechanisms available as a matter of course to hearing clients, such as AA, were rarely accessible. A1-Anon and Alateen groups were non-existent.

When analysing obstacles to treatment, the AID Project found the lack of available qualified interpreters was the problem most frequently encountered. Boros (1981) states that even with interpreters, much of the therapeutic milieu of a treatment centre is lost as only essential sessions and interviews are interpreted. McCune (1988) found that deaf adolescents on a hearing psychiatric ward experienced re-enactments of the frustrations of isolation, personal inadequacy and inability to share thoughts and feelings that results from linguistic isolation.

Boros (1981) says that to ascertain the relative benefits of integrated versus segregated treatment facilities, a comparative research programme would be required. Given the absence of segregated programmes, Boros says that the existing network of treatment facilities can be made accessible to the Deaf through skilled, knowledgeable intervention by advocacy workers. However, the Department of Alcohol and Drug Programs of California published a set of recommendations regarding drug services provided to disabled participants: 59% of the 569 services surveyed could not serve deaf and hearing-impaired clients (Erickson and Lowe, 1988).

A further study in Southern California surveying 27 treatment programmes found that 99.7% of them did not provide ASL interpreters (even though 45% of the programmes were required to do so) and most reported that interpreters would not be paid for by the treatment programmes or by the person's insurance (The Seed, 1987). Whitehouse, Sherman and Kozlowski (1991) found many services tended to use family members or volunteers to interpret, or used the written word and believed this often violated confidentiality and clients' rights.

Thus, whilst it may be possible to adapt general (hearing) services to meet Deaf people's needs, in reality it may not be happening. Rendon (1992), researching in Alameda County (USA) estimates that of the deaf people statistically expected to have problems with alcohol or drugs, only 1% have been part of 'traditional or non-traditional recovery programmes including Alcoholics Anonymous and Narcotics Anonymous'. Whitehouse, Sherman and Kozlowski (1991), in their survey, found that there was a gap between what was desirable and the provision that agencies were actually willing to implement. For example, over half of the agencies surveyed said they needed training on Deaf issues, but 60% said they did not need a textphone.

There are very few inpatient units in the USA specifically for deaf people with drug or alcohol problems (Larson and McAlpine, 1988). Many have closed due to insufficient funding, and others offer treatment only to patients from within the state or to those who have private insurance.

Whitehouse, Sherman and Kozlowski (1991) purport that 'The complexity of the disability and the isolation from the general population which Deaf people uniquely experience justify specialized services.' They add that mainstream services are ineffective and costly. They recommend specialized facilities, with staff well trained in sign language and Deaf culture, technological and structural adaptations such as flashing door bells, affirmative action to employ deaf staff, and additional staff available to tackle other complex needs of deaf people, i.e. a communication specialist and a teacher of the deaf.

There are no specialized inpatient facilities for deaf people with drug and alcohol problems in the UK at present, although plans are afoot in the south of England to develop a rehabilitation hostel.

In the UK there are three generic psychiatric services for the deaf (each with inpatient and outpatient treatment facilities) and a few voluntary Deaf agencies which provide some counselling facilities, e.g. the British Deaf Association (BDA) and the Royal Association in Aid of Deaf People (RAD). In 1987 the BDA established 'Aids Ahead', an organization focusing on issues of HIV/AIDS. Since 1991 the BDA renamed the service the Health Promotions Service and broadened its remit to include other areas of health need, such as drugs and alcohol. The accessibility of health services to deaf people was studied (BDA, 1995) and it was found that of the 112 people sampled, only 17.6% had ever had an interpreter present for consultation with their GP and only 19.6% had ever had an interpreter for a hospital or clinic stay or consultation. Most were unsure of their entitlement to an interpreter and none were clear who should or did provide one. In the USA the 'Americans with Disabilities Act' makes equality of access a requirement of law. In the UK, however, where the equivalent law is less assertive, interpreter provision is *ad hoc* and often determined by the goodwill of the service provider or the assertiveness of the customer.

If, as Rendon (1992) claims, only 1% of deaf people with drug and alcohol problems have engaged in treatment, we need to ask why. It may be that the services provided to deaf people are insufficient or that they are of the wrong type (integration was provided when, in fact, segregation was required or vice versa, and so on). Moser and Rendon (1992) acknowledge the lack of formal research but advocate that a choice in types of programme be available to deaf clients; e.g. mainstreamed, specialized or deaf-run. In the UK, a similar recommendation was made by Alcohol Concern (1987) that all clients should have some choice: that there should be enough services available to enable clients to choose between at least two different types of help. Until there are comparative data we cannot draw conclusions. However, just as a number of interacting factors created a deaf person who uses drugs or alcohol, so there will probably be a number of interacting factors preventing Deaf people from accessing and using treatment.

Factors leading to increased likelihood of drug use

An interplay of three aspects of a person's life determines what sort of choices they make concerning drug and alcohol use: the agent, the environment, and the host (see Figure 10.1).

The agent refers to the drug or drugs (or other behaviour in the wider addictive behaviour sense) that the person chooses to use. A number of factors will determine whether, and (if so) how, a drug is used. There are three that are most powerful.

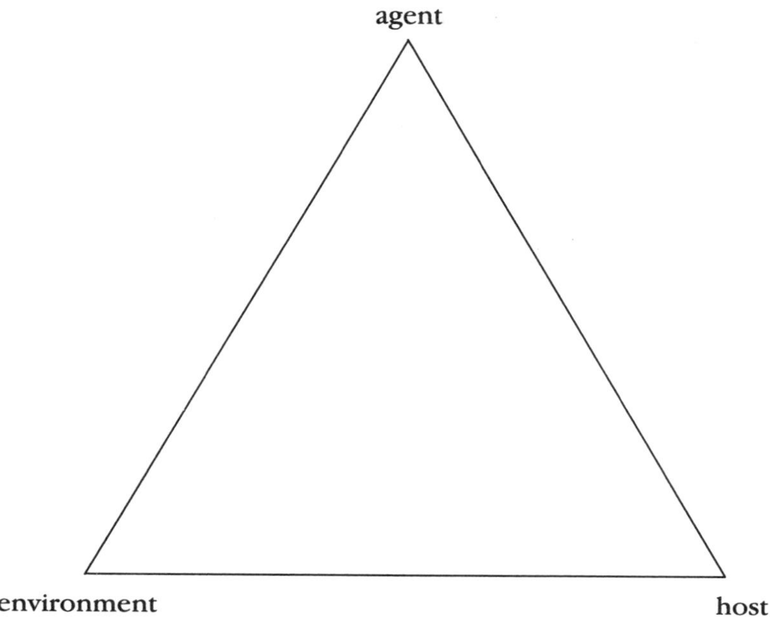

Figure 10.1

Factors for addiction

- **Pleasure** - the nicer and more pleasurable the drug is, the more addictive it will be. The major tranquillizers rarely become addictive as their effects are quite unpleasant. Whether the 'hit' is pleasurable will be affected largely by personal preference but also by the purity of the drug, the mixture of drugs taken, the psychological and physical disposition of the user, the expectation and experience of the user, tolerance or cross-tolerance to particular drugs, social setting and peer pressure, date of last use and knowledge of the various rituals associated with obtaining, preparing and using the drug (MacDonald and Patterson, 1991).
- **Immediacy** - the quicker a drug works the higher its addictive potential. The route of drug introduction determines the time it takes to reach the bloodstream and therefore the immediacy of the hit. Drugs which can be taken intravenously, intramuscularly, smoked or taken anally are the fastest acting. Drugs like antidepressants, which take two weeks to work, or depot injections of antipsychotics, which may take 4-5 weeks to work, are unlikely to become addictive. Immediacy is vital in addiction as it facilitates many very powerful behaviour reinforcers: *'I sniff this liquid I feel calm'* or *'I swallow this tablet then I feel happy'*. You are sure that the tablet gave you the pleasure as opposed to a slower-acting drug where you may not be clear what acted to provide the pleasure, i.e. in the case of an antidepressant, *'I took this tablet,*

went to work all week, met friends at the weekend, slept well, spoke to my doctor and felt better'.

- **Come-down** - the worse the 'Come-down' or withdrawal from a drug, the more addictive it is. Behavioural reinforcers (in some cases combined with physical craving) build connections between not taking the particular drug and feeling bad.

Thus, a combination of factors: a fast-acting drug which feels pleasurable when on it and feels dreadful when off it is a recipe for addiction. 'Crack' fits the description perfectly and its danger was once pointed out by a national newspaper using the headline '7 seconds to Heaven'.

Other factors affecting addictive potential are **availability** and **cost**.

The environment refers to the places and company in which a person uses drugs. For example, a Deaf club where activity revolves round the bar and a drinking culture will increase both availability and social acceptability of alcohol use. Social reinforcement affects both the type and amount of a drug used: an older person is unlikely to be socially reinforced to use solvents, whereas alcohol may be more acceptable. Some environments are such that drugs or alcohol may go unnoticed for a long time, e.g. staff in pubs or in the entertainment industry are forgiven for being disinhibited as it often entertains and benefits others.

Where a deaf person is mixing with hearing people, his or her intoxicated language behaviour may go unrecognized and be inadvertently reinforced. Steitler (1984) in the USA reports that there is widespread resistance among educators, parents and others to recognize warning signs of drug problems in deaf people. The BDA (1995) in the UK reports that social workers have been denying the scale of drug and alcohol problems.

Whilst parents and older people may not consciously reinforce drug use they may model drug-using behaviour. Many parents have admonished their child for drug use whilst smoking and drinking regularly themselves. Similarly, children brought up in families where there is heavy drug or alcohol use are more at risk of developing such problems themselves. Sociological theories claim that drug use provides escape from poor living conditions, unemployment and low expectations.

Watson, Boros and Zrimec (1979) believe that for a person with a drug problem, the Deaf community in America can be a barrier to recovery as it has severely stigmatized drunkenness as an unacceptable indication of sin and character weakness. As a result, the Deaf community has collectively denied any problem. Having got rid of the label of 'deaf and dumb' they do not now want to be labelled 'deaf and drunk'.

Issacs, Buckley and Martin (1979) said that attempts to establish formal recovery programmes had been met with denial by the Deaf community. Larson and McAlpine (1988) put this down to a lack of understanding of the disease model of chemical dependency resulting in moralistic attitudes which lead to people being fearful of admitting they have a problem (the first step to recovery in the 12-step approach) (Lane, 1989). Rendon (1992) says that such denial on the part of the individual and the community lays the groundwork for an increased incidence of drug use in the deaf community. Similar problems have not been identified in the UK deaf population. This may be for a number of reasons: that this area is as yet unresearched in the UK; that the British deaf population is less moralistic; that the British deaf population is better informed about the disease model (highly unlikely given the scarcity of specialized educational or treatment facilities); or that the 12-step model of abstinence, as exemplified by Alcoholics Anonymous, is less popular in the UK, making denial a less crucial concept. There is no evidence in the UK that drunkenness is particularly frowned upon in the Deaf community.

Westerlund (1993), writing on deafness and incest, points out that the Deaf world is small and that some potential clients avoid therapies as they fear that confidentiality will not be maintained or that they may accidentally meet their therapist socially.

Grant, Kramer and Nash (1982) warned that for those trying to control their drinking, or even abstain from drinking, their 'restricted social circle that may well include other Deaf alcoholics or heavy drinkers' will hinder recovery. If there are only a few other deaf people in your area then splitting from your friends and removing the only source of fluent communication is a great sacrifice.

Treatment services are most often designed for hearing people and run by hearing people. When deaf people approach there will be a meeting of two cultures: the Deaf and the Hearing. Rendon (1992) says that where the staff have no knowledge of the psychosocial aspects of deafness or sign language the result will be an encounter with confusion and ambivalence, which may cause them to avoid treatment agencies in the future.

The host Many books and articles have been written about the general (hearing) population and what sort of person with what sort of experiences may develop problems with drug or alcohol use. Theories covering individual personality dynamics, family dynamics, biological models and learning theory have been explored but are too numerous to cover here. Instead, we shall raise only issues that are more particular to deaf people. McCrone (1982) says that deaf people may use drugs to deal with their anger, a product of their experiences with hearing parents, teachers and others where they are scapegoated, infantilized and overprotected. Steitler (1984) says that deaf people may use drugs and alcohol to attain numbness and relief from their oppression. Garber and Seligman (1980) report that deaf people experience low self-concept and helplessness, which in turn creates difficulty in adjusting to deafness, and that the pain of these experiences is the core of problems with substance use. Garrison and Tesch (1978) report that deaf people have generally lower self-esteem than their hearing peers. However, it is a myth that deaf people use alcohol or drugs only to escape their deafness. This idea may be a projection of the care-givers.

Drug use is about increasing pleasurable feelings such as confidence, relaxation, happiness and/or decreasing unpleasant feelings such as sadness, anger, fear, or shame. Deaf people will share some experiences with their hearing peers and may have some that are unique and that lead to a higher prevalence (Issacs et al., 1979). Stewart (1983) says that deaf people suffer unique pressures of social isolation, loneliness, difficulties in personal relations, lack of education and inability to hold jobs.

Deafness can isolate individuals from mainstream society because of language and cultural differences. Drug use may be a way of coping with the discomfort and frustration of problems communicating with hearing people. Indeed, 95% of deaf people have hearing parents, which may create linguistic and cultural divides within families. Many deaf people were sent to boarding school at a very early age and experienced more loneliness and isolation (some were sent before they and their parents had sufficient shared language for the deaf child to comprehend where he was being sent, why and for how long). Rendon (1992) says that isolation and lack of information can increase the use of substance abuse in the deaf. Furthermore, where there is an inadequate parental relationship, drug dependency can become a substitute for the lacking healthy dependency.

Communication with hearing people who do not sign or lip-read in social situations can be an exhausting and often stressful situation. Some deaf people may drink socially to 'break the ice' and increase their perception of their success in communicating (in reality lip-reading skills decrease with alcohol). Breakwell (1986) suggested that marginalized groups may cope with stigma and threatened identity by adopting the strategy of 'passing'. The individual attempts to remove him or herself from the threatened position (i.e. being deaf) by gaining access to another group (i.e. hearing) under false pretences. Additionally, lack of positive deaf role models increases the risk of the deaf person's making efforts to 'pass' which may elevate the risk of drug use. Living a lie and living in fear of being found out results in constant stress and a feeling of inferiority. The isolation of deafness has been likened to the loneliness of alcoholism (Rendon, 1992), leaving the deaf alcoholic doubly isolated: isolated from the general population by deafness and isolated from the Deaf community by an alcohol problem.

Another use of drugs and alcohol is in covering psychological distress. Many hearing people with drug problems have experienced sexual or physical abuse. The drug provides a pseudo power (don't feel, don't talk, don't trust). In the USA incidence of sexual abuse in the general population is estimated at 25% of girls and 10% of boys (Finkelhor, 1986). However, in deaf children it appears that 50% of girls and 54% of boys reported having experienced sexual abuse (Sullivan, Vernon and Scanlon, 1987) (see Chapter 7). Such a traumatic history may increase the risk of the individual using drugs to cope with these experiences. Furthermore, both deafness and sexual abuse can lead to perceiving the body as defective and powerless and both can be associated with loss (of childhood, of ideal family, of hearing). This creates more distress to cover up with drugs.

Cohen (1979) says that increasing numbers of deaf children are being given psychoactive medication, mostly the drug, Ritalin, to treat supposed hyperactivity. It has been observed that diagnosis of hyperactivity is inaccurate and the problem is actually restlessness and disruptive behaviour as a result of communication problems. The children being medicated may begin to associate deafness with illness, and problems with medication. Later they see self-medication either by alcohol, street drugs or prescription drugs as the only way to cope with the ordinary problems of life. Cole and Edelmann (1991) found that deaf adolescents have the same concerns as hearing adolescents but that they assumed a particular significance in the presence of deafness: that is they believed that it was because of their deafness they did not have a girlfriend/boyfriend or they argued with their parents. Such a belief eschews an intractability which is very disempowering for the deaf person, implying that whatever they do will not solve the problem as they will still be deaf.

This powerlessness is addressed in the theories of Schlesinger and Meadow (1972), who found that hearing parents are more directive with their deaf children than with their hearing offspring. They are also more controlling, intrusive, inflexible, disapproving and over-protective. As a result, the deaf person can develop an external locus of control which has disadvantages related to drug use. Firstly, they may be more easily persuaded or pressured into drug use or drug-related behaviours. Secondly, the deaf person may feel less culpable for his or her actions. This affects motivation to work at recovery and reduces perceptions of the negative effects of drug use. For example, if they have upset someone or damaged something when drunk, the deaf individual may see that as a hazard of *being drunk* rather than accepting responsibility for having *become drunk*. Whilst some issues here are factors of the altered perception of a person with an external locus of control, they are also reinforced by the very real disempowerment of deaf individuals who are commonly protected from the disincentives of continued drug use. Families which are used to over-protecting a deaf member will find the boundary setting of 'Tough Love' (where users are made totally responsible for their behaviour) very difficult to implement. Very few deaf people are prosecuted for drink–driving and only a few convictions of deaf people ever reach court. Most cases are thrown out due to difficulties in arranging appropriate sign language interpreting of the proceedings, or just because people in the judicial system feel sorry for the Deaf criminal (see Chapter 9). Deaf drug dealers know that due to poor employment prospects they are unlikely to make the same money by working or claiming benefits as they can by dealing in drugs.

Education of deaf children about drug and alcohol use is generally poor. Adolescents frequently experiment with alcohol, drugs and sex (Haffner, 1988). Overprotection leads schools to refuse to use realistic information with children. Deafness creates barriers to many types of incidental learning, such as TV, radio, gossip and overhearing adults talking. Newspapers and other written material may be inaccessible due to the generally lower average reading skills. McCrone (1982) says that this can result in accidental drug overdose because the deaf person has not learned about drug tolerance, purity/impurity or drug interactions. In the absence of school education the result will be 'peer pressure education'.

Deaf youths are often away at boarding school or attend school a long way from home. In their home town they often have few friends of their own age and may 'hang out' with older siblings or the more 'visual' crowd of drug- and alcohol-using or party-going groups. The older sibling or other influential person is unlikely to have sufficient communication skills to build a genuine relationship and to explain fully the complexities of the drugs. The deaf sibling, possibly desperate for attention or acceptance, joins the experimentation without sufficient information to make healthy life choices.

Not all drug use is intended to increase pleasure or create a high: some drug use is motivated by a desire to decrease negative experiences. Just as hearing people do, deaf people may use drugs to 'self-medicate' for a variety of problems: that is to try to control their anxiety, depression, physical pain, or even schizophrenia. There is no evidence that deaf people have higher rates of any of these problems; however, lack of access to generic medical and psychiatric facilities may make a deaf person less likely to access formal help and more likely to self-medicate. Similarly, lack of access to information may lead a person to use a remedy which works in the short term but is detrimental in the long term. For example, tinnitus, experienced by both deaf and hearing people, can be very distressing and sufferers can get short-term relief by drug or alcohol use. However, in the long term, this is not an effective coping strategy.

Conclusion

It seems from most of the research that the prevalence of drug and alcohol use in the deaf and general population is similar. However, there is a lack of services that are truly accessible for deaf people. This dearth includes everything from education and prevention, to treatment programmes such as detoxification and relapse prevention. This lack of accessibility begs the question of whether the samples used to estimate prevalence were, in fact, an accurate representation of the whole deaf population. The dilemma is raised that, without accurate statistics, funding for appropriate services will not be provided.

Even given the present estimates of prevalence there are not enough services available to meet the needs of those deaf drug and alcohol users. There is, as yet, no consensus as to whether integrated or segregated services are preferable and there have not been any comparative studies. The recommendation that clients be offered a choice of treatment styles or recovery programmes does not seem to fit easily with either the paucity of funding and treatment facilities or with the desire to discover the one right type of treatment approach.

Whilst deaf people are vulnerable to all of the same risk factors as are hearing people, they may have some unique additional vulnerabilities that are connected to their deafness and their experience of being a deaf person in a predominantly hearing world. For equality of access, education, prevention and treatment facilities must embrace the chosen communication style of the deaf person and have an understanding of the psychological aspects of deafness.

Perhaps the relative lack of deaf services reflects society's attempt to sanitize that which may embarrass or shock. Paternalism would have us care for 'the deaf' so that they experience no additional difficulties. Professionals feel it is their responsibility to ensure that deaf people do not have drug or alcohol problems. We do not have the power to ensure this but we can pretend by the censorship of services and thus our very language. If there are few services for deaf drug users, there are fewer opportunities to discuss deaf people with drug problems. Thus we can pretend that deaf people do not have drug problems. It is so much easier than admitting our own powerlessness over others, even those we perceive to be less fortunate than ourselves.

Perhaps we are patronizing deaf people if we expect them to have fewer drug or drug-related problems than hearing people. As people, we should expect deaf youth to experiment recreationally with drugs; we should be prepared for a lesser number to develop more serious problems; we should not be surprised to meet deaf drug dealers or to hear of drug-related deaths. It is not wrong to want there to be fewer deaf people with drug or alcohol problems, but hope will not secure this. For this goal to be achieved, services are needed that not only equal but exceed those open to hearing people.

References

Adler EP (1983) Vocational rehabilitation as an intervenor in substance abuse services to deaf people. In Watson D, Steitler K, Peterson P, Fulton W (eds) Mental Health, Substance Abuse and Deafness. Silver Spring. MD: American Deafness and Rehabilitation Association.

Alcohol Concern (1987) Alcohol Services Information Pack.

Baker-Shenk C, Kyle JG (1990) Research with deaf people: issues and conflicts. Disability, Handicap and Society 5: 1.

BDA (1995) British Deaf Association: Survey of Deaf People's Health Habits. BDA Health Promotion Services Report.

Betros ES (1974) Drug Abuse Prevention: Report of the Temporary State Commission to Evaluate the Drug Laws. Albany, NY: NY State Legislative Document, No. 11.

BJ (1968) AA and the Deaf Mute. The Grapevine, December: 32–33.
Block MA (1965) Alcoholism: Its Facets and Phases. New York: Day.
Boros A (1979) Role of action research in services for the deaf alcoholic. Journal of Rehabilitation of the Deaf 12: 1–5.
Boros A (1981) Alcoholism intervention for the deaf. Alcohol Health and Research World Special Issue: The Multidisabled 5: 26–30.
Breakwell GM (1986) Coping with Threatened Identities. London: Methuen.
Cohen MJ (ed)(1979) Drugs and the Special Child. New York: Gardiner Press.
Cole SH, Edelmann RJ (1991) Identity patterns and self- and teacher perceptions of problems for deaf adolescents: a research note. Journal of Child Psychology and Psychiatry 32: 1159–1165.
Conrad R (1979) The Deaf School Child: Language and Cognitive Function. London: Harper & Row.
Dixon A (1982) Incidence of solvent use amongst young people in North London. Unpublished research.
Donovan DM, Marlatt GA (1988) Assessment of Addictive Behaviours. New York: Guilford Press.
Edwards G, Chandler J, Hansman C (1972) Drinking in a London suburb. Quarterly Journal of Studies on Alcohol (Supplement) 6: 69.
Erickson J, Lowe L (1988) Summary and Recommendations of the Alcohol and Drug Services Provided to Disabled Participants in California. Sacramento, CA: State of California Department of Alcohol and Drug Programs.
Ferrell R, George JD (1984) One community's response to alcohol problems among the Deaf community. Journal of Rehabilitation of the Deaf 18: 15–18.
Finklehor D (1986) A Sourcebook on Child Sexual Abuse. Beverey Hills, CA: Sage Publications.
Garber J, Seligman MEP (eds) (1980) Human Helplessness, Theory and Applications. New York: Academic Press.
Garrison WM, Tesch S (1978) Self concept and deafness: review of research literature. Volta Review, December, 457–466.
Glow BA (1989) Alcoholism, drugs and the disabled. In Lawson G, Lawson AW (eds) Alcoholism and Substance Abuse in Special Populations. Rockville, MD: Aspen Publishers. pp. 65–93.
Goodwill DW (1989) Alcoholism. In Kaplin HI, Sadock BJ (eds) Comprehensive Textbook of Psychiatry V. Baltimore, MD: Williams & Wilkins.
Gorey J (1979) Rational alcoholism services for hearing impaired people. Journal of Rehabilitation of the Deaf 12: 6–8.
Grant TN, Kramer CA, Nash K (1982) Working with deaf alcoholics in a vocational training program. Journal of Rehabilitation of the Deaf 15: 14–20.
Haffner DW (1988) Aids and adolescents: school health education must begin now. Journal of School Health. 58: 154–155.
Hetherington RG (1979) Deafness and alcoholism. Journal of Rehabilition of the Deaf 12: 9–12.
Israel J, Cunningham M, Thumann H, Arnos KS (1992) Genetic counselling for deaf adults: communication/language and cultural considerations. Journal of Genetic Counselling 1: 135–153.
Issacs M, Buckley G, Martin D (1979) Patterns of drinking among the deaf American. Journal of Drug and Alcohol Abuse 6: 463–476.
Johnson S, Lock R (1978) Student Drug Use in a School for the Deaf. Paper presented at the National Drug Abuse Conference, Seattle, Washington (1978).
Lane KE (1989) Substance abuse among the deaf population: an overview of current strategies, programs and barriers to recovery. Journal of the American Deaf Rehabilitation Assocation 22: 79–85.

Larson EW, McAlpine DE (1988) Treating the hearing impaired in a standard chemical dependency unit. Journal of Studies on Alcohol 49: 381–383.

MacDonald D, Patterson V (1991) A Handbook of Drug Training: Learning about Drugs and Working with Drug Users. London and New York: Routledge.

McCornell JV (1986) Understanding Human Behaviour. The University of Michigan: Holt, Rinehart & Winston.

McCrone WP (1982) Serving the deaf substance abuser. Journal of Psychoactive Drugs 14: 199–203.

McCune N (1988) Deaf in a hearing unit: coping of staff and adolescents. Journal of Adolescence 11: 21–28.

Moser N, Rendon ME (1992) Alcohol and drug services: a jigsaw puzzle. Journal of the American Deaf Rehabilitation Association 26: 18–21.

Orford J (1985) Excessive Appetites: A Psychological View of Addictions. Chichester: Wiley.

Pyke JM, Littman SK (1982) A psychiatric clinic for the deaf. Canadian Journal of Psychiatry 27: 384–389.

Rathod NH (ed) (1992) Substance Abuse – A Layman's Guide (second edition). Mid Downs Health Authority.

Release (1982) The Trouble with Tranquillizers. UK: Release Publications.

Rendon ME (1992) Deaf culture and alcohol and substance abuse. Journal of Substance Abuse Treatment 9: 103–110.

Royal College of Physicians (1987) (statistics on alcohol and medical admissions).

Schlesinger HP, Meadows KP (1972) Development of maturity in deaf children. Exceptional Children, February, 461–467.

Schuckit MA (1989) Drug and Alcohol Abuse: a Clinical Guide to Diagnosis and Treatment (third edition). New York: Plenum Medical Books.

Steitler KAL (1984) Substance abuse and the deaf adolescent. In Anderson GB, Watson D (eds) The Habilitation and Rehabilitation of Deaf Adolescents. Wagoner, OK: University of Arkansas Rehabilitation Research and Training Center on Deafness and Hearing Impairment.

Stewart LG (1983) Hearing impaired substance abusers. ALMACAN Newsletter, April.

Sullivan PM, Vernon M, Scanlon J (1987) Sexual abuse of deaf youth. American Annals of the Deaf, October, 132: 256–262.

The Seed (1987) Summer, 4–5.

Watson EW, Boros A, Zrimec GL (1979) Mobilization of services for deaf alcoholics. Alcohol, Health and Research World, Winter: 33–38.

Westerlund (1993) Thinking about Incest, Deafness and Counselling Nagler, Mark et al (eds) (1993) Perspective on Disability (second edition), Test and readings on disability, pp 341–344. Pal Alto, CA.

Whitehouse A, Sherman RE, Kozlowski K (1991) The needs of deaf substance abusers in Illinois. American Journal of Drug and Alcohol Abuse 17: 103–113.

Chapter 11
Acquired Deafness

KATIA GILHOME HERBST

Introduction

It is an example of the very imprecise nature of our language that someone who has slight to moderate difficulty with hearing in their later years, and someone who is profoundly hearing-impaired from birth, are still referred to as 'deaf' by the general public. For their part, the pre-lingually deaf community and those who are acquainted with their world use the term 'deaf' solely to describe deaf people whose usual way of communication is with sign.

This chapter is concerned with those people who totally or partially lose their hearing after the acquisition of language — those whose deafness is acquired and whose natural way of communication tends to remain the spoken word.

The imprecision in the meaning of the word 'deaf' is both the cause and the effect of much misunderstanding. Indeed, an Office of Population Censuses and Surveys (OPCS) study on public attitudes to deafness carried out in 1980 contributed little to the subject by virtue of the feeling of the researchers that:

> ... it would have been asking too much of informants to press them to distinguish between the different categories of deafness such as ... those deaf since birth and those who became deaf later in life after acquiring language. (Bunting, 1981, p. 3)

Society is far from neutral in its attitude to different disabilities. These attitudes are deeply rooted in our culture and not easy to understand. Deafness is a hidden disorder and very difficult to imagine. It tends to handicap the 'unafflicted' during social intercourse almost as much as it does the deaf. This can transform a deaf person into a frustrating and even a frightening companion and may substantially discomfit hearing people.

Acquired deafness is often used by playwrights and novelists to represent a breakdown in meaningful communication with the world and to depict the unimportant or slightly ludicrous. Not so blindness. Blindness is used to depict the tragic and romantic. A blind man may even represent trustworthiness and particular intellectual foresight. The 'none-so-deaf-as-those-who-will-not-hear' connotations of deafness are not paralleled by any proverb which accuses a blind man of peeping when he wants to see. This difference of attitude towards blindness and deafness is wonderfully described by Lesley Jones in a personal account, *Living with Hearing Loss* (Jones, 1987).

Our society mistrusts and dislikes acquired deafness which, unlike its sister handicap blindness, holds no poignant beauty and no heroic overtones. It is a disability that is not explicitly included in the targets for The Health of the Nation (HMSO, 1992). These refer almost solely to rehabilitation services for people with mental and physical disabilities. There is evidence to suggest that there may be one-third more people suffering from deafness than from visual impairment (Martin, Meltzer and Elliot, 1988). None the less, the incomes of those charities working for blind people exceed those of charities working for the deaf by a factor of eight (Charities Aid Foundation, 1993). People prefer to give money to blind people rather than to deaf people.

There are, of course, two further connotations of 'deafness' which make it very different from blindness. The first is the very apparent similarity between the symptoms of 'deafness' and those of some types of mental disorder. These symptoms often encourage people to talk to and treat deaf and hard-of-hearing people as if their cognitive abilities were impaired. The second is that it is commonly known to be associated with ageing — even used to depict or characterize old age. Indeed, in our profoundly ageist society, it could be argued that much of society's dislike of acquired deafness is derived from its very synonymity with old age and all its much stereotyped attendant frailties — including loss of intellectual capacity.

Denial of the presence of hearing loss in the face of obvious difficulties has for many years been noted by researchers and clinicians interested in the welfare of those with acquired deafness (Menninger, 1924; Berry, 1933; Wilkins, 1950; Townsend and Wedderburn, 1965; Humphrey, Gilhome Herbst and Faruqi, 1981; Hetu et al., 1990; Gilhome Herbst, Meredith and Stephens, 1991; Chmiel and Jerger, 1993).

Indeed, Hetu and colleagues both in 1990 and in 1996 confirm the suggestion of earlier researchers (Phillips, 1957; Goffman, 1963) that denying the presence of the disability is an essential protecting mechanism for those with acquired hearing loss (Hetu et al., 1990; Hetu, 1996).

The thesis of this chapter will rotate around the following premise. Acquired deafness is a socially hated disorder. Its prevalence is great — particularly amongst old people — and it is known to be age-related. It is largely kept hidden. There may be many reasons why it is concealed but probably one of the major ones — and the most intractable — is deliberate denial by the sufferer.

Such denial — although a natural defence mechanism against society's disapproval — compounds with the disabling and handicapping nature of the disorder to serious personal cost. Furthermore, those who do not acknowledge their difficulties, for whatever reason, are unlikely to request, or accept, deafness-specific services.

Prevalence

Until the 1980s, estimates of the presence of hearing loss were based upon a study carried out between 1946 and 1947 by the OPCS in order to estimate how many free hearing aids were likely to be required when the new NHS Act of 1946 was to come into force. As a secondary objective only, it was hoped that some assessment of the prevalence and incidence of deafness in the adult population would be arrived at (Wilkins, 1950). A seven-point scale was used, based upon a subjective, or self-estimate, measure of hearing difficulty. Since healthcare is a service provided primarily on demand — and since probable demand for hearing aids was the point of the study — this was a more or less satisfactory method.

The presence of hearing impairment in the elderly had been noted by many researchers since the early 1940s in their quest to assess the needs of elderly people that would have to be met by the new welfare state. The presence of the disorder was always established by self-report only. In this way, it was estimated that about 30% of all those of retirement age had some form of hearing loss (Gilhome Herbst and Humphrey, 1981).

Such estimates were frankly challenged by two community studies on elderly people, using audiometric techniques to establish the presence of hearing loss. One was undertaken in London (Gilhome Herbst and Humphrey, 1980). The other was carried out in Scotland (Milne, 1976, cited in Gilhome Herbst, 1983). Both these studies used audiometry and found that some 60% (and not 30%) of the retired population probably had some significant hearing loss. These findings were confirmed more recently by other researchers (also using audiometric techniques) investigating the presence of hearing loss amongst older people in the Welsh Valleys (Gilhome Herbst, Meredith and Stephens, 1991).

'Deafness' was defined in all three studies as an average loss over the speech frequencies at 1, 2 and 4 kHz of 35 dB or more in the better ear — a loss of 35 dB being generally regarded as reflecting a level of impairment sufficient to necessitate the use of a hearing aid (Table 11.1).

Between 1980 and 1986, the Institute of Hearing Research in Nottingham embarked upon the first large-scale national study of the prevalence of deafness which did not rely solely on self-report, the National Study on Hearing (NSH). Its findings are based upon data from 2708 people aged 18–80 years who underwent audiological investigation

Table 11.1 Prevalence of hearing impairment in older populations

	Inner London* (%)	Edinburgh** (%)	Welsh village*** (%)
Total population aged ≥ 70 years	60	68	77.5
Total population aged ≥ 80 years	82	94	93

*Gilhome Herbst and Humphrey (1980).
**Milne (1980) cited in Gilhome Herbst (1983).
***Gilhome Herbst, Meredith and Stephens (1991).

Table 11.2 Estimate of the prevalence of hearing impairment as a percentage of people in the UK aged 18–80 years, with different degrees of severity of hearing impairment in the better ear*

Severity of hearing impairment (dB HL)	Prevalence estimate	Low CI	High CI
25+	16.1	15.0	17.3
35+	8.2	7.4	9.1
45+	3.9	3.4	4.4
55+	2.1	1.7	2.5
65+	1.1	0.8	1.4
75+	0.7	0.5	1.0
85+	0.4	0.2	0.7
95+	0.2	<0.1	0.5
105+	0.1	<0.1	0.4

•Thresholds averaged over the frequencies 0.5, 1.2 and 4 kHz to obtain an average level of hearing impairment. The low and high 95% confidence intervals (CI) are also shown. $N = 2662$ (people with acceptable audiograms).
Source: Davis (1993b).

following initial contact by postal questionnaire. The results of this study have been published widely (Davis, 1983, 1993b, 1996). Probably the most readily digestible text is that of Davis (1993b). The more recent texts include projections of the likely prevalence of hearing loss amongst populations aged 81 and over.

Using an average loss of 25 dB HL (hearing level) and greater over the speech frequencies at 0.5, 1, 2 and 4 kHz in the better ear (the better ear average, BEA) as an index of impairment, the NSH found that 16.1% of the adult population in the UK aged between 18 and 80 years had some hearing loss (Davis, 1993). This compares with the estimates based on self-report made by Wilkins (1950) of 3.6%. If people aged 81 and over were included, the prevalence of hearing impairment for the whole adult population, aged 18 or over, would rise to 20% (Davis, 1996) (Table 11.2).

It was found that most of these hearing impairments (some 87%) were of a sensorineural rather than conductive type. But as severity of loss increased so the likelihood of there being a conductive overlay also increased. This finding is important when estimating the likely benefit to be derived from wearing a hearing aid for the more severely impaired. As severity increases, so prevalence decreases. But the NSH confirmed that the prevalence of hearing impairment is significantly age-related — as is severity of impairment (Table 11.3).

Subsequent studies have employed the same method used by the NSH and have also demonstrated that prevalence of acquired hearing loss increases with age. A team from the Welsh Hearing Institute, seeking to establish the presence of hearing disability in people aged between 50 and 65 in two different populations in the Afan Valley, found that 53% in one population and 46% in the other were hearing-impaired (Stephens et al., 1990).

Two points need to be made regarding these prevalence estimates.

The first is a definitional issue. The NSH takes as a level of functional disorder a BEA of 25 dB HL, yet practitioners generally accept that the level at which it is normally considered advisable to seek amplification from a hearing aid (i.e. when hearing function is impaired to such an extent that there is a blatant need for rehabilitation) is a BEA of 35 dB HL over the same speech frequencies.

The second issue concerns the statistic of 16% of the UK adult population having some form of hearing loss; the NSH study was restricted to adults under the age of 80 years. As shown in Table 11.1, three studies, even when using a more severe criterion of 'deafness' of 35 dB HL as the

Table 11.3 National estimates of acquired deafness showing the prevalence in each age cohort at a Better Ear Average (BEA) of > 25 dB HL as a function of age and median BEA, pooled over women and men

Age group (years)	Prevalence (%)	Median BEA (dB HL)
20–24	3.0	3.8
25–29	0.8	4.5
30–34	2.7	6.0
35–39	2.3	6.3
40–44	4.8	8.0
45–49	19.7	9.3
50–54	18.5	12.3
55–59	19.0	13.0
60–64	29.7	15.0
65–69	44.2	22.5
70–74	45.4	23.3
75–79	76.6	36.0

Source: Davis (1993).

BEA, demonstrate that it is precisely after the age of 80 years that the presence of hearing impairment is most marked (Gilhome Herbst and Humphrey 1980; Milne, 1980, cited in Gilhome Herbst, 1983; Gilhome Herbst, Meredith and Stephens, 1991). In mid-1991, the estimated number of people in the UK aged 80 years and over was just over two million (Eurostat, 1991), of whom it should be estimated that some 80–90% were hearing-impaired. This was recognized by the NSH — hence the later projections, based upon extrapolations from other studies, for the whole population, including those over the age of 80.

In 1990, extrapolating from statistics offered by the NSH, the Royal College of Physicians' Report on Health Services for Adults with Physical Disabilities, Edwards and Warren suggested that by taking an average hearing level of 35 dB or more over the speech frequencies as significant impairment, the prevalence of acquired deafness in the UK adult population is approximately 10%. This produces a figure three times that estimated by Wilkins in 1950. The Report further acknowledges that this figure rises to 75% in those aged 70 years and over.

Notwithstanding the caveats mentioned, the NSH provides the best available estimates in the UK for bilateral, severe and profound hearing impairments and they must be accepted for what they are. They produce a picture of sufficient bleakness for the Royal College to suggest that hearing impairment is one of the most widespread of all physical disabilities. This is amply confirmed by the survey of the prevalence of disability among adults conducted by the OPCS, which reports that hearing disabilities are the most common in the UK after locomotion disabilities, even when not using audiometric techniques to assess their presence (Martin et al., 1988).

Those studies which do use audiometry to assess the presence of acquired deafness underline the extent to which it is not noticed, or denied — or at least not accepted or volunteered — by the sufferer.

Other problems associated with acquired deafness

Ménière's disease and tinnitus sometimes accompany acquired hearing loss.

Tinnitus

Tinnitus is the term used to describe a subjective head noise of internal origin — which is very rarely, if ever, heard by others. Sufferers report sounds such as ringing, buzzing, steam escaping, clicking or even a sound comparable to that produced by a pure tone audiometer. These noises are to be distinguished from auditory hallucinations, which are ego alien and more complex, such as music or 'voices'. Tinnitus may be absorbed into a system of other hallucinations and delusions, with abnormal meaning ascribed to it. It should not be mistaken for autophony — hearing one's own breathing and other internal bodily functions.

It is well established that the presence of tinnitus is correlated to acquired hearing loss (Davis, 1993a). The findings of the NSH suggest that one in three adults report some experience of tinnitus, but only 10% of the population reports noises in the head which last for five minutes or more (Coles, Smith and Davis, 1990). The proportion of people reporting intrusive tinnitus increases with severity of hearing impairment, so that 15% of those with average losses in the better ear of 85 dB HL are afflicted in this way. It is a sad irony that people who are most severely hearing-impaired are those most likely to be troubled by internal head noises. Indeed, of all those who seek medical advice concerning any hearing impairment, about one-third do so on account of tinnitus. Thus the onset of tinnitus may draw an individual's attention to a previously unrecognized or unacknowledged hearing difficulty (Coles, Smith and Davis, 1993).

Whilst there seems to be a cure or treatment for very few types of tinnitus, and since it is considered unwise to undertake surgery of the middle or internal ear where the primary complaint is the tinnitus, increasing attention is now paid to the management of the problem by masking (Hazell and Wood, 1981; Coles, 1987) and by counselling (Hazell, Sheldrake and Meerton, 1987; Slater, 1987). The successes of counselling as a management or rehabilitation technique should be noted and examined. There being no easy solution to tinnitus, counselling has had to be used as a rehabilitative device, much as it may have been used for those with more standard hearing problems had the hearing aid not usurped the status of counselling by virtue of the ease and cheapness with which it can be dispensed.

Early observations about the social and psychological implications of acquired deafness

The RNID library holds a substantial collection of early books and manuscripts which recount the experiences of those who are losing or who have lost their hearing. Some advise fellow sufferers on how to cope with their deafness. They are particularly useful to this text because the opinions on, and attitudes to, deafness expressed in them are less sophisticated — less hindered by political correctness? — than they would be today. Recent 'How-to-Cope' books are more constrained and measured (Lysons, 1978). They come from three sources: autobiographical accounts; advice-giving texts (on how to cope); and personal letters and observations. The range and number of early writers is naturally restricted to those who were moved enough to document their experiences, and they come mainly from America.

As early as 1926, Peck, Samuelson and Lehman (three deafened ladies, and founder members of the New York League for the Hard of Hearing) attempted to make sense of the recurring pattern of reactions to acquired deafness. They suggested that there were four reactions:

- The 'truth-at-any-price-people'.
- The 'hermits'.
- The 'won'ts'.
- The 'panaseekers' (Peck, Samuelson and Lehman, 1926).

Twenty years later the psychologist, Knapp, made the same observation — that there were four most common reactions to acquired deafness (Knapp, 1948). The 'truth-at-any-price' people were considered well-adjusted. They are those who want to know the facts so that they can try to adapt themselves to their deafness in the full knowledge of it. The 'hermits' Knapp described as those presenting a maladjusted reaction by retreating from society. The 'won'ts' he suggested were those who denied their hearing loss, who over-compensated by speaking rather than listening and who generally commanded social situations. The 'panaseekers' Knapp defined as those who go on and on seeking the final solution, leaving no stone unturned and who sometimes exploit their disability to gain attention. Not surprisingly, this last group comprised 55% of his patients.

However anecdotal — and what follows is unashamedly anecdotal — some experiences do seem to be generally common to all those with acquired hearing loss. The first experience expressed by all the deaf writers — without exception — is the social rebuff, which seems to set in motion all the other reactions.

> 'It is not infirmity that society punishes, but inability that it recognizes — inability to meet it, to interest it, to charm it.' (Jackson, 1902)

> 'For my part I have come to realize that I am barred from terms of social equality with those who live in the kingdom of sound. I have come to be prepared for a certain amount of impatience and annoyance.' (Collingwood, 1923)

> 'There is no excuse whatsoever for a contemptuous attitude towards a cripple of any classification. Ethical teaching forbids it in all social strata. But every deafened person knows and knows well the sting of contempt.' (Peck, Samuelson and Lehman, 1926)

Two forces seem to be at work underlying this rejection. Firstly, the difficulty for hearing people to be at ease with deaf people. Secondly, perhaps consequently, the unforgivable treatment of the deaf by hearing people:

> 'Deafness threatens our vanity more than a blind eye or a lacking limb because people in general confuse hearing, a physical function, with understanding, a mental process. By this reasoning a person who hears poorly is held to understand or think poorly.' (Hays Heiner, 1949)

Of the consultants:

> 'Some simply shrugged and gave encouraging smiles; others treated me as if I were a congenital idiot and discussed my condition with Pauline ... lack of imagination led some people to feel superior, occasionally in curious ways.' (Ashley, 1973)

The 'hermits' (those said by Knapp to be exhibiting the maladjusted reaction), respond by withdrawing so as to protect themselves:

> 'So forgive me if you ever see me withdrawing from your company which I used to enjoy. Moreover my misfortune pains me doubly, for in as much as it leads to my being misjudged. For there can be no relaxation in human society, no refined conversations, no mutual confidences.' (Beethoven, 1802, in Gal, 1965)

> 'I am deaf and shall probably remain so for ever. No treatment, no doctors have helped. To this unspeakably sad fate come other worries, and thus it happens that I prefer not to write to you.' (Smetana, in a letter to a former pupil, 1877, in Gal, 1965)

The withdrawal of the 'hermits' however, leads to self-denigration, lowering of self-esteem — a bitter humility and feelings of inferiority. With this humility comes the shame and sense of stigma:

> 'I felt as if I were living in a twilight world. Deafness seemed a badge of shame.' (Ashley, 1973)

The 'won'ts' solve their problem of communication with the hearing world by commanding conversations and thus restricting and determining the responses of the hearing. Similarly, by reducing their hours of contact with hearing people they reduce their need to hear. Indeed, in 1946, Calkins went so far as to exhort people to work out how many hours in the day they are really deaf. On his calculation the average person is only handicapped by deafness for two or three hours per day — a mere trifle:

> '... even the deaf are not deaf all the time. They are not deaf when there is no occasion to hear.' (Calkins, unreferenced).

One of Bertrand Russell's biographers notes that in his old age, Russell fully recognized that by commanding the conversation, all parties involved were saved from the embarrassment caused by his extreme deafness (Crawshaw-Williams, 1970).

These experiences and strategies are commented on and explored by those with acquired hearing loss in a more recent book on adjustment to acquired hearing loss by Kyle (1987). They report no significant changes at all in the experience. They have more recently been confirmed by Hallberg and Carlsson (1991), using careful research techniques, who found that the hearing-impaired subjects in their sample used a variety of strategies to manage their disability — with preferences for either controlling or avoiding contact with the normally hearing (Hallberg and Carlsson, 1991). These researchers concluded that these kinds of coping strategies, whilst focusing on diminishing the disability (or functional loss), none the less increased the perceived handicap (or social disadvantage). Such analysis confirms — in a more systematic way — the anecdotal views and experiences of those with acquired deafness over many years. To some extent, these almost standard responses, or attitudes to hearing impairment, are now slowly being drawn into plans for rehabilitation (Hallam and Brooks, 1996).

Attitudes of hearing people

As early as 1941, Heider and Heider surveyed old scholars of a school for the deaf in the USA to assess their opinion of the attitude of hearing people towards them. They reported that:

> ... many of the deaf feel that the cause of their difficulty lies with the hearing. That they themselves are handicapped in a physical sense they recognise and accept, but that their deafness involves peculiar social problems they blame largely on the group of those who are not deaf. (Heider and Heider, 1941, p. 81)

Later these authors concluded that attitudes towards the deaf were so negative that:

> ... one may say that one of the grave difficulties that the deaf have to face in their adjustment to the world of hearing people is that of the stereotype which the hearing have for the need of them. (Heider and Heider, 1941, p. 93)

In 1953, Barker and colleagues (Barker et al., 1953) reported the results of their survey of jokes about handicap. Deafness came third highest on the list of the most-joked about physical defect — coming after having an unattractive face and fatness. Montgomery (1975) found that negative attitudes towards the pre-lingually deaf reduced their opportunities for finding work even within schools for the deaf. Such was the concern about the inference of negative social attitudes to deafness that a quarter of the addresses which fell within the remit of the Commission on Psychology, at the World Federation for the Deaf Seventh World Congress in Washington DC in 1975, were concerned with attitudes towards deafness.

These examples refer to early childhood deafness, but we have accepted that the attitude of society to the different types of deafness is probably similar.

Almost one-third of Kyle's (1987) book was dedicated implicitly (though not always explicitly) to the experience of the negative attitude of hearing people to their acquired hearing loss (Kyle, 1987). And more recently still, Woolley (1991), in an emotionally charged text, speaks freely of her need to deal with her loss of wholeness as well as of function, and her feelings of injustice and powerlessness in the face of the normally hearing:

> We 'acquire' the hearing loss we didn't ask for and most certainly did not deserve (Woolley, 1991).

Some authors mention the responsibilities that the hearing-impaired have to the hearing. In 1926, Peck, Samuelson and Lehman devoted one entire chapter to 'Putting the Hearing at Ease'. From Denmark, Vognsen (1976) reminds hearing-impaired readers of 'Hearing Tactics': that they must help the hearing understand them. This sentiment is repeated regularly by all writers — with compassion by some (McCall, 1992). Thomas (1984) wisely brings to an end his text by suggesting how much of the responsibility for helping hearing-impaired people must lie with the normally hearing. People with acquired deafness have two main problems to face — the first is the functional problem caused by the loss, the second is the attitude of others. It seems likely that it is the attitude of hearing people, rather more than the functional restrictions caused by the impairment, that leads individuals with acquired hearing loss to feel like handicapped people (Gilhome Herbst, 1983).

Internalizing the negative attitudes of society to their disorder causes a lowering of self-esteem and damage to the self-image and may be accompanied by personal maladjustment and, finally, depression. Little wonder, therefore, that denial of the disorder has recently been proposed as a natural and healthy response — a protecting mechanism (Kyle, Jones and Wood, 1985; Hetu et al., 1990; Hetu, 1996).

Denial

Researchers have now agreed that those with acquired hearing loss tend to attempt to 'pass', or deny their hearing impairment (Humphrey, Gilhome Herbst and Faruqi, 1981; Weinberger and Radelet, 1983: Hetu et al., 1990; Hallberg and Carlsson, 1991). The corollary is that there is felt to be something intrinsically shameful or unpleasant about the disorder which is worthy of being hidden — notwithstanding the fact that hearing impairment is one of the most prevalent of all disabilities (Martin et al., 1988) and is the norm not the exception in old age (Davis, 1993b). This merits further discussion.

Goffman's (1963) interpretation of the functioning of stigma will be used to form a paradigm from which to understand the perceived social strategies of those with acquired deafness in response to their deafness and to the normally hearing. Goffman's theory attempts to explain the negative social attitudes towards people who are physically handicapped and the responses of the handicapped people to these attitudes (Goffman, 1963).

To the sophisticated eye of the socially experienced, people who are different are usually quite clearly so. This is the essential ingredient of Goffman's stigma theory. This difference acts both to discriminate the dissimilar and subsequently to act as a cohesive force to those who see themselves as the same — in this case as stigmatized. Those with acquired deafness are different. There is no preparation for the outsider (whether he is hearing-impaired or not) for deafness. There is no evident mark which everyone recognizes as meaning 'that person is a deaf person', unless, that is, he or she should use their hands to sign or unless they are wearing a hearing aid.

The second essential ingredient of Goffman's theory, 'the pivotal fact' as he called it, is that people tend to hold prevailing social attitudes to their own disability. Consequently, Goffman suggests that a sense of shame arises from the individual's perception of his own attribute as a defiling thing and one he can readily imagine himself not possessing. This shame, Goffman suggests, is the motivating force behind most subsequent behaviour of the disabled when interacting with 'normal' people.

Acquired deafness is what Goffman (1963) would call a 'discreditable' problem. It is popularly known and recognized to be a stigmatizing defect but, as it is not immediately evident, it can be hidden.

Goffman's theory, so briefly expressed, provides a theoretical paradigm from which to understand — or even to explain — why those with acquired deafness may behave in certain ways. Many of the problems of those with acquired deafness stem from the ease with which they can control information about their hearing disability and 'pass' as a 'normally' hearing person.

There is some evidence to suggest that, concerning the feeling of being stigmatized, the experiences of those with acquired deafness differ little from those with pre-lingual deafness (Myklebust, 1964; Humphrey, Gilhome Herbst and Faruqi, 1981). This is attributed to two main factors. Firstly, to the marginality of those with acquired deafness in that their incapacity is less severe and therefore less identifiable and accepted by the normally hearing as a serious disability. Secondly, to the fact that there is much general confusion amongst the general population about the difference between pre-lingual and post-lingual deafness.

This capacity to deny or reject acquired hearing loss needs to be considered for three main reasons.

Firstly, because it is likely that those who deny it in themselves and strive to conceal it will succeed. In this way those who have lost their hearing may not recognize in others the problem that they have themselves. This may exacerbate feelings of aloneness — namely being the only one with a dreadful disability to cope with. And indeed, there are three studies (expressed in Table 11.4) which show how few other people with acquired deafness those who suffer from it themselves appear to know (Thomas and Gilhome Herbst, 1980; Humphrey, Gilhome Herbst and Faruqi, 1981; Gilhome Herbst, Meredith and Stephens, 1991). This table must be read while bearing in mind the true prevalence of the disorder in the age groups under consideration.

There is no reason at all to assume that, as members of society, people with acquired hearing loss should hold different attitudes to their disability than the rest of society. As long ago as the 1950s psychologists (Phillips, 1957) have been able to show that if people internalize and hold society's negative attitudes to a certain condition or state in life which they know and accept to be theirs (e.g. deafness or Blackness) they are more likely to be maladjusted than if they do not (Rosow, 1967). Denial of the 'condition' is thus a substantial protecting mechanism.

This possibility of hiding their disability in order to reduce the effect of societal disapproval (the stigma) is one of the major differences in experience between those who are deaf from early childhood and those who acquire deafness later. Since the former can less readily 'pass' as normally hearing, and less readily escape their identity as a 'deaf' person they belong unequivocally to a group of people with similar experiences. Their communication and lively culture binds them together. Ironically, though they may in medical terms be more severely disabled, deaf people may feel less isolated by virtue of their clearer identity. There is less question about their position within their group, or that they belong to one. As has been said, it seems as if it is the very marginality of those with acquired deafness that contributes to their unpleasant experiences.

The second reason why denying their deafness is important is because those who are unwilling to accept that they have a problem are equally unlikely to come forward for deafness-specific rehabilitation services. At the moment rehabilitation is likely to mean the issue of a hearing aid. Thomas and Gilhome Herbst (1980) found that 40% of their subject sample of people of employment age knew that they had had a hearing loss for 20 years or more before coming forward to seek an aid. Similarly, Humphrey and colleagues (1981) found that, in a sample of hard-of-hearing people over the age of 70 years who would admit to experiencing a hearing loss, 45% knew that they had had a loss since before retirement age, yet only 21% of the group possessed a hearing aid (Humphrey, Gilhome Herbst and Faruqi, 1981). Similar findings were reported by Gilhome Herbst and colleagues (1991), with the suggestion that general health education should inform the 'middle-aged' of what they may face in later life if they disregard a hearing loss whilst younger (Gilhome Herbst, Meredith and Stephens, 1991). The practical problems of detecting and servicing the large numbers of middle-aged hard-of-hearing people who tend to shun their hearing loss has been thoroughly explored by Davis and his colleagues in Wales (Davis et al., 1992). These authors found that during the course of their enquiry, 60% of those who had not previously used a hearing aid (but were deemed to 'require' one) accepted the offer of one.

Table 11.4 Proportion of total samples (%) of hearing-impaired people who express lack of awareness of, or denial of, hearing loss

	Inner London of working age*	Inner London aged 70+**	Welsh village aged 70+***
I don't know anyone else who has difficulty with their hearing	29	39	25
I know of one other person who has difficulty with their hearing	22	29	32
No — I don't tend to tell people about my hearing loss soon after meeting them (and their mean dB loss in the better hearing ear)	60	75 55.8 dB (SD 14.5)	72 53.2 dB (SD 14.9)
No — I have nothing wrong with my hearing (and their mean dB loss in the better hearing ear)	–	25 43.8 dB (SD10.0)	25 48.2 dB (SD 11.3)

*Thomas and Gilhome Herbst (1980).
**Gilhome Herbst and Humphrey (1980).
***Gilhome Herbst, Meredith and Stephens (1991).

The third reason why it is important to explore denial of deafness is its role or function within the rehabilitative process, a subject recently revived and extended by researchers in Holland (van den Brink et al., 1996). The conventional principles of rehabilitation demand acceptance of the problem before therapeutic intervention can either take place or be effective. As already said, this was already accepted by Knapp in 1948. Little wonder that rehabilitation of those with acquired hearing loss is still, relatively speaking, in its infancy. Indeed, interventions other than the hearing aid are relatively rare in the UK (Field and Haggard. 1989). All the indications suggest, however, that given the very complex responses to those with acquired hearing loss, simply issuing a hearing aid will rarely be sufficient to achieve satisfactory rehabilitation. This was, of course, foreseen by the planners of the early NHS hearing aid service, who always envisaged that extra support would be essential (Ewing, Ewing and Littler, 1937). But counselling and individual attention by a specialist to help with the social problems encountered by those with acquired hearing loss has never been universally available. In the UK, attempts were made to ameliorate this situation in the mid-1970s with the creation of a new class of worker, the hearing therapist (DHSS, 1978). In practice, however, their work has been largely swallowed up by low-level activities designed to get people to wear their hearing aids more frequently (Hegarty, Pocklington and Crowe, 1983).

Hearing Tactics — a term people used to describe behavioural methods to help hard-of-hearing people manage the disability and handicap they experience — although regularly accepted by 'the wise' as essential and effective, are only rarely systematically in use as a rehabilitation tool (Vognsen, 1976; Abrams et al., 1992; Lindberg et al., 1993; Jordan et al., 1993).

Loneliness and isolation

From what has been discussed so far, it appears that the position of hard-of-hearing people in society is ambiguous. They do not belong to any Deaf community in which common experiences, common language and communication desires and needs bind people together. Rarely do they have any specific deafness-related links with others with similar problems. Very few people belong to hard-of-hearing clubs. They are perforce alienated or estranged from the hearing community — of which they were once a part. Loneliness and isolation is the most commonly noted social effect of acquired hearing loss in adults.

The *Concise Oxford Dictionary* defines 'lonely' as meaning 'solitary', 'companionless', 'isolated'. Other dictionaries add 'depressed for lack of friends'.

In practical usage, loneliness is normally understood to denote an unwanted feeling of being alone — which arises either from a lack of companionship *per se*, or from a lack of companionship of the desired kind.

These two constituents of loneliness need to be considered separately. Firstly, there is the feeling which arises from an impoverished number of social contacts. This is generally known as 'social loneliness' or 'social isolation'.

Secondly, there is an unpleasant feeling of loneliness which may have nothing to do with the frequency or variety of social contacts, but stems rather from a lack of empathy with others. This is generally known as 'emotional loneliness or 'emotional isolation'.

The distinction is useful in our discussion about those with acquired hearing loss. The concept of 'social isolation' has now become firmly embedded in British empirical research — typically research on older subjects — as founded upon an objective assessment of insufficient contacts with family and community, based upon precise annotated accounts (Townsend, 1957).

Thomas and Gilhome Herbst (1980) found that the overriding social effect of acquired deafness in adults of employment age was (emotional) loneliness. The hearing-impaired of employment age in their study suffered significantly more from feelings of loneliness than did the control group of hearing adults. Indeed, extreme loneliness (feeling lonely all the time, or very often) was found more often amongst hearing-impaired people of employment age than has been found by researchers concerned to ascertain the prevalence of loneliness in populations of the retired and elderly. The stress associated with such loneliness — or lack of kindred spirits — is illustrated by the finding that 60% of those who felt that way were assessed during the study as being psychiatrically disturbed.

Whilst finding significant loneliness amongst hearing-impaired people of employment age, Thomas and Gilhome Herbst (1980) found no significant isolation in this population.

The reverse was true of a later study, on the social and psychological implications of acquired deafness in older people. Here it was found that hearing impairment in older people was linked to isolation — but not necessarily to loneliness (Gilhome Herbst, 1983).

Social isolation emerged as the principal handicap associated with acquired deafness in a study by Stevens (1982). Indeed, Stevens (1982) went further to report that many of those in his study experiencing severe deafness for a number of years mentioned that they were no longer able to cope with social situations, the implication being they were so isolated that they were out of practice (p. 455).

In 1991, Eriksson and Carlsson reported on the stress experienced by the 'middle-aged' hearing-impaired. They found that insecurity in social settings, which caused a perceived loss of social control (an important deafness-management technique, as we have seen) was implicated in somatic stress conditions.

Loneliness has long been understood to be stressful (Weiss, 1973) and has been referred to frequently as implicated in the onset of depression — particularly in populations of older people.

Thus these findings support the suggestions of psychiatrists investigating the possible social causes of mental illness in middle and older age, that deafness of onset in early adult life may be the most pernicious in its effect on the social and psychological well-being of people in their later years. Deafness in middle age may cause or exacerbate long-standing reductions in sociability and create a tendency to loneliness and isolation, and subsequently a predisposition to mental disorder in later life.

In a recent review of research on mental health and acquired hearing loss, Jones and White (1990) concluded that the only reliable and consistent effect of acquired hearing loss on mental state was social stress, isolation and depression.

Mental disorder and acquired hearing loss

The previous discussion suggests that the social effects of hearing loss, though diverse, stem from two sources: the *disability* — namely the functional restriction caused by the impairment — and the *handicap* — the unpleasant results of society's attitude. When combined, it may be argued that the major social effects of acquired hearing loss are a greater tendency to experience loneliness and isolation than do normally hearing people and a greater tendency to experience feelings of low self-esteem, shame and frustration. The extent to which the socio-somatic imbalances associated with acquired hearing loss may produce or contribute to more serious psychological disturbance must now be considered.

It is inappropriate simply to discuss all hearing-impaired people as if their experiences were the same. Research suggests that time of onset (whether during employment age or in retirement) rather more than severity of impairment is important in determining the experiences associated with acquired hearing loss. Indeed, systematic enquiry now shows quite conclusively that degree of deafness (the impairment) is only remotely associated with disability, and even less with the handicap — in both younger and older sufferers (Thomas and Gilhome Herbst, 1980; Gilhome Herbst, 1983; Hetu, Lalonde and Getty, 1987; Mulrow et al., 1990). Consequently, the experiences of older people will be discussed separately — but not the experiences of people with different degrees of hearing impairment.

The literature on the association of acquired hearing loss and mental disorders deals mainly with depression — both in people of employment and of retirement age; paranoia in those of employment age and (more commonly) paranoid psychoses in older people; and organic brain syndromes or cognitive function in older people alone.

Depression

It is generally presumed and accepted that psychiatric illness arises through the interaction of predisposing factors (for example, genetic characteristics) and fundamental life experiences (such as physical illness and emotional stress). Clinicians and researchers interested in the effects of acquired hearing loss tend towards the notion that it may be a precipitating factor in its association with affective disorders, encouraging those whose mental state may or may not have been predisposed to mental disorder to be more prone to such experiences.

The mechanisms or processes whereby acquired hearing loss may function as a precipitating factor have already been discussed earlier in this chapter. They are discussed again here from a different perspective.

In a particularly useful text, Newton (1988) reminds the reader that similarities between grief and depression have held a central role in the development of psychoanalytic theory. In 1917, Freud proposed that loss was central to both these states. Subsequently, the importance of loss and low self-esteem to depression has been generally accepted. Loss is central to Bowlby's theories — though here it is loss early in life that produces the vulnerability to psychiatric disorder (Bowlby, 1969; 1980). Beck's (1973) cognitive theory of depression centres on the development of a negative view of oneself and life in general, which can lead to depression. Seligman (1975) has suggested that a maladaptive style of thinking — 'learned helplessness' in particular — may predispose a person to depression, in particular perceived loss of control.

These researchers and clinicians talk of the same *precursors*, or factors significantly associated with depression, which we have seen are the experience of many of those who suffer from acquired hearing loss: grief, loss, lowered self-esteem, helplessness and loss of control. To this we must add the tendency to isolation or loneliness which is the experience of so many with acquired deafness.

Studies which aim to assess the presence of clinical depression in general populations now report with reasonable consistency an average rate of 4.8% across the whole adult population: 6.4% in women and 3.2% in men (Paykel, 1989).

An association between deafness and depression in people of employment age has been constantly reported by psychologists and psychiatrists over the years (Menninger, 1924; Ingalls, 1946; Knapp, 1948; Ramsell, 1966; Mahapatra, 1974; Denmark, 1976). However, reviewers (Cooper, 1976; Rosen, 1979; Jones and White, 1990) have pointed out that until recently this association was an assumption based primarily on clinical observation and not upon systematic research on unbiased samples. Thomas and Gilhome Herbst (1980) saw their study as one of the first to fill this gap since it investigated the social and psychological implications of acquired deafness on an unbiased hearing-impaired sample possessing NHS aids, and used psychological measuring techniques which were not likely to mis-classify deaf people. Moreover, as has been stated, their results were stringently controlled on a hearing population. In that study, they confirmed the association between deafness and depression. They estimated that deaf people of employment age were four to five times as likely as hearing people to suffer from anxiety and depression (Thomas and Gilhome Herbst, 1980).

Both Paykel (1989) and Murphy (1989) report that, in contrast to the stereotypical view of old age as a time of sorrow and despair, the prevalence rates of depression amongst elderly people are similar to — or at least not markedly higher than — younger cohorts (Murphy, 1989). Recent research suggests a steady prevalence of depression of between 10% and 13% of all age groups amongst elderly people living at home (Morgan, Dallosso and Arie, 1987; Lindsay, Briggs and Murphy, 1989). This is in contrast to earlier community studies which suggest a prevalence of depression in community-based populations of persons of retirement age of between 20% and 30% (Kay, Beamish and Roth, 1964a; Blessed, 1979).

Community studies have observed a specific relationship between deafness and depression in old age (Goldberg, 1970; Charatan, 1975; Garland, 1978) but they did not use audiometric techniques to establish the presence of deafness. Nor was this association established on the basis of systematic enquiry. Gilhome Herbst and Humphrey's (1981) study assessed the presence of depression by using the depression scale taken from the CARE schedule (Gurland et al., 1980), and assessed the presence of hearing loss using audiometry. In their study on older people living at home, the same authors found a significant relationship between deafness and depression in older people, even when adjusting for age and poor general health (Gilhome Herbst and Humphrey, 1980).

Similar findings have subsequently been repeated by a range of researchers in a range of locations, for example in Wales (Jones, Victor and Vetter, 1984), in Italy (Carabellese et al., 1993) and in Japan (Ihara, 1993). However, in America, Mulrow and colleagues (1990) were not able to document an association between hearing loss and depression after adjusting for potential confounders such as age and visual acuity. Work concerning the implication of poor sight coupled with poor hearing in old age needs to be developed.

As has been mentioned, in the summary of their review of mental health and acquired hearing impairment, Jones and White (1990) report that the only area in which there seems to be some consistent agreement amongst researchers is in the association between acquired hearing loss and depression — for both younger and older adults.

Paranoia

Paranoia — generally categorized as a functional psychosis — is a relatively rare condition. Patients suffering from paranoia are characterized by delusions of persecution accompanied by excessive suspiciousness and sometimes by delusions of grandeur. In less florid cases, it may be difficult to distinguish paranoia from socially acceptable degrees of suspicion and eccentricity.

The early studies of Myklebust (1964) and of Thomas and Gilhome Herbst (1980) failed to find any association between paranoia and acquired hearing loss in those of employment age. The evidence, reviewed exhaustively by Cooper (1976) suggests that, on balance, there is unlikely to be an association between acquired deafness and paranoia.

On the other hand, Nett (1960), in a methodologically unsound study, suggests that deafened persons of employment age are more likely to be paranoid. Mahapatra (1974), also reporting on a study of questionable methodology, reported a number of cases of paranoia in a hearing-impaired sample, but his sample was restricted to people with conductive losses awaiting surgery, and his interviews were conducted on the day before their operations.

The relationship between deafness and late paranoid psychosis or later paraphrenia appears to have been well-accepted for some time (Post, 1966; Roth, 1974). Indeed, Bromley (1988, unreferenced) suggests quite firmly on late paraphrenia that 'partial or total deafness is thought to occur more frequently than in other psychiatric groups of the same age, but physical health is not greatly impaired'.

There was a great deal of interest in the relationship of deafness with paranoid psychosis in the elderly in the 1970s, as can be seen by the quantity of research on this matter stemming from the Medical School at Newcastle upon Tyne (Cooper et al., 1974; Kay et al., 1976; Cooper and Curry, 1976; Cooper, Garside and Kay, 1976; Cooper, 1978). In their examination of evidence regarding a 'psychosis of the deaf' Cooper, Garside and Kay (1976) remind the reader that:

> ... an association between deafness and paranoid psychosis in later life has often been reported, but few comparisons have been made of the clinical and other characteristics of deaf and non-deaf patients. (p. 532)

The 'other' characteristics of deaf and non-deaf patients investigated by the team are singled out here from research on the matter because they contribute to existing knowledge concerning the influence of deafness on social life and show how it, in turn, affects mental state.

Cooper, Garside and Kay (1976) confirm the earlier finding of Houston and Royse (1954) that paranoid patients who are also deaf exhibit less constitutional predisposition and have fewer hereditary factors which might predispose them to psychosis than do the non-deaf. They further identify an important sub-group for whom this is particularly true, namely patients with deafness of onset in middle or early age. From this they conclude that deafness, working in its role as an isolating agent over a long period of time, may be capable of exerting pathogenic effects of its own (Cooper, Garside and Kay, 1976). At the same time, the team could find little evidence to suggest that deafness, even of long duration, produced any consistent personality changes which might have resulted in an increased liability to psychotic illness. They recommend that the presence of deafness is a useful diagnostic tool to discriminate between patients with paranoid and affective psychoses. Moore (1981), in a retrospective case note study, found deafness to be less common in a depressed group than in the general mental health population and more common in paranoid groups. As recently as 1993, Stein and Thienhaus also recommended that hearing impairment should possibly be considered as a potential risk in the development of psychoses in elderly people (Stein and Thienhaus, 1993).

In their exploration of the role of social isolation as a factor in the causation of late schizophrenia, Kay and Roth (1961) suggest that the isolated circumstances of a high proportion of such cases (in their study) 'must be attributed to some extent to accidental factors such as deafness'. Indeed, these authors found that 40% of their paraphrenic cases were deaf — a proportion far in excess of those with affective disorders, although they note that 'assessments (of deafness) were made by rough methods only'. This greatly reduces the reliability of their work — rendering it almost without value.

So, the debate about the association of acquired hearing loss and paranoia, which has been raging for the past 30 or so years, goes on. The reviews of Thomas (1984), Meadow-Orlans (1985) and Jones and White (1990) are consistent in their observations that any association between acquired hearing loss and paranoid illness needs further work before it can be confirmed or refuted.

Organic brain syndrome

The proportion of old people aged 65 years and over living in the community suffering from organic brain syndromes has been assessed consistently over the years at around 5% — increasing exponentially with age (Kay, Beamish and Roth, 1964a; Lindesay, Briggs and Murphy, 1989). Equally consistently, and by the same researchers, the prevalence rate for moderate to severe cognitive impairment in those aged 80 years and over has been assessed at about 20%.

Whether there is any association between hearing impairment and organic brain syndrome in older age is still unclear. That it may be related to cognitive decline seems to be more widely accepted.

Let us first consider the issue of an association between acquired hearing loss and organic brain syndromes.

Two major early UK studies exploring the social and medical aetiology of dementia in old age noted that those with organic brain syndromes were up to twice as likely to be hearing-impaired than those who were not exhibiting any dementia (Kay, Beamish and Roth, 1964b). Kay and colleagues (1964b) went so far as to suggest that:

> It is possible that those defects of sight and hearing may have sometimes played a part in the production of the mental symptoms by reducing the subjects' contact with the outside world; for the association of sensory defects with organic mental state seemed to be too strong to be wholly explicable by the advanced age of the subjects. (p. 676)

In their study of the relationship between mental disorder and deafness in the elderly living at home, Gilhome Herbst and Humphrey (1980) found an apparently closer association between deafness and dementia, finding that 79% of those suffering dementia in their study were also deaf. They further reported a significant association between severity of dementia and severity of deafness, so that as people get deafer they are significantly more likely to be demented and the severely demented are significantly more likely to be deaf. However, their results do not support the suggestion made by Kay and colleagues (1964b) that the connection between deafness and dementia is 'too strong to be wholly explicable by the advanced age of the subjects'. Gilhome Herbst and Humphrey (1980) report that, once age is controlled for, the apparent relationship between deafness and dementia is lost. They suggest that deafness and dementia are merely contiguous conditions, both being a function of age.

A simple explanation for the discrepancy between this finding and those of other researchers is to be found in the fact that no audiometry was performed in any previous studies looking at the possible aetiology of dementia. Albeit Gilhome Herbst and Humphrey (1980) found an apparently closer relationship between deafness and dementia than other studies, they also showed that deafness is the norm, and not the exception, in all those over the age of 80.

The work of Gilhome Herbst and Humphrey (1980) suggests that at least a third of the deafness found in the elderly is probably of onset in middle age (see also Stephens et al., 1990). It is still possible that there is some causal link between deafness and dementia derived from a complicated interweave of cause and effect of time of onset, type of deafness and type of dementia. As a strong component of organic brain syndrome is poor memory recall, it is not possible to determine in any accurate way duration of deafness amongst those with dementia without recourse to longitudinal studies.

Gilhome Herbst and Humphrey's (1980) suggestions have subsequently been confirmed by Eastwood and colleagues studying comorbidity in older people (Eastwood et al., 1985) and by Vesterage and colleagues in Denmark (Vesterage, Soloman and Jagd, 1988).

However, in an American study on 38 patients with senile dementia of the Alzheimer's type, and using pure tone audiometry to assess hearing loss, Peters, Potter and Scholer (1988) found cognitive decline more rapid in those with dementia and hearing impairment after follow-up 6–16 months later (even when age was controlled for) and concluded that there is an interaction between acquired sensorineural hearing loss in later life and Alzheimer's disease. Three possible mechanisms for this more rapid decline in hearing-impaired patients were proposed:

- That hearing declined during the study period and that the lower scores were simply a result of reduced ability to respond to verbally presented neuropsychological tests.
- That auditory sensory deprivation accelerates cognitive loss in patients suffering dementia.
- That there is a disease–disease interaction between presbyacusis (old age deafness) and Alzheimer's disease.

All these suggestions need to be further researched.

The disease–disease interaction theory is discussed usefully by Oyer and Solberg (1989) and is supported more recently by Sinha and colleagues (1993), also studying the observed consistent pattern of degeneration in the auditory system of sufferers from Alzheimer's disease.

With regard to the effects on cognitive function of acquired hearing loss in older age, a slightly clearer picture is now unfolding — but leaving ample room for further work.

In 1986 an important special report of the *Danish Medical Bulletin* dedicated to hearing problems and the elderly claimed that:

> ... to the best of our present knowledge such changes in central discrimination functions/cognitive functions are not the result of deafness and can in no way be regarded as part of a dementia syndrome, but must be seen rather as a result of different types of cerebral micro-insults (Salomon, 1986, p.12)

New research suggests otherwise. By 1989, Uhlmann and colleagues were able to show that the diminished cognitive performance in older people associated with mild to moderate hearing loss is not necessarily an artefact of cognitive testing — in that it is largely based upon verbal tests (Uhlmann et al., 1989). Similarly, Blessed and colleagues working from Newcastle upon Tyne in the early 1990s found that cognitive function scores were markedly affected by hearing — in addition to other variables, of course — including visual deficits, age and dementia, but not depression (Blessed et al., 1991). Finally, in a review of the literature on the subject, Gennis and colleagues (1991) rather helpfully pointed out that they had come to the view that hearing ability is related to cognitive status in those with organic brain syndromes but that there is little to suggest that in the normal elderly, hearing impairment leads to cognitive decline. Once again, the precise nature of the interplay between hearing impairment and cognitive functioning is unclear — leaving ample room for further research.

Conclusion

This chapter began by considering society's general distaste for acquired hearing loss. The prevalence of the disorder was discussed, and the considerable discrepancies in prevalence to be found when assessed by self-report and when assessed by audiometric techniques. Some suppression, or denial, by sufferers was proposed as one reason for this discrepancy.

The attitude of hearing people to deafness was considered and found, generally, to be wanting in understanding and sympathy by those with impaired hearing. Anecdotal evidence about attitudes to acquired deafness, to be found in relatively early texts on acquired hearing loss, was explored and found to be reflected in later, more systematic research on the subject. The most common responses of those with acquired hearing loss were found to be denial of, or suppression of knowledge about, deafness, and controlling behaviour in order to manage social situations and minimize unexpected encounters.

Goffman's theory of stigma (Goffman, 1963) was used to explain the concepts lying behind the perceived strategy of many people to deny their hearing loss. It was even suggested that such denial had been found to be important in protecting the individual from the harmful effects of the attitudes of other people (Hetu et al., 1990). Denying the disorder was found to carry forward further problems — not least the feeling of not knowing anyone else with the problem and thus feeling even more alone and isolated.

Indeed, those of employment age with acquired hearing loss were found to be significantly more lonely than were people of the same age with normal hearing. However, similar degrees of loneliness were not found in the elderly — where the effect of acquired deafness is more likely to be isolation — a reduction in social contacts *per se*.

The association of depression and deafness in all ages was noted and proposed as the only association with a mental disorder on which there is common agreement by researchers and clinicians. Further research needs to be undertaken to assess whether there is any association between acquired hearing loss and paranoia, late paranoid psychosis, or the dementias. The association between cognitive decline in old age and acquired hearing loss is also not conclusive.

Those who do not acknowledge their acquired hearing loss — for whatever reason and with whatever result — are less likely to request rehabilitation services.

References

Abrams HB, Hnath-Chisolm T, Guerreiro SM, Ritterman II (1992) The effects of intervention strategy on self perception of hearing handicap. Ear–Hear 13: 371–377.

Ashley J (1973) Journey into Silence. London: The Bodley Head.

Barker RG, Wright BA, Myerson L, Gonick MR (1953) Adjustment to Physical Handicap and Illness: a survey of the Social Psychology of Physique and Disability (second edition). Social Science Research Council, Bulletin 55, New York.

Beck AT (1973) The Diagnosis and Management of Depression. Philadelphia: University Pennysylvania Press.

Berry G (1933) The psychology of progressive deafness. Journal of the American Medical Association 101: 1599–1603.

Blessed G (1979) Depression: Assessing the patient behind the mask. Geriatric Medicine May: 29–32.

Blessed G, Black SE, Butler T, Kay DW (1991) The diagnosis of dementia in the elderly. British Journal of Psychiatry 159: 193–198.

Bowlby J (1969) Attachment and Loss. Vol 1: Attachment. London: Hogarth Press.

Bowlby J (1980) Attachment and Loss. Vol 3: Loss, Sadness and Depression. London: Hogarth Press.

van den Brink RHS, Wit HP, Kempen GIJM, van Heuvelen MJG (1996) Attitude and help-seeking for hearing impairment. British Journal of Audiology 30: 313–324.

Bunting C (1981) Public Attitudes to Deafness. Social Survey Division of the Office of Population Censuses and Surveys. London: HMSO.

Carabellese C, Appollonio I, Rozzini R, Bianchetti A, Frisoni GB, Fratolla L, Trabucchi M (1993) Sensory impairment and quality of life in a community elderly population. Journal of the American Geriatrics Society 41: 401–407.

Charatan FB (1975) Depression in old age. New York State Journal of Medicine 75: 2505–2507.

Charities Aid Foundation (1993) Charity Trends 1993 (16th edition). Tonbridge.

Chmiel R, Jerger J (1993) Some factors affecting assessment of hearing handicap in the elderly. Journal of the American Academy of Audiology 4: 249–257.

Coles RRA (1987) Epidemiology of tinnitus. In Hazell J (ed) Tinnitus. Edinburgh: Churchill Livingstone.

Coles R, Smith P, Davis A (1990) Tinnitus: its epidemiology and management. In Jensen JH (ed) Presbyacusis — and Other Age Related. 14th Danavox Symposium, Danavox Jubilee Fdn., Copenhagen.

Collingwood HW (1923) Adventures in Silence. Distributed by the Rural New Yorker.

Cooper AF (1976) Deafness and psychiatric illness. British Journal of Psychiatry 129: 216–226.

Cooper AF (1978) Paranoid psychosis and late hearing impairment. In Montgomery G (ed) Deafness, Personality and Mental Health. Scottish Workshop with the Deaf.

Cooper AF, Curry AR (1976) The pathology of deafness in the paranoid and affective psychoses of later life. Journal of Psychosomatic Research 20: 97–105.

Cooper AF, Curry AR, Kay DWK, Garside RF, Roth M (1974) Hearing loss in paranoid and affective psychoses of the elderly. Lancet ii: 851–854.

Cooper AF, Garside RF, Kay DWK (1976) A comparison of deaf and non-deaf patients with paranoid and affective psychoses. British Journal of Psychiatry 29: 532–538.

Crawshaw-Williams R (1970) Russell Remembered. Oxford: Oxford University Press.

Davis A (1983) The epidemiology of hearing disorders. In Hinchcliffe R (ed) Hearing and Balance in the Elderly. Edinburgh: Churchill Livingstone.

Davis A (1993a) The prevalence of deafness. In Ballantyne J (ed) Deafness. London: Martin & Martin.

Davis A (1993b) Hearing in Adults: the prevalence and distribution of hearing impairment and reported disability. In the MRC Institute of Hearing Research National Study of Hearing. London: Whurr Publishers.

Davis A (1996) Epidemiology. In Stephens SDG (ed), Kerr A (gen ed) Otolaryngology Volume 2: Adult Audiology. Edinburgh: Churchill Livingstone.

Davis A, Stephens D, Rayment A, Thomas F (1992) Hearing impairments in middle-age: the acceptability, benefit and cost of detection (ABCD). British Journal of Audiology 26: 1–14.

Denmark JC (1976) The psychological implications of deafness. Modern Perspectives in Psychiatry 7: 188–205

Department of Health and Social Security (1978) Health Service Development. Appointment of Hearing Therapist. Health Circular HC (78) 11.

Eastwood MR, Corbin SL, Read M, Nobbs H, Kedward HB (1985) Acquired hearing loss and psychiatric illness: an estimate of prevalence and co-morbidity in a geriatric setting. British Journal of Psychiatry 147: 552–556.

Edwards FC, Warren MD (1990) Health Services for Adults with Physical Disabilities: A Survey of District Health Authorities 1988–1989. London: Royal College of Physicians of London.

Eurostat (1991) Basic Statistics of The Community. Luxembourg (28th edition).

Ewing AWG, Ewing IR, Littler TS (1937) The Use of Hearing Aids. Report IV of the committee upon the Physiology of Hearing. Medical Research Council Special Report Series No. 219, London: HMSO.

Field DL, Haggard MP (1989) Knowledge of hearing tactics: (1) Assessment by questionnaire and inventory. British Journal of Audiology 23: 349–354.

Freud S (1917) Mourning and melancholia. In Strachey J (ed) Completed Psychological Works, vol. 14. London: Hogarth Press.

Gal H (ed) (1965) The Musicians World: Great Composers and their Letters. London: Thames & Hudson.

Garland MH (1978) Depression and dementia. Hospital Update June: 313–319.

Gennis V, Garry PJ, Haaland KY, Yeo RA, Goodwin JS (1991) Hearing and cognition in the elderly. New findings and a review of the literature. Archives of International Medicine 151: 2259–2264.

Gilhome Herbst KR (1983) Psycho-social Consequences of Disorders of Hearing in the Elderly. In Hinchcliffe R (ed) Medicine in Old Age — Hearing and Balance. Edinburgh: Churchill Livingstone.

Gilhome Herbst KR, Humphrey CM (1980) Hearing impairment and mental state in the elderly living at home. British Medical Journal 280: 903–905.

Gilhome Herbst KR, Humphrey CM (1981) Prevalence of hearing impairment in the elderly living at home. Journal of the Royal College of General Practitioners 31: 155–160.

Gilhome Herbst KR, Meredith R, Stephens SDG (1991) Implications of hearing impairment for elderly people in London and in Wales. Acta Otolaryngologica (Suppl.) 476: 209–214.

Goffman E (1963) Stigma: Notes on the Management of a Spoilt Identity, Harmondsworth: Penguin.

Goldberg EM (1970) Helping the Aged. National Institute of Social Work. Training Series 19, London: George Allen & Unwin.

Gurland B, Dean L, Cross P, Golden RR (1980) The epidemiology of depression and dementia in the elderly: the use of multiple indicators of these conditions. In Cole JO, Barratt JE (eds) Psychopathology in the Aged. New York: Raven Press.

Hallam RS, Brooks DN (1996) Development of the Hearing Attitudes in Rehabilitation Questionnaire (HARQ). British Journal of Audiology 30: 199–213.

Hallberg LR-M, Carlsson SG (1991) Hearing impairment, coping and perceived hearing handicap in middle aged subjects with acquired hearing loss. British Journal of Audiology 25: 323–330.

Hays Heiner (1949) Hearing is Believing. Cleveland and New York: World Publishing Co.

Hazell JWP, Wood SM (1981) Tinnitus masking — a significant contribution to tinnitus management. British Journal of Audiology 15: 223–330.

Hazell JWT, Sheldrake JB, Meerton LJ (1987) Tinnitus masking — is it better than counselling alone? In Feldmann H (ed) Proceedings of 3rd International Seminar. Karlsruhe: Harsch Verlag, pp. 239–250.

Hegarty S, Pocklington K, Crowe M (1983) The Making of a Profession. Uxbridge: The National Foundation for Educational Research.

Heider F, Heider GM (1941) Studies in the Psychology of the Deaf. Psychological Monograph Series. Evanston, IL: American Psychological Association.

Hetu R (1996) The stigma attached to hearing impairment. Scandinavian Audiology (Suppl.) 43: 12–24.

Hetu R, Lalonde M, Getty L (1987) Psychosocial disadvantages associated with occupational hearing loss as experienced in the family. Audiology 216: 141–152.

Hetu R, Riverin L, Getty L, Lalande NW, St-Cyr C (1990) The reluctance to acknowledge hearing difficulties among hearing impaired workers. British Journal of Audiology 24: 265–276.

HMSO (1992) The Health of the Nation: A Strategy for Health in England. (Cm 1986). London: HMSO.

Houston F, Royse AB (1954) Relationship between deafness and psychotic illness. Journal of Mental Science 100: 990–993.

Humphrey CM, Gilhome Herbst KR, Faruqi S (1981) Some characteristics of the hearing impaired elderly who do not present themselves for rehabilitation. British Journal of Audiology 15: 25–30.

Ihara K (1993) Depressive states and their correlates in elderly people living in a rural community. Nippon Koshu Eisei Zasshi 40: 85–94.

Ingalls GC (1946) Some psychiatric observations on patients with hearing defects. Occupational Therapy and Rehabilitation 25: 62–66.

Jackson AW (1902) Deafness and Cheerfulness. Boston, MA: Little, Brown and Co.

Jones L (1987) Living with hearing loss. In Kyle JG (ed) Adjustment to Acquired Hearing Loss. Bristol: University of Bristol, Centre for Deaf Studies.

Jones DA, Victor GR, Vetter NJ (1984) Hearing difficulty and its psychological implications for the elderly. Journal of Epidemiology and Community Health 38: 75–78.

Jones EM, Victor GR, Vetter NJ (1990) Mental health and acquired hearing impairment: a review. British Journal of Audiology 24: 3–9.

Jones EM, White AJ (1990). Mental health and acquired hearing impairment. A review. British Journal of Audiology, 24 (1): 3–9.

Jordan FM, Worrall LE, Hickson LM, Dodd BJ (1993) The evaluation of intervention programmes for communicatively impaired elderly people. European Journal of Disorders of Communication 28: 63–85.

Kay DWK, Beamish P, Roth M (1964a) Old age mental disorders in Newcastle upon Tyne. Pt. I: A study of prevalence. British Journal of Psychiatry, 110: 146-158.

Kay DWK, Beamish P, Roth M (1964b) Old age mental disorders in Newcastle upon Tyne PtII. A study of possible social and medical causes. British Journal of Psychiatry 110: 668–682.

Kay DWK, Roth M (1961) Environmental and hereditary factors in schizophrenias of old age. Journal of Mental Science 107: 649–686.

Kay DWK, Cooper AF, Garside RF, Roth M (1976) The differentiation of paranoid from affective psychoses by patients' pre-morbid characteristics. British Journal of Psychiatry 129: 207–222.

Knapp PH (1948) Emotional aspects of hearing loss. Psychosomatic Medicine 10: 203–222.

Kyle JG (1987) Adjustment to Acquired Hearing Loss. Bristol: University of Bristol, The Centre for Deaf Studies.

Kyle JG, Jones L, Wood PL (1985) Family and Adjustment to Acquired Hearing Loss Final Report PEI School of Educational Research Unit University of Bristol.

Lindberg P, Scott B, Andersson G, Melin L (1993) A behavioural approach to individually designed hearing tactics training. British Journal of Audiology 275: 299–301.

Lindesay J, Briggs K, Murphy E (1989). The Guys/Age Concern Survey. British Journal of Psychiatry 155: 317–329.

Lysons CK (1978) Your Hearing Loss and How to Cope with It. Newton Abbot: David & Charles.

McCall R (1992) Hearing Loss? A Guide to Self Help. London: Robert Hale.

Mahapatra SB (1974) Deafness and mental health: psychiatric and psychosomatic illness in the deaf. Acta Psychiatrica Scandinavia 50: 596–611.

Martin J, Meltzer H, Elliot D (1988) The Prevalence of Disability Among Adults OPCS surveys of disability in Great Britain Report 1 OPCS Social Survey Division. London: HMSO.

Meadow-Orlans K (1985) Social and psychological effects of hearing loss in adulthood: a literature review. In Orlans H (ed) Adjustment to Adult Hearing Loss. London and Philadelphia: Taylor & Francis.

Menninger KA (1924) The mental effects of deafness. Psychoanalytic Review 11: 144–155.

Montgomery GWG (1975) Looking after our own? Hearing 30: 107–111.

Moore N (1981) Is paranoid illness associated with sensory defects in the elderly. Journal of Psychosomatic Medicine 25: 69–74.

Morgan K, Dollosso HM, Arie T (1987) Mental health and psychological well-being among the very old living at home. British Journal of Psychiatry 144: 135–142.

Mulrow CD, Aguilar C, Endicott J, Velez R, Tuley MR, Charlip WS, Hill JA (1990) Association between hearing impairment and the quality of life of elderly individuals. Journal of the American Geriatric Society 38: 45–50.

Myklebust HR (1964) The Psychology of Deafness. New York: Grune & Stratton.

Murphy E (1989) Depression in the elderly. In Herbst K, Paykel ES (eds) Depression: An Integrative Approach. Oxford: Heinemann Medical Books.

Nett EM (1960) The relationship between audiological measures and handicap. A project of the University of Pittsburg School of Medicine and the Office of Vocational Rehabilitation US Dept of Health Education and Welfare.

Newton J (1988) Preventing Mental Illness. London: Routledge and Kegan Paul.

Oyer HJ, Solberg LC (1989) Audiological rehabilitation of older people: visual and vibrotactile considerations. British Journal of Audiology 231: 33–37.

Paykel ES (1989) The background: extent and nature of the disorder. In Herbst K, Paykel ES (eds) Depression: An Integrative Approach. Oxford: Heinemann Medical Books.

Peck A, Samuelson E, Lehman A (1926) Ears and the Man: Studies in Social Work for the Deafened. Philadelphia: Davis Co.

Peters CA, Potter JF, Scholer SG (1988) Hearing impairment as a predictor of cognitive decline in dementia. Journal of the American Geriatrics Society 36: 981–986.

Phillips BS (1957) A role theory approach to adjustment in old age. American Sociological Review April: 212–217.

Post F (1966). Persistent Persecutory States of the Elderly. Pergamon Press, Oxford.

Ramsell DA (1966) The psychology of the hard of hearing and the deafened adult. In Davis H, Silverman SR (eds) Hearing and Deafness (revised edition). New York: Staple Press.

Rosen JK (1979) Psychological and social aspects of the evaluation of acquired hearing impairment. Audiology 18: 238–252.

Rosow I (1967) Social Integration of the Aged. New York: Free Press.

Roth M. (1974) Hearing loss in paranoid and effective psychosis of the elderly, Lancet, ii: 851–854.

Salomon G (1986) Hearing Problems and the Elderly. Danish Medical Bulletin Gerontology Special supplement Series No 3.

Seligman MEP (1975) Helplessness: On Depression, Development and Death. San Francisco, CA: Freeman.

Sinha UK, Hollen KM, Rodriguez R, Miller CA (1993) Auditory system degeneration in Alzheimer's disease. Neurology 434: 779–785.

Slater R (1987) Guest editorial: On helping people with tinnitus to help themselves. British Journal of Audiology 21: 87–90.

Stein LM, Theinhaus OJ (1993) Hearing impairment and psychosis. International Psychogeriatrics 5: 49–56.

Stephens SDG, Lewis PA, Charny MC, Farrow SL, Francis M (1990) Characteristics of self reported hearing problems in a community survey. Audiology 29 (2): 93–100.

Stevens JM (1982) Some psychological problems of acquired deafness. British Journal of Psychiatry 17: 175–181.

Thomas AJ (1984) Acquired Hearing Loss: Psychological and Psychosocial Implications. London: Academic Press.

Thomas AJ, Gilhome Herbst KR (1980) Social and psychological implications of acquired deafness for adults of employment age. British Journal of Audiology 14: 76–85.

Townsend P (1957) The Family Life of Old People. London: Routledge and Kegan Paul.

Townsend P, Wedderburn D (1965) The Aged in the Welfare State. Occasional Papers on Society. Admin No 14, London: G Bell and Sons Ltd.

Uhlmann RF, Teri L, Rees TS, Mozlowski KJ, Larson EB (1989) Impact of mild to moderate hearing loss on mental status testing. Journal of the American Geriatrics Society 37: 223–228.

Vesterage V, Solomon G, Jagd M (1988) Age-related hearing difficulties. II Psychological and social consequences of hearing problems — a controlled study. Audiology 27: 179–192.

Vognsen S (ed) (1976) Hearing Tactics. Copenhagen: National Council of Health Education.

Weinberger M, Radelet M (1983) Differential adaptive capacity to hearing impairment. Journal of Rehabilitation 4: 64–69.

Weiss RS (1973) Loneliness: The Experience of Emotional and Social Isolation. Cambridge MA: MIT Press.

Wilkins L (1950) The Prevalence of Deafness in England, Scotland and Wales. Acta-oto-laryngologica, Stockholm, 90: 97–114.

Woolley M (1991) Acquired hearing loss: acquired oppression. In Taylor G, Bishop J (eds) Being Deaf: The Experience of Deafness. Milton Keynes: Open University. p 224.

Section B: Management and Intervention

Chapter 12
Mental Health Workers: Deaf – Hearing Partnerships

HERBERT KLEIN AND NICK KITSON

Introduction

Why is it worth writing a chapter on this subject? Deaf people have been discriminated against in education, training and the workplace. With a few exceptions (e.g. Lane, 1990; Sacks, 1990) books by hearing authors tend to highlight the failings and needs of Deaf people rather than their achievements. This is of course true in some ways of this book. Partly this is inevitable, as it focuses on the mental health needs of Deaf people. Books by Deaf authors, on the other hand, tend to celebrate Deafness and Deaf people's achievements, (e.g. Jackson, 1990). Redfearn (1996), a Deaf professional, calls for praise for the Deaf people, 'really doing good work'.

In the UK the employment of Deaf mental health workers in mental health services for Deaf people is 'new technology'. The London service at Springfield University Hospital, now the South West London and St George's (SWLSG) National Deaf Mental Health Services, for example, was run entirely by hearing staff from 1971 to 1986. It had a majority of mental health experts with limited Deaf expertise and a minority of Deafness experts, including a social worker, an educational psychologist and a priest. '*The Deaf are...*' was a common defence by the 'Deaf experts' as was '*...mental health is the priority...*' from the mental health experts. Occasionally advice and voluntary work was sought from Deaf people, though only in the fields of entertainment and recreation. Visits to American Deaf mental health services had shown that Deaf mental health workers and professionals could be employed, though there remain very few worldwide. In the UK there were a few Deaf qualified social workers, who also provided an example, but there were no Deaf specialist mental health workers. SWLSG National Deaf Services' first Deaf worker in 1986/7 was 'lent' by an education authority, in view of the requirement that the authority provided education to a 14-year-old child, who was admitted to the service. These experiences, as well as rare calls in the literature for deaf paraprofessionals and professionals and their training (Harris, 1981), led to superficial recognition of the value and potential of Deaf mental health workers. A policy was adopted that the service should aim for at least half of its clinical staff to be Deaf. This policy was a leap into an unknown world, based on the simple belief that it was right for Deaf patients to be treated by Deaf staff. Too little thought had been given to the preparation and training of hearing staff, patients and the new Deaf staff. Initially, three Deaf staff were appointed in 1988. This number has expanded progressively to include about one-third of the 45 staff of the service. This proportion has remained relatively static since about 1991. The need for a majority of qualified staff in a mental health service, coupled with poor access for Deaf people to qualifying training, has made it extremely difficult to increase numbers further. By encouraging contract support services to employ Deaf staff the service has achieved a 50% Deaf: hearing staff ratio. The remaining challenge is the training of qualified Deaf mental health professionals.

The employment of Deaf people in mental health services for Deaf people has become official policy of the European Society for Mental Health and Deafness (Kitson and Monteiro, 1991) (See Appendix C). Now all three mental health services in the UK and many aftercare settings for Deaf people have relatively high proportions of Deaf mental health workers. It appears that the UK leads most countries in the systematic employment of Deaf staff in Deaf mental health services. Other countries, notably the USA, but also some European countries, appear to have better education and training opportunities for Deaf people. In those countries, those few who are employed in mental health services are usually qualified professionals.

Training

Training of mental health staff in deafness and communication has been emphasized (Denmark and Warren, 1972). It is also necessary to train those with Deaf expertise in mental health. Attempts at accessing qualifying training for Deaf people have met with obstruction, mostly based on ignorance, attitude and lack of finance. In 1989 the first counselling certificate course in Sign Language for Deaf trainees in the UK was started by the Westminster Pastoral Foundation in association with Springfield University Hospital, London (Redfearn, 1991). The courses had the added benefit of informing the larger Deaf community of the possibility of counselling and help for less severe mental health problems. Deaf graduates of the courses have joined the teaching staff since 1991. Similar courses have followed in other British cities such as Manchester. Such courses have been available at Gallaudet University in Washington for many years. In 1993 a voluntary agency, Sign Campaign, together with the SWLSG Service in London, pioneered National Vocational Qualifications for Deaf people (Vaughan, 1996). These qualifications are recognized nationally and will provide access to, or accepted alternatives to, registered mental health qualifications. They are largely practical and work-based and so are ideal for able Deaf people who have difficulties with written language.

Deaf sign language users with formal mental health qualifications remain rare internationally. Most mental health degree and diploma-awarding bodies expect good oral and written skills. As a result, in the UK, Deaf staff are usually in less powerful and unqualified roles, and there is a need for Deaf qualified staff in the mental health services. There is a clear need for better access to higher education. Recognized training — adapted for and available to Deaf people — is also needed so that able Deaf people with limited English skills can gain access to qualifications. In the UK some progress has been made with the nursing authorities (Wright and Kellet, 1994) and there appears to be little resistance in the area of occupational therapy.

Why Deaf workers?

Although the original employment of Deaf staff was based on a fairly simplistic view, from our experience there are clearer reasons.

Communication is fundamental to psychiatric practice, to both diagnosis and treatment. Deaf and hearing people brought up in Deaf families have a natural advantage of sign language as a first language, and a deep understanding of the culture and predicament of Deaf people (Kitson and Monteiro, 1991). Deaf people, through a lifetime's experience, tend to have a greater natural flexibility in the use of visual and tactile communication.

> A patient with a history of extreme violence was transferred from a maximum security hospital to the open hospital ward of the SWLSG Deaf mental health service. Minor slips in signed conversation could result in yet another violent outburst. With the help of a clinical psychologist, a detailed anger management programme was devised for the patient. This was administered in a highly visual fashion by use of charts, sliding scales, colour and pictures. The whole staff team was encouraged to respond similarly to the patient's problem outbursts. He was encouraged to confront his problems on the ward, and used a wide range of visual metaphors to communicate his feelings. The use of standard mental health expertise, translated into Deaf language and culture, was very successful. The patient is now living independently, mixing freely and happily with his local Deaf community, and continues to have warm and friendly informal contact with the service (Austen and Klein, 1996).

Deaf staff tend to be much better communicators with deaf people with limited or odd communication. They 'code switch' naturally, especially those with Deaf parents themselves (Hoffmeister and Moores, 1987), resulting in improved communication for patients both with fluent sign language and with limited or disordered communication. This also relieves frustration and its consequences. Again, consider the following example.

> A patient with severe impulsive behaviour problems, including assaults, appeared to be suffering autism in the context of moderate learning disability. She had attended a Deaf school in a far distant region until the age of 16 years, when she was institutionalized and had remained in that hearing world for 30 years. A hearing psychiatrist with past experience of the Deaf mental health service took over responsibility for the patient's care and immediately transferred her to the London service. She was observed to sign in a very repetitive distressed fashion with little evident meaning. In London, Deaf staff could communicate with her only a little more fluently than hearing staff. Contacts in the Deaf world were utilized to explore the sign language that would have been used in the patient's school over 30 years previously. Using this newly acquired vocabulary, we were able to communicate fairly fluently. The patient was enabled to express many stories of pain and grief and as well to relieve her frustration in the here and now. Her behaviour improved markedly, but remained odd. Increased access to her experience and language enabled a diagnosis of schizophrenia to be made. Deaf staff had enabled her language and so also her schizophrenic thought disorder to be available to staff. Additionally, a Deaf researcher (together with hearing professionals) had enabled the analysis of thought disorder in sign language that was used in the diagnosis of this patient. Specific treatment of the mental illness improved her condition further.

Deaf people have the advantage of continuing personal experience of deafness and greater credibility with Deaf clients or patients (Kitson and Monteiro, 1991). This can be used in specific Deaf therapy aimed at cultural awareness and enhanced self-esteem and identity as a Deaf person (Sims, 1989). The 'Deaf way' clearly cannot be achieved without Deaf people. Deaf people provide appropriate role models (Kitson and Monteiro, 1991) through both their professional behaviour and social lives. They show demotivated patients that Deaf people can achieve, have families and the usual variety of interests and life-styles. They may also dispel some Deaf patients' prejudices about Deaf people.

> A patient with visible physical disability was referred for depression, frustration and isolation. He had been teased and bullied by his peers at his Deaf school. He assumed this to be typical of Deaf people, so immersed himself in the hearing world for 20 years after he left school. His depression brought him into contact with a social worker for Deaf people, who referred him to the specialist mental health service for Deaf people. He was surprised to find Deaf people amongst the staff and patients who treated him with respect. Slowly his attitude to Deaf people changed and he was introduced to the Deaf community, where he eventually flourished. No specific mental health treatment was necessary.

Other Deaf patients, although not specifically prejudiced against Deaf people, will have experienced only hearing people in positions of power and authority. Often they have an unconscious assumption that Deaf people, including themselves, cannot achieve. We recall the surprise and suspicion of patients, when Deaf members of staff were first employed. Initially patients did not approach the Deaf staff and questioned their ability, as they felt safe with the hearing staff, whom they saw as 'clever, skilled and confident'.

Deaf staff enable patients (and hearing staff), by example, to access the activities of the local Deaf communities. The experience of Deaf staff (and other Deaf mental health trainees) demystifies and destigmatizes mental health (Rebourg, 1991) through their social contacts in the wider Deaf world. They will be able to present modern Deaf mental health services to counter the reputation gained from the mental health institutions that have admitted Deaf people in excessive numbers in the past. When Deaf staff were first employed they took Deaf patients into the Deaf community, for example, visiting Deaf clubs. At first the Deaf community was very wary of Deaf patients, and the patients of them. Mutual understanding was slow at first but both groups grew in confidence and patients became motivated and took it upon themselves to visit instead of being led by staff.

Deaf people provide fundamental learning experiences for hearing staff. Again, when Deaf staff were first employed, they found themselves in the middle, torn between hearing staff and Deaf patients. Slowly the gap has narrowed so that even in the temporary absence of Deaf staff, patients have the confidence that the hearing staff will be 'Deaf aware' and accept Deaf people as equals.

If they had had Deaf colleagues, would psychiatrists for Deaf people (as recently as the mid-1980s) have over-generalized from their Deaf patients to say that deaf people exhibit concrete thinking, rigidity, decreased empathy, projection of responsibility on to others, lack of insight or self-reproach, unrealistic views of their own abilities, increased demands and impulsivity with poor control of rage? Would others (Evans and Elliott, 1981) have argued that the first rank symptoms of schizophrenia were too dependent on the use of sound, subsequently shown not to be the case in a setting with many Deaf staff (See Chapter 4)?

Through a lifetime's experience, Deaf people tend to have greater visual observation and reporting skills — which are core mental health nursing skills (Kitson and Klein, 1995). In Deaf mental health services either the psychiatrist or the patient may have difficulty with sign language and the psychiatric interview is likely to be impaired. Detailed nursing observation is all the more important. Experience shows that the best hearing nurses (mostly qualified and experienced) give clear sequential descriptions, but with some inference. The best Deaf nurses (none are qualified) give clear three-dimensional accounts, with much descriptive detail, but little inference. It is in the nature of Deafness to be more visually observant. It is in the nature of sign language, particularly in role shifts, to include moods and responses, with detailed descriptions of interactions. So it appears that Deaf people tend to have one of the core nursing skills without training. For the diagnostician, full clear description without inference is more useful, although the inferences of qualified experienced staff can form useful shorthand, where time is pressured.

Deaf people are also the natural experts and judges of the success of environmental and technological aids and of the needs of their less able fellows, who might not be able to fend for themselves.

Attitudes to Deaf Staff

The following are condensations of multiple views expressed about deaf staff.

- **Deaf patients won't trust members of the gossiping back stabbing Deaf community.** Anxieties among service users about maintaining confidentiality for Deaf professionals in the small Deaf world are expressed by both Deaf and hearing people. This anxiety seems greater in the smaller Deaf communities of Europe. In the UK it is known, through employing and training significant numbers of Deaf mental health workers in health, residential and social services that, when Deaf people learn professional codes of behaviour, they gain the respect of their clients. Confidentiality remains a problem only for a small minority of Deaf patients, many of whom have unresolved negative attitudes to their deafness, which is projected on to the Deaf community as a whole.
- **Deaf patients should integrate.** Criticism of a ghetto mentality has been made, as most long-term Deaf mental health service patients live and work in a Deaf signing environment. The services can be criticized for neither normalizing nor integrating, but they do follow Deaf people's choices. Ninety per cent of deaf people, though born to hearing parents, marry deaf partners (Rainer and Deming, 1963) and they seek each other's company in Deaf clubs and centres (Phoenix, 1988). Patients with all their disabilities and handicaps secondary to mental illness, need the best communication in their first/preferred language and an appropriate culture to ensure a good enough emotional life.
- **Deaf staff will over-identify with patients ... and split staff.** Life experience may be the motivator to help other Deaf people, but may lead to over-identification with the patient and loss of professional behaviour. A therapeutic distance allowing critical reflection is necessary (Rebourg, 1991). Similar motivation also exists among hearing staff. Why have they chosen to work in a setting where they are usually more powerful?
- **Deafness is not mental health training, and untrained deaf people have no place in staffing a psychiatric hospital.** The unqualified Deaf mental health worker is in danger of being undervalued and/or

overvalued. Lack of qualification might lead to assumed lack of ability, but Deaf experience might lead to assumed ability. A Deaf mental health worker's greater fluency with patients might lead to an exclusivity in relationships which is damaging to the team approach (Rebourg, 1991). For example, a newly recruited Deaf nursing assistant was the first to be secretively told by a patient, with symptoms of borderline personality, of the patient's suicidal intent and detailed past abuse. Fortunately the nurse had the backing of experienced Deaf work colleagues and a qualified nursing team and so was enabled to share her experience with supportive staff. Had she been the only Deaf employee the risk of exclusivity would have been much greater and may have reinforced the idea that Deaf staff might split teams.

The communication handicap of hearing staff, in a profession largely reliant on communication, is highlighted by the fluency of the Deaf staff member, leaving them feeling deskilled. Hearing staff are at risk of maintaining 'superiority' by aggrandizing and avoiding sharing mental health skills or denying their communication handicap. This can lead to defensive separate groupings of Deaf and hearing staff.

- **Deaf staff just dump their 'emotional baggage' on to hearing people, especially staff.** Deaf staff may inflict negative 'emotional baggage' from their past experience on to hearing staff, who represent past hearing oppressors. They may be expecting discrimination or may even create it. Of course, all staff carry 'emotional baggage'. Such behaviours, which are not uncommon in Deaf/hearing settings, need extra staff support and staff groups with an independent facilitator. Ideally, of course, the facilitator should be independent of the Deaf/hearing issues, but this can really be obtained only by having facilitators from both cultures. In practice, supply determines that the facilitator is usually a hearing psychotherapist who has a limited knowledge of Deafness.
- **Deaf staff will not hear the noise of crises or shouts of staff for help.** In fact, the number of serious incidents of 'explosive rage' said to be characteristic of deaf people (Altshuler, 1971) has fallen (Figure 12.1). In any case, the visual and vibration sensitivity of deaf staff and technology can enable an appropriate response to be made.
- **Partially deaf/hearing and oral deaf users are at a disadvantage with Deaf staff.** Although deaf people may need special help, Deaf staff are usually better at code switching. Hearing staff may be better able to understand those Deaf people who use limited sign, but have useful vocalizations. In a clear demonstration that little can be taken at face value in Deaf mental health, it is not at all uncommon for deaf people, including those with virtually no sign language, to communicate more fluently with members of the Deaf community. It would not

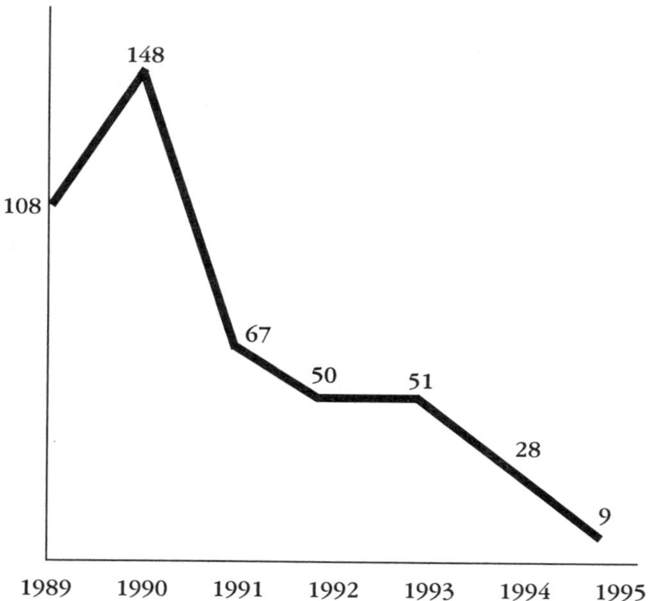

Figure 12.1 Seclusions per year resulting from serious incidents (1989–1995).

be sensible to have a mental health service run totally by Deaf staff, if it serves other deaf people and operates within a larger hearing world. All other things being equal, it would be better for patients' self-esteem if their services are led by Deaf people.

- **Deaf staff (or people) are rude.** Some Deaf people are rude, as are some hearing people. Mostly this statement is based on misunderstanding of cultural differences between Deaf and hearing people. Deaf and hearing people clearly have different communication and environmental awareness needs. For example, an attempt was made to challenge a domestic supervisor, who was sitting in the Deaf patients' lounge of the Service speaking casually to hearing staff from behind a newspaper. The domestic supervisor was abusing the patients' lounge, and worse was rudely communicating in a language largely unavailable to the patients, whose lounge it was. The domestic supervisor initially ignored polite remonstrations, but when the newspaper was removed, a formal complaint was made about rudeness. We would regard it as rude for a visitor to sit on our sofa in our lounge at home and chat in a language foreign to us. To add insult to injury, in a Deaf context, a visible line of communication was cut off by the paper. Who was rude to whom? Fortunately there is a positive side to such incidents. Deaf patients were able to observe, through the action, how a Deaf person might appropriately assert themselves against discrimination. In our workplace there are policies against such inappropriate behaviour by visiting staff, though of course they still occasionally occur through ignorance.

- **Deaf staff are lazy...always off sick...do not want to serve patients.** Of course, like hearing staff, some are. Employing Deaf staff who do not have a general or mental health work experience is more risky and more mistakes are made. It is easier for hearing-dominated services to gain information on prospective hearing staff who have had to pass exams and have more work experience, and the grapevine is easier. At present the majority of those who select staff are hearing. The Deaf grapevine can easily be ignored. It is particularly important with some new Deaf recruits, depending on past experience, to inculcate the basics of work and care ethics before giving them responsibility for patients. This comes best from experienced Deaf staff, or jointly with hearing staff. Disciplining Deaf staff also has difficulties, as the senior staff outside the Service and appeals bodies do not have a knowledge of Deafness. They are as likely to overprotect as to reject Deaf staff, neither of which is helpful.

Attitudes to hearing staff

- **Mental health training is hearing-orientated and irrelevant to work with Deaf patients.** This view implies Deaf people are special and not human. Mental health training should take into account different cultures and its principles should be appropriate to all humans. Experience shows that Deaf people have much the same mental health needs as hearing people. The treatments are the same, but need to be given in the context of Deaf culture and language.
- **Hearing staff are pursuing their careers at the expense of Deaf patients and staff.** Of course this is partially true. The jobs would not exist without patients. The careers of hearing staff can be advanced by working with the Deaf, but they can also be hindered. The main question for all staff is whether they are doing significantly more good than harm to their patients.
- **Hearing staff are not sensitive to Deaf patients' needs.** In any particular situation this may be true, or it may be that the Deaf observer is too sensitive and is overprotecting the Deaf patient due to over-identification with the patient's problems or lack of mental health experience and training. However, Deaf staff are more likely to be appropriately sensitive to Deaf patient's needs.
- **S/he is not mentally ill, hearing staff have not understood.** It is relatively common for new Deaf staff who have not worked with mentally ill patients before to assume the illness is anger at hearing staff who do not understand. They find out later that the same patient shows paranoid beliefs about Deaf people also. On the other hand,

there is a long history of misdiagnosis of Deaf patients and the views of Deaf mental health workers are vital to multidisciplinary assessment and decision-making, including diagnosis.

- **Hearing people are not direct and straightforward.** That is, Deaf people are. Of course, neither are fully direct, open and honest. We all, some of the time, cover up our real feelings to avoid conflict or problems. It does appear there is a cultural difference. Deaf people do appear to express themselves more openly and expansively in sign language when compared to the relative reserve of professional British hearing people. Hearing people from different cultures are probably more like Deaf people. Often, the apparent directness of Deaf people is about superficial things. We have experienced Deaf counselling trainees being surprised to realize, through group therapy experiences, their own unconscious covering up of feelings and attitudes.
- **Hearing staff cannot communicate as well as Deaf staff and should not interview without Deaf staff assistance.** In many situations, hearing staff with good signing can undertake mental health tasks alone, and in very rare situations can understand Deaf patients better than a Deaf staff member (e.g. when a patient is mentally ill and the hearing staff has much experience of Deafness and mental health). In most situations, however, a combination of a hearing Deafness mental health expert and an experienced Deaf staff member will result in the most accurate assessment. In the future, when enough Deaf people have mental health training and experience, they will be most likely to provide the most accurate assessments for patients.

Mutual hostility and paranoia between Deaf and hearing staff can develop, and has developed. Maybe it is inevitable, though it can be the ready scapegoat for other staff splits. Austen and Klein (1996) point out that either/or splits between Deaf unqualified or hearing qualified staff are unhelpful. They encourage the either/or (concrete) thinking too commonly ascribed to Deaf patients in the past.

The emotional support measures generally necessary for good team work are more important. It is necessary to consider technological and human aids, which will enable Deaf and hearing people, individually and jointly, to be fully involved in all aspects of care. A communication policy is essential. The SWLSG's service signing policy is based on the principle that all staff should sign/voice off in the sight of a Deaf person.

Conclusion

Deaf people should lead and provide the services for Deaf people, but not as a right. This should be achieved by relevant training, qualifications and experience (Kitson and Monteiro, 1991). Deaf history shows that Deaf people are capable of achieving in the highest professions, given the chance. Too many people see the deafness, not the Deaf person with potential. A rock may look worthless, but when opened reveals a diamond ready for cutting, polishing and becoming a precious, valuable stone.

References

Altshuler, K (1971) Studies of the Deaf. Relevance to psychiatric theory. American Journal of Psychiatry: 127(11) 1521–1526.

Austen S, Klein H (1996) The last straw that broke the camel's back: cognitive behavioural approaches to 'psychopathy'. In Laurenzi C, Ridgeway S (eds) Progress through equality: New perspectives in the Field of Mental Health and Deafness. British Society for Mental Health and Deafness (BSMHD) Publications, pp 63–67.

Denmark J, Warren F (1972) A psychiatric unit for the deaf. British Journal of Psychiatry 120: 423–428

Evans J, Elliott H (1981) Screening criteria for the diagnosis of schizophrenia in deaf patients. Archives of General Psychiatry 38: 787–790.

Harris R (1981) Mental health needs and priorities in deaf children and adults: a deaf professional's perspective for the 1980s. In Stein LK, Mindel ED, Jabaley T (eds) Deafness and Mental Health. New York: Grune & Stratton, pp 219–250

Hoffmeister R, Moores DF (1987) Code switching in deaf adults. American Annals of the Deaf 132: 31–34.

Jackson P (1990) Britain's Deaf Heritage. Edinburgh: Pentland Press Ltd.

Kitson N, Klein H (1995) Deaf services by Deaf people? European Society for Mental Health and Deafness. 3rd Congress proceedings.

Kitson N, Monteiro B (1991) Policy on Deaf Mental Health Professionals. European Society for Mental Health & Deafness.

Lane H (1990) When the Mind Hears: A History of the Deaf. New York: Random House.

Phoenix S (1988) An Interim Report on a Pilot Survey of Deaf Adults in Northern Ireland. Northern Ireland Workshop with the Deaf.

Rainer J, Deming W (1963) Demographic aspects: number, distribution, marriage and fertility statistics. In Rainer J, Altshuler M, Kallmann F, Deming E (eds) Family and Mental Health Problems in a Deaf Population. Department of Medical Genetics, New York State Psychiatric Institute, Columbia University, pp 13–27.

Rebourg F (1991) Minutes of the meeting on the training of deaf professionals in mental health work. Proceedings of the Second International Congress of the European Society for Mental Health & Deafness.

Redfearn P (1991) Deaf students learn counselling skills. British Deaf News 22: 5.

Redfearn P (1996) Deaf professionals — a growing stream. In Laurenzi C, Ridgeway S (eds) Progress Through Equality: New Perspectives in the Field of Mental Health and Deafness. British Society for Mental Health and Deafness (BSMHD) Publications, pp 81–84.

Sacks, O (1990) Seeing Voices: A Journal Into the World of the Deaf. New York: Harperperennial.

Sims J (1989) Breaking the silence. Nursing Times 84: 116–117.

Vaughan J (1996) Health and social care training for deaf professionals. In Laurenzi C, Ridgeway S (eds) Progress Through Equality: New Perspectives in the Field of Mental Health and Deafness. British Society for Mental Health and Deafness (BSMHD) Publications, pp 69–74.

Wright D, Kellet J (1994) Deaf persons' access to nurse education. Proposal to the English National Board for Nursing, Midwifery and Health Visiting.

Chapter 13
Interpreters in Mental Health Settings

JOAN TURNER, HERBERT KLEIN AND NICK KITSON

Introduction

Interpreting in any language means translating the meaning and concepts as represented in one language to another. Clearly it is not possible to be 100% accurate, particularly when interpreting nuances or where there are no generally accepted translations for complex ideas. Interpreting in a mental health setting can be fraught with difficulties. There are no absolutes, and situations vary greatly from one setting to another, as do the people involved. The setting may be within a service specifically for deaf people where specialist staff, both deaf and hearing, are involved; it may be a child-based service, again with specialist staff experienced in working with deaf children. As there are only three adult services and one children's service in the UK, it follows that many Deaf people seeking, or being referred to, mental health services may find themselves facing mental health professionals who have no (or very limited) knowledge of deafness or methods of communication with deaf people. In some areas there may be a specialist social worker with deaf people involved and an interpreter with some knowledge of mental health. The possibility — indeed, in some areas the probability — of no specialists in the field of deafness being involved and an interpreter with no training or experience in mental health is very real. The scenario which would cause the greatest concern would be one where no specialist worker with deaf people was involved and there was no competent interpreter to help the patient. Ebert and Heckerling (1995) found that even doctors who understand the issues usually do not use an interpreter.

Not only do situations vary so much, but so do people who are deaf. 'Deafness' is a blanket term which covers everyone from the elderly person who is losing hearing acuity due to age, to the baby born profoundly deaf. In between are those who are born hearing, partially hearing, severely deaf and those who lose some or all of their hearing at some time during their lives. Deafness in any degree may occur in infancy, childhood, adolescence, as an adult, in middle age or in the elderly. All these people need some allowance made for their hearing loss, with an understanding on the part of the professionals of the effect of this loss on the individual's ability to cope in an interview. In addition, awareness is needed of the influence the hearing loss has had on lifestyle, relationships, self-image and the confidence of the individual. However, for the majority of these people, an interpreter will not be necessary, although in some cases a lip speaker and/or a willingness to write by those interviewing may be essential. Users of a mental health service requiring an interpreter will, in the main, be those people who were born deaf or who became deaf in infancy or early childhood, before the acquisition of language. The lucky ones will have been born to a Deaf environment and acquired sign language. In addition, there will be those who identify with the Deaf community, who may have received their education in a school or unit for deaf children and who use signing, with or without speech and speech reading as their usual or preferred mode of communication. The use of an interpreter in mental health, as in other settings, should result in improved communication and comprehension between the deaf and hearing people involved. How the interpreter is used will vary according to the situation. Perhaps the most common situation occurs when an interpreter is called upon to interpret between a hearing mental health professional and a deaf service user. It may be at a mental state examination or with a view to compulsory admission to hospital under mental health law.

Responsibility of interpreters

Whatever the situation, the responsibility of the interpreter is great. Where the professionals have no knowledge of deafness, it is likely they will pose questions in a manner outside the comprehension of the deaf person. Concepts may be propounded which are not understood. There is a risk that the deaf person's intelligence may be underestimated. How should the interpreter behave? Impartiality, non-involvement, independence, are all demanded by the British Interpreters' Code of Practice (CACDP, 1994). But how are they to react in a situation where the deaf person's differences are not known or recognized? Until such dilemmas are resolved and appropriate strategies developed and put into practice, the interpreter should be able to make the mental health professionals aware of the linguistic and cultural aspects involved. This is implied (see Chapter 9) in the Code of Practice to the Mental Health Act 1983 (Department of Health and Welsh Office, 1993). Great care is essential in these circumstances. Moving outside the specific role of interpreter, albeit for legitimate reasons, presents difficulties for all parties. The deaf person may or may not be able to consent to this shift of role. The professionals may choose to ignore any advice offered or resent it as interference. They may ask for further information from the interpreter—which may be inappropriate, beyond their area of competence, and perhaps contrary to the ethic of confidentiality. Any deviation from interpreting should occur only in the full knowledge of the possible consequences and where there is no alternative at the time. Both deaf and hearing parties must be made aware of this stepping out of role, as far as this is possible, and the interpreter should not express an opinion about the mental state of the patient. Where the mental health professionals have no experience of working with deaf people, even with a skilled interpreter, the consultation may be conducted in a way which leaves the deaf person confused or not having fully understood what has transpired. When facing a new experience some deaf people need much explanation and reinforcement before they understand what has been said and the implications of the interview. Should it then be the responsibility of the interpreter to spend some time going over what has been said to ensure as much understanding as possible, if the deaf person wishes this? Certainly it should be the responsibility of the interpreter to ensure that the mental health professional is aware of the circumstances required to allow full interpretation. Within the deaf population seeking mental health care, there are those whose level of comprehension may preclude full understanding. There are those with minimal communication skills, in any mode, to whom it may be impossible for an interpreter to give or receive clear responses to the questions posed, or their account of their situation. 'Deaf and hearing people tend to use sign language differently which can lead to mutual misunderstandings or judgments.' (Stokoe and Battison 1981).

When faced with a situation that challenges the interpreter's competence, it is important that another interpreter becomes involved. The American Register of Interpreters of the Deaf (Solow, 1981) states that the interpreter shall use, ' . . . language most readily understood by the person served'. In these circumstances it may be preferable to use a deaf person, whose first and preferred language is sign and who shares the same culture as the patient, as a relay interpreter. Deaf staff tend to be much better communicators with deaf people with limited or odd communication. They 'code switch' naturally, especially those with deaf parents themselves (Hoffmeister and Moores, 1987). This is not always so.

> The route to BSL (British Sign Language) usage varies from child to child. A small number of deaf children may acquire BSL through exposure to the language at home and in contact with the Deaf community; others may develop BSL through contact with signing peers, while others may not learn BSL until their teens or they have left school. Such varied paths to competence in BSL may lead to specific variations in language use and possibly even differences in assimilation into the Deaf community. (Brien, 1992, p. 3).

In areas where there is no easy access to specialist mental health services for deaf people, or in crisis situations, an interpreter is of vital importance to ensure that the communication needs of the deaf patient are met and to provide them with access to appropriate services. A skilled interpreter will help the professional to make an assessment by interpreting the deaf person's version of events impartially. Without this impartiality, mistaken diagnoses could easily be made — and have been made many times in the past. There are, however, few interpreters available. At present, there are no special training facilities in the UK for interpreters to learn about mental health issues. In the normal course of events, interpreters are not frequently involved in this type of work and do not develop expertise by constant practice. Some basic training should be available, if only to help to develop an awareness of some of the particular difficulties and pitfalls. Others will need intensive training and experience. Phelan and Parkman (1995) provide a useful review for the health professional of the use of any interpreters in any setting. Their comments about non-local spoken languages are at least equally applicable to deaf patients.

Bilingual health workers are the ideal option

Trained interpreters are the next best option. Interpreters are skilled in interpreting the sense and intent of what is said. Other options have major disadvantages. Written English is generally not helpful for deaf patients. Using someone close to the patient may not stop their own views colouring their translation, maybe even to hide abuse. In the hearing world it is likely that the 'interpreter' will be more or less fluent in the non-local language. In the deaf world this is rare. Most deaf patients' relatives have little or no sign language. Worse still, some think they have. Bilingual mental health workers have observed relatives who insist on interpreting, because they 'can communicate better', and who misinterpret in a fashion that suits their own views or is inept. Sadly, some who claim to be interpreters in non-BSL/SSE manual forms of communication have also been observed to claim more fluent communication, when this can be observed not to be the case. Assisted oral communication still has some advocates — of whom mental health workers should beware.

It is not uncommon for registered interpreters to be close or known to their clients. This should be avoided where practical, but the deaf world is small and often the most fluent and flexible interpreters are hearing members of Deaf families, who have been brought up in sign language. Untrained volunteer 'interpreters' may have some understanding of what is required, but may be inept. If untrained interpreters are to be used, their level of signing skill should be understood and taken into account by all parties. In the UK the Council for the Advancement of Communication with Deaf People stages of communication skill, tested at examination, can provide a guide. When any unqualified 'interpreter' is used, the service provider should ensure that the 'interpreter' understands and agrees to follow the relevant codes of behaviour (CACDP, 1994) expected of qualified interpreters. In mental health settings the code of confidentiality is especially important. Phelan and Parkman (1995) suggest that the interpreter should be asked if there are any specific cultural factors that may have a direct bearing on the interview. Roe and Roe (1991) confirm that the interpreter can impart such information if it will ease communication, despite the code of the American Register of Interpreters of the Deaf (Solow, 1981) which states that interpreters shall not counsel, advise, or interject personal opinions. For deaf patients this means allowing the interpreter (as far as is practical for the health activity) to control the setting. The use of sign language interpreters involves different positioning, so that the interpreter is beside and slightly behind the interviewer, both of whose fronts should be in good light that does not shine in the patient's eyes. Additionally, in most settings, and definitely in mental health settings, it is important for the interpreter to meet the patient before the interview and ascertain their particular variety of sign and identify and resolve any communication difficulties between interpreter and patient. Some patients attending mental health services will have limited or idiosyncratic sign usage. It is not the role of the interpreter to assess and provide comment on the patient's communication ability, but it is their role to comment on client–interpreter communication problems and, if necessary and practical, to recommend another interpreter. For example, a psychiatric specialist member of a Mental Health Tribunal, hearing an appeal by a deaf patient against a specialist psychiatrist for deaf people's compulsory detention order, asked the interpreter about the intelligence of the patient. Fortunately for the interpreter, the social worker for deaf people and the psychiatrist for deaf people, who were also present, contested this action.

Interpreters will only rarely be so fortunate as to have other deaf experts present. They should contest any misuse of their skills. This can be difficult in judicial and quasi-judicial situations, which in general are not designed to put those present at ease. It is also incumbent on the chairing authority to put the interpreter at ease and to invite the interpreter to comment on the communication process as it affects their role or the patient's communication, at any time during the proceedings. Roe and Roe (1991) support the view that referral to a signing therapist should be the first option, but point out that signing counsellors may be unable to provide the therapy needed; they may have others present and in such a situation cannot both interpret and be effective counsellors simultaneously. The deaf person may need more choice; he or she may be unable to understand a particular person's sign language. Roe and Roe (1991) point out other challenges when interpreters are used:

- Deaf clients may wonder whether interpreters will maintain confidentiality.

- Therapists may wonder whether interpreters are communicating exactly what is said.
- Interpreters may unintentionally relate their own feelings about what is happening.

Interpreters' skill levels, like those of mental health workers or any other professionals, vary greatly.

Unintentional psychodynamics

Although interpreters should avoid becoming overt figures in mental health situations, it should be recognized that they might unintentionally do so in the eyes of the client or the therapist. Both interpreter and therapist should be aware of this possibility and take corrective action if this starts to occur. This is likely to be a common and expected part of any psychoanalytically orientated therapy, and it is for the therapist, not the interpreter, to instigate corrective action. If the interpreter suspects any psychodynamics are occurring, of which the therapist is unaware, and that are interfering with communication (as they almost inevitably will) then the interpreter should make the therapist aware of the problem. This should occur outside the interview and not in front of the client, so the therapist is always left to control the situation. This situation can be minimized with therapists and interpreters who are used to the interpreting effects on interviews. Less deaf-aware therapists are likely to be unsure of the interpreter, for example where only a few signs are needed to convey a long spoken message (Roe and Roe, 1991). Sign language interpreting is usually simultaneous, but Roe and Roe (1991) report consecutive interpreting, during which the therapist talks to the patient without interpretation, followed by interpretation, to allow the patient to 'read' the body language of the therapist. This may be acceptable in a highly structured interview or therapy with short questions or statements, but is likely to be a considerable obstacle during counselling or most psychotherapies, which rely on spontaneity.

Interpreters in counselling

There is a danger of 'communication' as interpreted taking priority over the therapeutic process. Roe and Roe (1991) suggest that where there is any doubt about what is being communicated, the therapist should restate what is intended, and question or clarify as often as is needed. We would not always agree, as the nature of misunderstandings can be the stuff of psychotherapy and timing of interventions, including such clarifications, can be crucial. Roe and Roe's (1991) subsequent suggestion that such clarifications should be given 'using techniques the therapist would use with a hearing client' is more acceptable. In the USA, interpreters' involvement in counselling is regarded as being as much legally privileged as the counselling session itself, that is the interpreters cannot be ordered by a court to disclose or act as witnesses to the information gained in a counselling session. This is not the case in the UK. Hearing professionals may misdiagnose a deaf patient because they do not understand that the structure of BSL is different from written or spoken English. They also may not appreciate why some concepts are difficult for some deaf people to understand, why words may be misspelt, and so on. Care is needed so that the apparent bizarre 'English' structure or lack of vocabulary for abstract concepts are not mistaken as being symptomatic of psychiatric disorder. A good interpreter will be a safeguard here. On the other hand, there may be a danger of 'over-interpreting', trying to make sense in sign language of disturbed content which has little or no meaning and may be indicative of mental illness. It is possible to miss thought disorder and unwittingly mislead the mental health professionals (see Chapter 4).

Using an interpreter allows the person conducting the interview, consultation or therapy, whether deaf or hearing, to concentrate on the requirements of their role, without the added difficulty of using another language. In mixed family or group situations the deaf therapist, like the deaf patient, has the disadvantage of needing to concentrate on the interpreter, though this is compensated for by fluent direct communication with deaf patients and a clear demonstration to the hearing people present of the abilities and potential status of deaf people. Hearing and deaf people with speech, when communicating with deaf and hearing people together, cannot use BSL and spoken English simultaneously. The structure and grammar of the two languages differ so much as to make this impossible. In British deaf specialist mental health services, many professionals are skilled users of BSL but, without an interpreter, most of what is communicated in such a group would have to be spoken and then signed, or vice versa, thus detracting from the impact of what is said, seriously slowing down the proceedings and interrupting or changing the dynamics of the situation.

Discussing interviewing, Harry (1986) concludes from his review of the literature that techniques used with hearing people fall short during the evaluation of deaf people because their communication processes are quite different. Among the users of deaf mental health services are those people whose problems stem from, or are exacerbated by, poor communication within the family. Hearing parents of deaf children may have been counselled not to use signs but to concentrate on speech and speech reading only. For most prelingually profoundly deaf children, this is totally inadequate but parents usually accept the advice of professionals. As the child grows older, communication within the family may be restricted or stressful, leading to family problems. Using an interpreter in such a family situation can often prove to be the first time both deaf and hearing members have had an opportunity of freely expressing their thoughts and feelings to each other. It also gives an opportunity for the family to see other professionals in the field of deafness who recognize and respect the value of sign language, so helping them to modify their attitude. Harvey (1982), exploring the role of interpreters for deaf people in family therapy, points out that the interpreter's presence challenges the family's denial of deafness and challenges the family myth of the deaf child's helplessness. People who are deaf in a hearing family often feel left out, miss everyday exchanges and information. Many situations have been experienced where deaf people within a hearing family have been unaware of important events. For example one young man of 17 years of age did not know his sister was due to be married the following week, although others (hearing) in the family had known the date for months. They had assumed he had heard. Being fully included with other family members by use of an interpreter can assist in redressing the balance and provide a model for hearing people. It is not infrequent that important aspects of a family's activities or history are not known by the deaf member and these gaps may be filled during family sessions. The effect of poor communication can lead to isolation, alienation, depression, poor self-image and so on. The use of an interpreter recognizes the needs and rights of deaf and hearing people to understand and be understood. Such acknowledgement and the resultant improvement in exchange of information can, in itself, be therapeutic. Not only does the deaf person benefit, but hearing members of the family begin to 'hear' the deaf person's views and opinions. Angry outbursts can ensue as a result of years of frustration when the Deaf person says it is the first opportunity she or he has had of being heard. The parent's lament in this situation is often 'if only we had known'.

Stansfield and Veltri (1987) posed the question, 'Who does the interpreter belong to?' They maintained, 'the interpreter, as a professional service provider, is impartial and as such does not work for the client or therapist'. The client, however, may see the interpreter as someone 'on my side', depending on his or her past experiences with interpreters. The seating arrangement, with therapist and interpreter close together, may give the impression they are teaming up against the client, who may feel left out. Alternatively, the client may feel a closer bond to the interpreter because of communication. Because these perspectives may be only partly conscious, the client may need special help to differentiate the interpreter's role from that of the therapist.

Although an interpreter can be invaluable in enabling communication between the professional and the patient, there are also drawbacks to the situation. A third person being present in what would normally be a one-to-one therapeutic relationship will skew this relationship. Using an interpreter may interfere with eye contact between therapist and patient and make rapport more difficult to establish. Hoyt, Siegelman and Schlesinger (1981) found that an interpreter could 'dilute or distort the dyadic therapeutic relationship' and be seen as the centre of authority who 'understands' the deaf person. Care is needed that the therapist maintains eye contact with the interviewee, and directs speech to the person, not in the third person to the interpreter. This of course applies to all hearing people in interpreting situations.

The London Deaf Mental Health Service, part of SWLSG Mental Health NHS Trust, until its recent move to the community, based at Springfield University Hospital, consists of an Adult service (see Chapter 19), a Children's service and a Family Therapy Team (both unique in the UK) which comprises staff from both adult and children's teams and from the Family Therapy Clinic. Most of the hearing staff have good signing skills, and approximately one-third of the staff are Deaf fluent sign language users. All staff are expected to aim for fluency in sign language, though some relatively new members and most trainees have limited signing skills. Part-time interpreters are employed in the Unit on a sessional basis. Within the Unit, interpreters are used in a variety of settings. As all staff members are expected to be able to sign, priority is given to interpreting meetings which include both deaf, hard-of-hearing and hearing people, in case conferences etc, and in all other sessions where the multi-disciplinary team members meet.

Although a member of the team, the interpreter remains impartial, and should be able to understand and use the varied communication methods used within the service to allow all parties the opportunity to access information in an appropriate way. This also includes interpreting written material from English into sign language or vice versa, telephone calls and other business matters. The presence of an interpreter helps in increasing awareness of the necessity for all staff to develop good communication skills.

There are conflicting views, which are discussed from time to time, about the use of an interpreter at all meetings. One opinion is that hearing staff will not develop fluent communication skills if they depend on an interpreter. The focus of deaf staff has to be on the interpreter, so missing non-verbal signals of hearing speakers, especially in big meetings where it is difficult to scan all the faces in the room. These problems are overcome when all staff can and do use BSL during meetings. On the other hand, it is difficult for most hearing staff and some hard-of-hearing people to think as creatively in a second language; also, new staff with no or limited knowledge of signing would not be able to participate, and those learning may not feel sufficiently confident to sign in such a setting. When learning, some staff express the view that it helps them to improve their signing skills by watching the interpreter, though they are then not concentrating on the meeting and may be learning an appropriate interpreting model, but not an appropriate day-to-day sign. Hearing staff often prefer to be able to concentrate on the content of what they wish to say, and feel inhibited if they have to sign all the time during meetings. Deaf staff may similarly prefer to communicate with the consistent standard of communication provided by the interpreter. In practice, interpreters are normally used but when no interpreter is available, staff with sufficient hearing who are fluent signers have to interpret for those who cannot sign. This leads to confusion and a conflict of roles. Progress is also slower. An interpreter relieves the professionals of the need to communicate in a mode different from their own, whether they are deaf or hearing. Working in a mental health unit gives the interpreters an opportunity to develop some knowledge of mental health issues, terminology, and so on. This in turn helps both deaf and hearing professionals to feel confident that the interpreter is properly matching the spoken and signed language. Contributing to this are deaf mental health workers, who are involved in generating and developing sign vocabulary to express concepts in mental health and its specific jargon.

The Unit interpreters also work for staff and service users if the users do not attend with their own interpreters — an option given when meetings are being arranged. This is a difficult situation and one interpreter may not be adequate, even when adequate breaks are provided. Some deaf people with minimal communication skills may have developed idiosyncratic signing; there may be a strong dialect in sign; they may use special name signs or signs linked with a special school, and all of these factors could be overlaid by a mental illness or disorder. Signing is also contextual and patients find themselves in a strange situation trying to explain and understand concepts that are outside the current situation and outside the interpreter's knowledge. It is useful in such circumstances if a deaf sign language user is available to assist in communication. Understanding the culture, they are frequently better able to switch to different modes of communication and discover what the patient is trying to express. They are able to impart information in a more natural manner than even the best hearing interpreter. Sometimes a relative, friend or professional who knows the patient and his or her circumstances well, may have developed an insight and understanding of idiosyncratic signing and can be of great help in the interpretation. It is important to be aware that untrained 'interpreters' may not appreciate the necessity only to interpret and not to attribute meaning not expressed or add information from their experience.

In family therapy, all people present are given an opportunity of signing and/or speaking for themselves. The interpreter can be used solely for communication between deaf professionals and the hearing people present. In some families, one or two (or all) hearing members may prefer to sign themselves to their deaf child, parents or partner. This leaves the interpreter with the task of signing or voicing for the professionals only.

A therapist can find this helpful in recognizing some of the dynamics within a family: which member communicates with whom and how? Who is excluded? Who does not sign? Therapy can also be aided by simple example, such as positioning for more comfortable communication, by recognizing that only one person speaking/signing at a time can be understood. In the rough and tumble of family life, such details — so important to deaf people — may be missed, ignored or neglected. This leads to greater frustration or resentment, which is not conducive to good mental health. By experiencing the discipline of using an interpreter, the difficulty is highlighted and may lead to a change in communication behaviour outside the clinical setting. At the very least the problem may begin to be acknowledged.

The clinician can also use the positioning of an interpreter to modify group dynamics. By positioning the interpreter, the therapist can manipulate the visual contact of members in the group. Participants may find this different from their everyday experience when they have more control of where they sit and with whom.

The presence of the interpreter and positioning can restrict information gained, by the family taking up their own chosen positions and communicating in their way of choice. This can lead to a loss of information and therapeutic opportunities. The possible conflicts of therapist's and interpreter's roles in these situations need resolution with or without the family before the session.

In a Deaf–hearing situation, it is easy for the hearing people to dominate the discussion with a hearing clinician, thus excluding the Deaf people present. A similar situation may arise with deaf dyads, now that there are more deaf clinicians. Exclusion of either party is less likely with an interpreter present. It is not unknown for a professional to be told by a hearing person, 'don't tell him/her, but...' An interpreter will interpret everything and this is made clear at the onset of the session.

The therapist and team have to be aware of the influence of the presence of the interpreter. Having to position the interpreter to ensure the most effective communication can restrict the possible use of positioning for other therapeutic purposes. Deaf members of a family, where the therapist is hearing, may try to make an alliance with the interpreter or try to discuss matters directly with him or her. The interpreter has to avoid being drawn, without alienating the Deaf members. There may be feelings of frustration when questions or comments are not readily understood and which may affect the therapy. These may be rightly or wrongly attributed to the interpreter, leaving the therapist to judge. Harvey (1982) states, 'the psychological lack of identity of the interpreter encourages participants to exhibit the ego defense mechanisms of projection and displacement or transference'. Hearing family members may have feelings of guilt, anger, frustration or sadness if they perceive themselves as lacking in ability to communicate with their deaf members, an inability which is highlighted by the use of an interpreter. This may lead to feelings of resentment or hostility towards the therapist and/or the interpreter. The very presence of an interpreter tends to highlight the Deaf/hearing divide and signing, which may mask less overt communication and other difficulties within the family.

An interpreter can also make it possible for deaf mental health workers to work in situations where there are both deaf and hearing service users: deaf children with hearing parents, a deaf person with a hearing partner, etc. The low status and recognition afforded to deaf people in the past has not contributed to their mental health. Using interpreters in this way, enabling deaf staff members to integrate in deaf mental health service staff teams and to gain access to mental health training, goes a little way towards redressing the balance.

Children have special needs when an interpreter is being used. Very few deaf children have experienced using an interpreter. Their age, educational attainments, degree of hearing loss and the type of education they are receiving, will all determine the mode and level of communication they use and understand. Some may have only an extremely limited vocabulary of signs, mainly nouns and verbs. Others may have a sound BSL structure but with limited content and lack of knowledge of everyday ideas. There will be those whose educational and family experience of communication will have been oral/aural and whose speech may be difficult to follow, particularly for those meeting the child for the first time.

If clinicians are unable to communicate with the child, or if a few people are involved, an interpreter is essential and the interpreter should have special skills in dealing with children. Preferably, they should have had experience of being with Deaf children in schools, units and social centres and have developed an understanding of their culture and method of education. This can vary from one school or unit to another depending on the school's philosophy and communication methods used.

With young children, as with some adults with poorly developed communication skills, the interpreter may have to introduce drawing, models, mime and other visual aspects of communication to try to understand and be understood. Here again, the boundary between the interpreter and therapist may be blurred by the interpreter's necessary reliance on inference.

If a child has been educated in a rigid oral/aural environment, he may show hostility to signing or find it embarrassing. This is particularly so if the child has been punished or strongly criticized for signing. Where the interviewee or therapist is also deaf, a positive role model is provided for the deaf child which may subsequently help in overcoming the reluctance to use an interpreter. The interpreter while signing for the deaf professional must also be sensitive to the interpreting needs of the child and try to meet them.

Interpreting for deaf children is a special skill, requiring sensitivity, understanding and flexibility of an even greater degree than when interpreting for adults. A paper discussing abuse of deaf children asserts 'If the subtleties of deaf communication, and the link between the development of language and development of ideas are not fully understood, care provided will be inadequate' (Dixon 1989).

Conclusion

There is a need to look further into the role of interpreters in mental health. Frequently, far more than an interpreter is required. There is a need for more information and preparation to be given before many deaf people can benefit from therapy. There is a need for de-briefing and reinforcement following consultation to ensure the deaf person has understood what has transpired and what is expected of them subsequently. Sessions must be short, where a deaf person needs to be able to concentrate visually on new and difficult concepts. New concepts may need to be introduced in a staged fashion to give time for them to be assimilated. Someone should be able to make these factors known to mental health professionals. Is this the role of an interpreter? Perhaps interpreters in a mental health setting should undergo additional training and become interpreter/advisers. Deaf people should be trained in mental health issues to enable them to be used more often as interpreters, with an advisory role. It is vital that any advisory role relates only to actual current communication and not, for example, comments on language pathology. Either the adviser should be another person or the interpreter should overtly step out of role and explain to both parties the advice, each in their own language.

Ideally, in a one-to-one setting in mental health services, clinicians should be able to communicate directly with their patients. In the specialist services this is the case, but outside these few special provisions deaf people have to use services which are inadequate to their needs. Interpreters, deaf advocates, and so on, can go some way to alleviating some of the difficulties. Full access to mental health services will not be available to deaf people until sufficient numbers of practitioners, deaf and hearing, who are competent to deal directly with deaf people, with a knowledge of their culture and a skill in their language, are trained. This would leave interpreters to operate in the more formal situations where deaf and hearing colleagues meet. They could be used in other situations where more than two or three people are present who are unable to use fluent BSL, or the preferred method of communication of the deaf participants.

References

Brien D (1992) The Deaf community and its language. In Dictionary of British Sign Language. London: British Deaf Association.

CACDP (1994) Code of Practice for Sign Language Interpreters. Council for the Advancement of Communication with Deaf People, Pelaw House, School of Education, University of Durham, Durham DH1 1TA.

Department of Health and Welsh Office (1993) Code of Practice: Mental Health Act 1983. London: HMSO.

Dixon R (1989) Silent sufferers. Nursing Times 85: 33.

Ebert D, Heckerling P (1995) Communication with deaf patients: knowledge, beliefs, and practices of physicians. Journal of the American Medical Association 273: 227–229.

Harry B, (1986) Interview, diagnostic and legal aspects in the forensic psychiatric assessments of deaf persons. Bull Am Acad Psychiatry Law 14: 147–162.

Harvey M (1982) The influence and utilization of an interpreter for Deaf persons in family therapy. American Annals of the Deaf, December: 821–827.

Hoffmeister R, Moores DF (1987) Code switching in deaf adults. American Annals of the Deaf 132: 31–34.

Hoyt M, Siegelman E, Schlesinger H (1981) Special issues regarding psychotherapy with the deaf. American Journal of Psychiatry 138: 807–811.

Phelan M, Parkman S (1995) Work with an interpreter. British Medical Journal 311: 555–557.

Roe DL, Roe CE (1991) The third party: using interpreters for the deaf in counselling situations. Journal of Mental Health Counselling 13: 91–105.

Solow S (1981) Sign Language Interpreting: A Basic Resource Book. Silver Spring, MD: National Association of the Deaf.

Stansfield M, Veltri D (1987) Assessment from the perspective of the sign language interpreter. In Elliott H, Glass L, Evans JW. Mental Health Assessment of Deaf Clients: A Practical Manual. Boston, MA: Little, Brown and Co.

Stokoe WC, Battison RM (1981) Sign language, mental health, and satiafactory interaction. In Stein L, Mindel E, Jabaley T, Deafness and Mental Health. New York: Grune & Stratton, pp 179–194.

Chapter 14
Educational Interventions: Prevention and Promotion of Competence

MARK T. GREENBERG

Introduction

The social, emotional, linguistic and cognitive development of deaf children can be understood only in the larger context of the ecology that surrounds the growing child. From the point of diagnosis onward, the deaf child and his family are greatly affected by prevailing assumptions and beliefs in the fields of medicine/audiology, psychology and education. Further, to understand how these ecologies influence the child and family, it is necessary to take a developmental perspective. Having a significant hearing loss may have *radically* different consequences for the child and his family, depending upon factors such as:

- The hearing status of the child's parents.
- The aetiology of the deafness.
- The age at which deafness occurred.
- The type of communication approach(es) adopted by the family.
- The type of schooling that is selected for the child.
- The nature of the school programme.
- The amount and nature of contact that both the deaf child and his parents have with other deaf children and adults.

All of these factors (and more) will influence how the child and family perceive deafness and its consequences socially, educationally and vocationally.

As a group, deaf children and adolescents are at risk of a number of adverse outcomes. These include low academic achievement, delays in some cognitive and social-cognitive processes, as well as higher rates of social maladaptation and psychological distress and disorder (Greenberg and Kusche, 1989; Marschark, 1993). However, not all deaf children develop adjustment problems, and the impact of deafness is mediated and moderated by several factors, including the quality of family environment, parental adaptation to deafness, family coping, the nature of school and community resources, as well as the child's own characteristics and transactions with his ecology.

This chapter presents a developmental framework for understanding the development of both social competence and maladjustment as it affects the growing deaf child. In doing so, findings and future directions are discussed concerning preventive and promotive interventions that involve education, psychology and the socio-cultural world of deafness. Interventions will be discussed at three different developmental phases of childhood in order to improve the holistic development of deaf children. However, before discussing the role of educational and psycho-educational interventions, it is necessary to discuss (1) the changing nature of deafness and deaf education and (2) social competence and factors that influence its development in deaf children.

Unique features of the ecology of deafness

Most deaf children and their families are presented with a unique dilemma. That is, that over 90% of deaf children are born to hearing parents. Further, most deaf parents bear hearing children. This intergenerational discontinuity in deafness leads to a significant dilemma faced by most deaf children; they are likely to become part of a clearly defined minority culture in which there are no other members in their family. This 'recognition' that deaf children of hearing parents are like 'minority' children, who will belong to their own culture and have their own language, has broad implications for education and supportive environments for both the deaf child and hearing parents. In their family-of-origin, most deaf children have no other minority members to show them that culture and language. Further, to be a successful member of society and gain full access to its richness and opportunities, they will need to learn to live at least to some extent in both worlds, that of the hearing and that of the deaf.

The changing nature of schooling

For over two centuries deaf people have been educated in unique school facilities in which language and culture are transmitted. Regardless of whether native sign language and culture were promoted, tolerated or banned, the residential school provided the ecology for the cultural socialization of younger deaf children by older deaf children and adults. Thus, deaf children who had little understanding of their deafness except that they wore hearing aids and had difficulty speaking, when placed in a residential school were introduced to a world which provided them with a unique and valued identity; one that could not be bestowed by their hearing parents. Thus, a great deal more than traditional educational subjects was attained at these schools. Of equal value was a sense of belonging and identity born of a new-found language, cultural history and, with these new tools, a revised perception of 'hearing' culture and how it might be circumvented and/or accommodated.

However, during the past two to three decades there has been a dramatic shift in the nature of schooling for deaf children. These shifts in schooling have led to new and more important roles for parents in the educational development and social–emotional adjustment of their children, and thus highlight the importance of the family's coping/adjustment to deafness. Three major shifts in educational policy have altered educational placement. The first is the 'revolution' in deaf education, which has led to the use of some form of manual communication as a central component of schooling. This has, in some cases, led to significant improvements in family communication (Marschark, 1993; Calderon and Greenberg, 1997). As a result, parents have become more involved with their deaf children and their education. As parents feel more competent to communicate, and as local schools offer programmes that utilize Total Communication (in one of its many forms), there have been less compelling reasons for sending children in early and middle childhood to distant locations to be educated (e.g. residential schools).

The second change in policy in most countries has been the notion of normalization or mainstreaming. Either by law or policy shifts, local schools, regardless of their size or number of deaf children, have been given greater responsibility for the education of deaf children. Regardless of the variations in quality and service that this has produced, a major effect has been to place more responsibility on the local schools, and especially families, in the social and academic development of deaf children.

Increasing numbers of children are now being educated in neighbourhood schools and are remaining at home rather than residing in state residential schools in the UK, USA and elsewhere (Moores, Cerney and Garcia, 1990). There has been a significant decrease in residential school enrolment for deaf children. In the USA approximately 70% of deaf children now attend local schools. For most elementary school-aged children, the deaf school institution and staff are no longer the child's 'home and family'. Deaf children remain in the 'hearing community' and are residing with their hearing families much longer, and fewer deaf children are being introduced into the 'deaf community' through the cross-generational process of attending a residential state educational institution.

In spite of significant improvements throughout the world in the education of deaf children, there is little doubt that many deaf children experience communicative and social deprivation that affects both cognitive and social development. As a result, there is an unusually high incidence of deaf children who experience communicative delays, and these, in turn, may lead to psychosocial disorders that range from poor peer relations to more serious behavioural and emotional difficulties. At present there is a disproportionately high number of deaf children with adjustment problems, as well as serious mental health problems (Meadow and Trybus, 1979; Hindley et al., 1994).

Keeping our eyes on the prize — competence as a developmental outcome

Explicit goals are an important component of the development of any model for education or mental health, and are especially important in the mission of preventing maladjustment or disorder. Although in some cases these goals might be viewed as the absence of difficulties (absence of psychiatric disorders, school drop-out, or substance abuse), for many preventive interventions, central outcomes are not the prevention of social or personal ills, but instead the promotion of healthy growth and development (having healthy relationships, managing stress effectively, self-efficacy). In the field of deafness, there have been few attempts at preventive interventions, and this has been especially so in the period of middle childhood.

There have been numerous conceptualizations of competence in childhood. Although some have been primarily an enumeration of skills (Anderson and Messick, 1974), there is considerable agreement that competence has broad features that cross developmental periods as well as competencies that arise or recede in importance in different developmental epochs. Further, not only can we posit certain competencies for children, but we can similarly identify both the different adults or groups who are most important to supporting these developments. Following Waters and Sroufe (1983), competence is defined here as 'an integrative concept that refers to the ability to generate and co-ordinate flexible, adaptive responses to demands and to generate and capitalize on opportunities in the environment' (p. 80). Implicit in this working definition is a recognition of components that draw primarily from the individual as well as opportunities supplied by the environment. Furthermore, competent functioning is associated with the ability to co-ordinate affect, cognition, communication and behaviour (Waters and Sroufe, 1983; Greenberg, Kusche and Speltz, 1991).

Below, we present exemplary competency models for each developmental period followed by an integrative model of social competencies. We then apply this model to preventive interventions in early childhood, middle childhood and youth.

The early years

During early childhood, a number of developmental outcomes signal competency. They include being:

- Self-confident and trusting.
- Intellectually inquisitive.
- Able to use language to communicate effectively.
- Physically and mentally healthy.
- Able to relate well to others.
- Empathic toward others.

(Carnegie Task Force on Meeting the Needs of Young Children, 1994).

Further, these competencies are seen as the result of a loving, caring interaction with the child's parents that leads to healthy attachments and early experiences with adult caregivers, which provide the building blocks for intellectual and communicative competence. As parents (the primary socializing agents) model healthy ways to relate to the child as well as others, teach acceptable behaviour, guide healthy habits and routines, and help the young child to manage his impulses, these competencies will unfold. As almost all deaf children are first diagnosed as having a hearing loss during the first five years, the quality and nature of support for the caregiver(s) and family are especially crucial for early social, cognitive and communicative outcomes.

Middle childhood

In the early and middle years of schooling there are vast changes in the child's cognitive and social-cognitive growth as well as the powerful microsystem's influences of the peer group and the school. An excellent exemplar of a model for promoting competency is that developed by the WT Grant Consortium on the School-based Promotion of Social Competence (1992). Although this model encompasses all school grades, it provides particular emphasis on the middle childhood years. It proposes that skills be developed in the competencies of emotions, cognitions, behaviours and their interrelations as applied to the following six domains of functioning: personal development, family life, peer relations, school-related skills, community/citizenship and event-triggered stressors.

In our own model of social competence (Greenberg and Kusche, 1993) we include the following processes and outcomes:

- Good communication skills.
- The capacity to think independently.
- The capacity for self-direction and self-control.
- Understanding the feelings, motivations, needs and so forth of oneself and others.
- Flexibility in appropriately adapting to the needs of each particular situation (which includes the ability to take multiple perspectives in any situation).
- The ability to rely on and be relied upon by others.
- Understanding and appreciating both one's own culture and its values as well as those of the cultures of others.

- Utilizing skilled behaviours to maintain healthy relationships with others and to obtain socially approved goals.

Social competence also includes at least two other critical characteristics. The first of these involves the ability to tolerate frustration (Freud, 1981; Mischel, 1983). The second additional characteristic has been termed 'tolerance for ambiguity' (Loevinger, 1976). This includes the ability and willingness to consider multiple perspectives of reality, not just one's own point of view, and the capacity to be flexible rather than rigid in adapting to varying circumstances. Tolerance for ambiguity also includes the ability to transcend the concrete polarities of good versus bad and the capacity to tolerate the frequent ambivalence in one's own feelings, cognitions and internal structures (Folkman, Schaefer and Lazarus, 1980). Finally, we believe that all the above aspects of social competence are directly or indirectly related to the ability to show adaptive coping under varying levels of stress (Greenberg, Lengua and Calderon, 1997).

From middle childhood onward, being socially competent requires good communication skills (Hamilton, 1982) and the use of complex cognitive strategies, including skills such as foresight, anticipation, reflection and imagination. These abilities help the individual to understand oneself and others more adequately, to plan and execute behavioural plans more effectively, and to receive and interpret the continual feedback from both intrapsychic and environmental sources. Social competence is not a static trait, but should be conceptualized as a dynamic and changing process that is affected by a variety of both internal and ecological variables. However, certain patterns of cognitive-affective awareness are more likely to be associated with social competence across different contexts.

Adolescence, competence and identity

The teen years provide new developmental challenges for all children. Connell, Aber and Walker (1995) have provided a comprehensive framework for understanding the competencies needed during the teen years. The desired outcomes are grouped into three gross domains: economic self-sufficiency, healthy family and social relationships, and good citizenship practices. Although economic capacity and opportunity, community demography, and the existence of social institutions (e.g. youth organizations) are seen as important factors, they place crucial emphasis on the density of bonds and networks among community participants (parents, neighbours, teachers, etc.) in taking responsibility for healthy youth development. Interactions between adult community members and youth are perceived as the building blocks and supports for healthy outcomes, while recognizing that cultural supports of healthy parent-teen interactions will facilitate these processes. These processes are especially critical for deaf children as they are compounded by the issues of bi-culturalism and stigma, as elaborated below.

Childhood deafness and social competence

As we have noted in previous reviews of social-cognition in childhood (Greenberg and Kusche, 1989), deaf children are (a) often delayed in language development, (b) tend to show greater impulsivity and poorer emotional regulation and (c) have an impoverished vocabulary of emotion language. As Benderly (1980) stated, 'Many deaf children lack expressive communication supple enough to contain their curiosity, let alone their anger. So the latter may remain violent, physical, and unchecked' (p. 64). Thus, for some deaf children, as well as for other individuals who have experienced delays in language or who have been deprived of sufficient language-mediated experience (Feuerstein, 1980), the inability spontaneously to mediate experience with linguistic symbols and label aspects of inner emotional states may be one important factor leading to increasingly serious gaps in social-emotional development.

In addition to the issue of delays in language and communicative ability, there are other important factors to be considered in understanding obstacles faced by deaf children in developing social and emotional competence, which have direct implications for educational interventions. Several of these areas will be discussed below.

Incidental learning

We believe that much of the understanding of ourselves, our culture, rules for how people and families communicate and so forth, are strongly influenced by incidental learning. Unfortunately for the deaf child, there are many types of messages that are difficult to make visible, e.g. parental or teacher discussions, problem-solving, arguments when children are out of sight but not out of hearing range, television and radio in the background environment, phone calls with relatives or friends, private conversations that are 'accidentally overheard', praise or disciplinary procedures directed towards a sibling, classmate and so on. To be understood, all communications must be directed specifically to deaf children and they, in turn, must also pay close visual attention. This can be a tiring process for these children, as well as for others communicating with them, and at times may also interfere with their ongoing activities. Thus, we believe that deafness itself limits some avenues of incidental learning commonly experienced by hearing children.

Although the use of Total Communication has provided the potential to create a variety of positive changes for both deaf children and their families (Greenberg, 1983; Greenberg, Calderon and Kusche, 1984), the signing deaf child nevertheless often experiences significant isolation within the family context (Freeman, Malkin and Hastings, 1975). Additionally, it is important to remember that the use of Total Communication is not a panacea for *all* the difficulties related to deafness. Although it provides an important vehicle for communication, a Total Communication approach does not ensure the quality, consistency, fidelity, affect or value of the communications expressed. Furthermore, although a Total Communication environment, or exceptional oral skills, undoubtedly enrich deaf children's knowledge and understanding, these children still miss out on the wealth of incidental learning that hearing children acquire by overhearing communications between other people. As a result, we believe that programmes to promote social and emotional competence should be used with all deaf children, not only those who are manifesting problems, in order to help remediate understanding that may be missed or distorted through gaps in incidental learning.

Parenting styles and their consequences

A variety of obstacles in parenting accompany the significant communication problems that are often found between deaf children and their hearing parents (Schlesinger and Meadow, 1972; Gregory, 1976; Schlesinger and Acree, 1984). When deaf children misbehave, they are often either removed from the situation or physically disciplined (Schlesinger and Meadow, 1972; Greenberg, 1978). Parents frequently report that because their deaf children do not understand them, they have no other options available for socializing their children. As a result, some deaf children have fewer learning experiences in which they learn (1) what they did wrong and why it was wrong, (2) how their behaviour affected others, and (3) what alternatives they could have chosen instead. Moreover, their parents are more likely to model avoidance and physical action as methods for solving problems. Similarly, parental frustration due to communication barriers often leads parents to 'take on' their children's problems; deaf children are then afforded little opportunity to learn from and resolve their own difficulties. Quite simply, the effect of limited explanations and restricted experiences *denies* to many deaf children their rightful opportunity to learn to understand others.

Linguistic overprotection

In addition to the other factors already discussed, we believe that other, more subtle factors are also involved in the constellation of immature behaviours that are frequently noted with deaf children. For example, with many (if not most) adults living and working with deaf children, manual/sign communication is a second language that has been acquired later in life and is never as 'natural' as their native spoken language. Therefore, in addition to the deaf child's communication difficulties, there is also an issue of lack of skill and insecurity on the part of many adults. As a result, when communicating with a deaf child, many hearing individuals (parents, therapists, vocational counsellors, etc.) have a great fear of being misunderstood or not understood at all. This (often unconscious) fear, as well as less than optimal communication skills, often leads us to 'talk down' to or reduce the linguistic and cognitive complexity of our communications with deaf children. For example, a word/sign such as 'good' might be substituted for 'proud', although the latter would teach a new and critical concept. In addition, some important concepts and feeling words that are commonly used with hearing children do not have signs in the existing contrived sign systems and often the hearing adults (teachers, parents) do not know the American Sign Language (ASL) equivalent of the concept. Because of this, certain concepts are either not introduced, must be fingerspelled, or are imprecisely represented by another sign that does not adequately express the concept.

This combination of fear of misunderstanding and/or being misunderstood, and communication deficiencies in adult role models results in an insidious form of 'linguistic overprotection'. Moreover, there is an obvious circularity in this process; a lack of linguistic exposure results in deaf children having more limited vocabularies. Due to their more limited comprehension, speaker/signers offer them less complex and mature communications. As a result, we believe that deaf children often appear immature because they are typically exposed to simplified as well as limited communications. For this, as well as many other reasons, it is critical that deaf children are exposed to fluent communicators during their early development. To do so requires extensive and extended sign training for teachers. Further, it is critical that parents as well as the child receive regular exposure to deaf adults as well as ongoing family support and education programmes (Greenberg and Calderon, 1987).

Culture, stigma and identity

At the societal level, Meadow and Nemon (1976) have elaborated the myriad ways in which stigma (Goffman, 1963) may affect or 'spoil the identity' of deaf individuals. As Emerton, Hurwitz and Bishop (1979) have noted, on an interpersonal level, stigma leads to deaf people receiving differential (prejudicial) treatment ranging from pity and over-concern to anger and disgust. Additionally, as a result of the differential (lower) expectations by the majority culture, deaf individuals may limit their own personal goals, develop negative self-concepts, or internalize cognitive attributions of helplessness, failure and inferiority.

Many deaf children and adults are socialized by a hearing society in such a way that they come to believe that 'Because I'm deaf, people will take care of me. I don't need to learn to take care of myself'. Lurking behind this idea there may also be the beliefs that, 'Since I am deaf, I am not responsible' or 'I am not skilled enough to be responsible'. A systemic sense of powerlessness and helplessness experienced by many hearing parents, educators and other persons who work with deaf children can be transmitted to deaf children (Gregory, 1993; Schlesinger and Acree, 1984). When they are treated differently (e.g. obtain free entrance to activities) and do not experience the natural consequences of their behaviours (which is very common in law enforcement situations), deaf children often receive the unfortunate and discriminatory message that they do not have to be responsible for themselves.

Although there are undoubtedly many levels and perspectives at which to understand the deficient or delayed social competence of deaf children, we feel that a viewpoint that combines environmental theory, social-cognitive models, and an understanding of dynamic educational and behavioural problems is contributed to by:

- Deficits in social understanding (Cates and Shontz, 1990; Weisel and Bar Lev, 1992).
- Misattributions of the causes and effects of one's own and others' behaviours.
- Inadequate cognitive skills for reflective thinking and planning (Luckner and McNeill, 1994).
- Insufficient symbolic skills with which to understand oneself.
- Inferior communicative skills with which to express one's feelings and attitudes to others.

Most deaf children have not been taught, and thus have not learned, how to harness linguistic and cognitive skills to understand and resolve both intrapersonal and interpersonal experiences and difficulties. Although some aspects of these potential deficiencies may be due to a lack of cultural understanding of deafness, others are due to the absence of developmentally structured educational opportunities that consider the 'whole child'.

Family intervention as a component of education-based prevention

Effects of early intervention

Recent reviews of the somewhat sparse literature on the effects of early intervention with deaf children conclude that it produces significant communicative growth (Greenberg and Calderon, 1984; Meadow-Orlans, 1987; Goppold, 1988; Calderon and Greenberg, 1997). However, we know very little about how programme variations affect outcome. In our work, we have shown that, compared to a less comprehensive approach, children and families involved in a comprehensive, family-focused model using Total Communication demonstrated significantly increased communication development, improved social behaviour, and lower maternal stress (Greenberg, 1983; Greenberg, Calderon and Kusche, 1984). In addition, Watkins (1987) found significant higher language abilities and achievement, better social-emotional functioning, and more positive parent attitudes between those children who were provided with both home and centre-based services compared to those who were offered only centre-based services.

In spite of these and other positive findings regarding the effect of early intervention, there has been little documentation of what kinds of intervention for the child, parents or family are most likely to lead to positive social adaptation and competence for both the child and family across the child's development, and thus prevent later mental disorders or family dysfunction (Howell, 1992). Although the primary goal of early intervention is for families to develop satisfying and rich communication, usually using a combination of speech and some form of manual communication, in our work we have noted a number of other factors that facilitate family adaptation. Firstly, in many or most cases, fathers are usually not targeted as a critical feature of intervention. Thus, home visiting usually occurs at times that are inconvenient and, as a result of both family dynamics and programme focus, fathers usually gain most of their information and experience regarding deafness from their wives. As a result, father–child communication is often poor and this places added strain on family roles and responsibilities. In our own experience, the use of programme components such as evening home visits by teachers, which include family sign language instructions, occasional groups for fathers to discuss their roles and concerns, and family learning vacations, have been very productive in facilitating both father–child relationships as well as the paternal role in the family's experience of, and adaptation to, deafness (Freeman, Boese and Carbin, 1981).

The second innovative area of early intervention programming is early and continued contact with deaf people (Hill, 1993). Early contact with a variety of deaf people usually has the effect of 'normalizing' deafness for families. That is, parents begin to see that deaf people vary widely in their personalities, skills and interests. Nevertheless, many deaf people share pride in both their history and language as well as their close subcultural ties. As contact occurs, parents see that deaf people can be a great aid in helping them to understand their deaf child and see his potential. Of course, such contact can be effectively guided by early interventionists who can create a variety of opportunities to meet deaf people in professional as well as non-professional roles. For example, innovative early intervention programmes employ deaf professionals in a variety of roles, including the director, teacher, home visitor and sign language instructor. Although the role of deaf people is much discussed in the early intervention process, and is likely to have a powerful effect in helping parents to 'depathologize' deafness, there is no research examining its effect.

Provision of support to parents following early intervention

Although much has been discussed about the role of parents in early intervention, there has been little focus on effective parent/family education and involvement in the later preschool or school years. The usual scenario is that a family (but really only the mother) receives significant emotional support and educational assistance during the infant and preschool years. However, by the time of school entry the family is left behind and is not considered a central part of the child's education. This leads to a number of currently negative effects on both the child and the family. Firstly, although the child continues rapidly to develop communication skills at school, the skills of parents reach a plateau at an inadequate level. This seriously affects family communication. Secondly, as new developmental stresses and crises arise, there is little assistance to help prevent major problems from developing. A variety of studies during middle childhood have found that parent attitudes, social support, expectations, and problem-solving skills are related to the academic and social development of deaf children (Bodner-Johnson, 1986; Watson, Henggeler and Whelan, 1990; Calderon, Greenberg and Kusche, 1991; Calderon and Greenberg, 1993). Thirdly, a significant rift is felt both on the part of the parents and the school, which leads to each blaming the other when things go wrong.

As a result there is a need for schools to see the crucial role of the parent educator who works directly with families with children and adolescents (Clarke, 1993). It is critical to understand that assistance to the family is essential for the child's social and academic growth and that a partnership needs to develop and be maintained. Although this problem is well known (Greenberg and Calderon, 1987), and a variety of models exist for parent education, most schools do not supply sufficient preventive family services to forestall the development of later difficulties.

Role of the school

From the perspective of the promotion of social competence, many educational and mental health professionals have considerable frustration with the traditional focus of most educational efforts with deaf children. There often appears to be a lack of clarity concerning both the intended goals of education and the procedures needed to obtain them in the classroom. Although the general intention of education is to prepare young people to reach their highest potential as well as to transmit the norms and values of society, we believe that awareness of the rationales and risks discussed above necessitates a re-examination of current practices in deaf education. Most instructional time in the classroom (as well as preparatory teacher training experiences) is spent on academic subjects (the three Rs), speech and communication skills. Yet, if one examines the 'big picture' of life-span outcomes we find that both rehabilitation counsellors and mental health professionals who work with deaf adults recount that many of the vocational difficulties experienced by deaf adults which lead to unemployment, underemployment and lack of advancement are accounted for by social and interactional difficulties stemming from poor self-concept, lack of appropriate assertiveness and poor social comprehension. These factors that affect the development of the interpersonal or social self have often been called the 'hidden curriculum'. The independent thinking (problem-solving) skills that are necessary for understanding and solving problems in interpersonal contexts are quite similar to those that also lead to greater success in academic subject areas (Feuerstein, 1980). However, teaching problem-solving alone, without also teaching social and emotional comprehension and emotional regulation is not sufficient for adaptive functioning. In short, we believe that teaching the 'whole child' involves viewing personal growth and understanding as critical educational goals.

As we have recently suggested elsewhere (Greenberg and Kusche, 1989), the absence of effective curricular programmes for deaf children is related to current issues in both teacher training and research/knowledge dissemination. At present, there is a wide gap between basic knowledge about deaf children and curricular practices and models of schooling. Global knowledge (e.g. that deaf children often show impulsivity or have difficulties with memory) is generally transmitted to practitioners, but this information is seldom translated to specific applications in the classroom. Moreover, teacher training programmes in deaf education often do not require sufficient coursework in the areas of cognitive and personality/social development; as a result, most graduates of such training programmes do not have state-of-the-art knowledge on how this knowledge translates into specific instructional techniques. Moreover, in-service training in school programmes is frequently inadequate to teach new skills. This latter problem has been increased as a result of the implementation of mainstreaming and normalization due to the development of many smaller, geographically dispersed programmes. Such programmes have few teachers and often no administrator, curriculum specialist or even psychologist who works solely with the hearing-impaired. Thus, the leadership necessary to implement new curricula and to attract appropriate in-service programmes is frequently lacking (Moores, 1987; Committee on the Education of the Deaf, 1988).

It should be noted here that communication deprivation, especially in the areas of affective life, is not limited to the home, but may also be exacerbated by the child's educational experience. It is not our intention to assign 'blame' to any one ecological niche of the child's life, and certainly it would be far too simplistic to do so. Further, to the extent that families and/or schools are not effective in promoting the personal and emotional development of deaf children, these problems should be considered systemic; these types of systems issues call for a re-examination of the objectives and priorities for the education of deaf children from the day of diagnosis onward.

If this challenge of promoting social-emotional competence is to be taken seriously, it raises numerous questions, and some of them are of a specific nature; others raise the role of the purpose of education, and others raise serious practical concerns. For example: can we teach children to be more socially competent? When should we begin? How? Are there developmental stages of social competence? How does social competence affect educational achievement, vocational adjustment and achievement? Is teaching social competency skills an important role for teachers? Should other specialists be teaching these skills? If promoting social competence is an important goal, how do we integrate aspects of social competence as curricular goals? If curricular implementation is to occur, how should teacher training proceed? What kind of ongoing support best facilitates teacher effectiveness? What is the role of parent involvement and education in this process? And finally, what type of evaluation should be conducted to lead to improvements in curricular implementation?

Our experience is that in most school systems there are very fragmented attempts to tackle these issues and objectives. Usually when solutions are being attempted they are either very short term (weekly discussion groups in special classes or led by support staff), respond only to emergencies (like the AIDS education crisis or the issue of teenage pregnancy), or are due to the vision of an unusual teacher, principal or administrator.

Promoting social competence in deaf children through curricular innovation

For the past 15 years, I and my colleagues have been involved in developing and implementing mental health prevention programmes in schools for deaf and hearing children.

In 1982, we began a series of studies and field tests on the use of a school-based curriculum, PATHS (Promoting Alternative Thinking Strategies), which was designed to improve the social competence and reduce the behavioural difficulties of deaf children (Kusche and Greenberg, 1995). The curriculum is grounded in a theory of development and change: the ABCD (affective-behavioural-cognitive-dynamic) model (Greenberg and Kusche, 1993). The goals of this programme are to teach children how to develop and maintain self-control, increase their awareness of and ability to communicate about feelings, and to assist them in conflict resolution through improving their problem-solving skills. Lessons are taught by teachers on a regular basis throughout the elementary years and there are extensive methods of generalization to help build and solidify these skills outside the classroom context.

Using a design that included the random assignment of classrooms to intervention and Wait-List Control Status: assignment occurred after pre-testing (Year 1 assessment), the curriculum assessment involved a sample of 70 severely and profoundly deaf children who were involved in three consecutive years of longitudinal data collection. The children ranged in age from 6 to 13 years. All of the children had hearing parents and attended self-contained classrooms in a local school which utilized Total Communication (operationalized as the simultaneous use of signs and speech). All of the children had an unaided hearing loss of at least a 70 dB (better ear); the average loss was 92 dB. The PATHS curriculum consisted of a 60-lesson manual that was used daily in the classroom for 20–30 minutes over a period of six months. The teachers and their assistants received three days' training prior to the school year and then received weekly observations, group supervision and individual consultations. During the second year, the children in the wait-list control group (and new children who entered the classrooms) received a revised version of the curriculum which had been expanded to include approximately 15 more lessons. At each assessment time (pre-test, post-test, follow-up), a variety of measures were utilized to assess social problem-solving, emotional understanding, academic achievement, and teacher and parent ratings of behavioural adaptation.

The results generally indicated significant improvements, with an overall effect size (across measures) of 1.1 (see Greenberg and Kusche, 1993 for an extended discussion of measures and results). Results of social problem-solving interviews indicated significant improvements in role-taking, expectancy of outcome, and means-end problem-solving skills. Intervention children also generated a significantly higher percentage of prosocial solutions, and a lower percentage of both neutral and negative solutions. Similar improvements were found on both emotional recognition and the reading of emotion labels. Teacher ratings indicated significant improvements in emotional adjustment and frustration tolerance. These improvements in both behaviour and social cognition were maintained up to two years post-intervention. Further, very similar findings were found for an independent replication sample, as well as in a smaller sample of oral-only educated children. Thus, teaching self-control, emotional understanding and problem-solving skills, led to changes in these skills themselves, as well as to improved behaviour. In addition, a change score analysis indicated that increases in affective–cognitive understanding appear to be related to behavioural improvements. We believe that the direction of 'causal' effects is likely to go from social-cognitive integrations to behaviour. Not only does our model hypothesize this direction, but we also believe that it is unlikely that changes in observed behaviour would lead to changes in the integration of social–cognitive and linguistic skills.

As a result of these early, brief field trials, we expanded the scope and duration of the curriculum through later field testing in day and residential schools. The present form of PATHS (Kusche and Greenberg, 1995) is planned as a multi-year model adaptable to the first years of schooling (approximately ages 6–12). It is currently being used with deaf (as well as hearing) students in Australia, Belgium, Canada, the Netherlands, the UK and the USA.

Although curricular-based interventions appear promising for improving the social competence of deaf children (Luetke-Stahlman, 1995) it is clear that such intervention needs to be teacher-based and sustained across grades. This is indicated by results of short-term, experimental demonstrations. For example, Regan (1981) utilized a shortened nine-session version of a well-known self-control training programme with a small sample of children and found no effects on behavioural impulsivity. Similarly, Lytle (1987a) evaluated an intervention curriculum which combined a behavioural social skills approach with social problem-solving in a residential setting over an eight-week period. The sample included 16 deaf high school students (and matched control subjects). Although the residential staff rated the intervention, and children improved in social skills and problem-solving, there were no differences on a normed measure of behaviour problems and social competence (MKSEAI, Meadow, 1983). At post-test there were no group differences in problem-solving skills, social self-efficacy ratings or perceived competence by the students. Thus, although Lytle's model (1987b) was promising, its brief duration and lack of integration with the classroom are likely to explain some dilution of effects.

Although there are a variety of issues that might lead to different interventions for middle and high school students, teaching both social skills and social problem-solving is still viewed as developmentally appropriate (Weisel and Bar Lev, 1992). Barrett (1986) effectively used role play with a small sample of deaf adolescents and found significant short-term effects on social adjustment; there was no long-term follow-up. Lou and colleagues (Lou and Charlson, 1991; Gage, Lou and Charlson, 1994) reported the effects of a short-term pilot programme to enhance the social-cognitive skills of deaf adolescents. Although they found no effects on the level of person conceptualization there were significant increases in role-taking ability between pre- and post-test. There was no assessment of behaviour or social competence and no control group or follow-up assessment reported.

Both operant and social-learning model treatment programmes have been widely used in secondary prevention and in treatment programmes for children who have been 'identified' as isolated, shy, aggressive, impulsive and so forth. These programmes focus primarily on short-term skills training for clearly identified behaviours that are hypothesized to increase positive social interactions. At the risk of doing an injustice to the variety of techniques and procedures and to the rich character of the numerous case-studies in the extant literature, the following simplified conclusions are offered. Firstly, behavioural techniques are often quite effective in showing demonstrable short-term behavioural changes (Bierman, 1989). Secondly, in most cases generalization of these behavioural changes to other settings has been found to be poor. Thirdly, in a high percentage of cases, behavioural changes are *not* maintained after the treatment programme has been discontinued (Meichenbaum, 1977). Fourthly, most behavioural outcome measures are focused on the target behaviours of interest and do not assess the child's self-perceptions or the broader domain of emotional and social adjustment.

Critics of behavioural approaches ascribe the lack of generalization and maintenance to the fact that such treatments do not alter the child's internal self, i.e. they do not alter the child's cognitive or affective understanding or his intrapsychic conflicts. However, it is important to emphasize that classroom management techniques are important for providing order, rules and consistency in the school. Clarity of rules and their applications may be especially important when teachers are using group instruction.

Behavioural approaches to social skills development have become popular for use with disabled children, especially those with severe behavioural disorders, developmental disorders, and pervasive developmental delays. Examples include the ACCEPTS Curriculum (Walker et al., 1983) and PEERS (Hops, Walker and Greenwood, 1979). Such programmes have shown similar strengths and weaknesses to other behaviourally-oriented treatments (Gresham, 1981; Hops, Finch and McConnell, 1985) and they have not been used successfully with deaf children.

Recently, a number of investigators have applied behaviourally-oriented social skills training to hearing-impaired and deaf children with behavioural and interpersonal difficulties. In two studies, Schloss and colleagues (Schloss, Smith and Schloss, 1984; Smith, Schloss and Schloss, 1984; Schloss and Smith, 1990) demonstrated the effectiveness of time-limited social skills training for increasing the social responsiveness and appropriateness of emotionally disturbed hearing-impaired orally-educated adolescents. Similarly, Lemanek et al., (1986) reported positive effects for behavioural social skills training with four case-studies of adolescents. Finally, Rasing and colleagues in The Netherlands have shown significant short-term effects of behavioural training programmes for individual social skills in language-disabled deaf children (Rasing and Duker, 1992, 1993; Rasing et al., 1994). There were no control groups or long-term follow-up in any of these projects and no assessments were made of the children's general social competence.

Developmental issues in prevention during adolescence

With the advent of adolescent development, the effects of both identity development and social networks are likely to play an increasingly important role in the adaptation of deaf youth (Cole and Edelmann, 1991). Although the development of a healthy identity is likely to result in part from healthy adaptation, new developmental forces complicate the picture (Greenberg, Lengua and Calderon, 1997).

Both one's intimate attachment to parents and peers as well as a feeling of belonging to a social network are important in healthy identity development in adolescence. One's social network might include a variety of individuals, including relatively close friends, members of one's extended family, co-workers or classmates, neighbours, casual acquaintances, and members of organizations or groups in which the adolescent actively participates. This 'less intimate social support' can be a powerful influence on mental health and coping ability. Both intimate attachments and/or one's social group can be invaluable resources for coping with stress by providing a variety of functions, including emotional support, information, advice, feelings of solidarity and actual physical or financial assistance. As more deaf children are educated in mainstream settings and thus have fewer early and adolescent experiences with deaf adults, the nature and function of the deaf adolescent's social network may be of particular importance for the following three reasons. Firstly, a social network provides a sense of connection or feeling of belonging to *some* type of 'community'. For a deaf person it could be either the 'deaf' world or the 'hearing' world or both. However, given that most deaf children grow up as a 'minority' with few or no role models to help them establish their identity, the feeling of belonging is both quite important and in some cases difficult for the individual to establish (Reagan, 1990).

The second function that certain types of social support may provide is to control the meaning of events. That is, events that an individual may appraise as very stressful or problematic may be reappraised as natural and not 'crazy'. Through the network interactions the individual comes to realize that 'I'm not the only one who has this problem'. This function is dependent upon the individual having access to other individuals who share similar issues, identities and concerns. In the area of deafness, such groups have been effectively utilized for hearing parents and for deaf children. However, there has been little or no use of such groups for deaf adolescents living in hearing families, especially in mainstream settings.

The third and related function of such network groups is to open up new channels of information for the individual, and thus provide the individual with more coping options, e.g. different alternative solutions to problems. Individuals who are isolated or have 'deficient' social networks are likely to be less able to deal adequately with stress for the variety of reasons mentioned above. Traditionally, the deaf adolescent's network developed through attendance at a residential school, as well as through special summer camp experiences, participation in athletic, activity-based and fraternal networks involving other deaf adolescents and adults. As enrolment at residential schools has declined dramatically, deaf adolescents are at greater risk (especially in rural areas) as they may not have access to social networks where they feel they belong, and which can help to 'normalize' the experience of being 'an outsider in a hearing world'.

With the exception of one study (Mertens, 1989) there has been little exploration of how school placement, social support networks or intimate relations affect adaptation in adolescents who are deaf. As adolescence is believed to be a time of significant risk, as well as a critical time for the formation of identity, such information is essential for the development of effective programmes to strengthen identity and adaptation. In this regard, there is a need to pay special attention to the potential role of deaf adults in affecting these developmental processes. Such information would provide direction for prevention programmes focused on later developmental periods.

Critical roles of deaf people in education and identity processes

There has been much discussion in the past few years of the importance of deaf adults to the education of deaf children. The Gallaudet Revolution and similar mini-revolts have served notice that the period in which deaf persons were discriminated against is over. In dealing with the topic of a healthy deaf identity, the understanding of deaf people is essential to the development of healthy school and community programming. Surely, deaf people need to be involved in education as teachers, psychologists, directors of schools, support staff and in every other conceivable position! Not only should they be employed at all levels in education but it is essential that deaf individuals become members of the school advisory board and other decision-making bodies. In addition, there are other roles for deaf people that may not be considered standard teaching positions. For example, hiring deaf individuals as professionals to offer ASL and deaf culture/history classes to deaf children, parents and teachers — including the art of storytelling.

As importantly, the schools need to reach out to the deaf community. Creating better ties between the school, the parents, deaf organizations and the deaf community should be a very high priority. For example, holding joint meetings, picnics, inviting deaf people specifically to events at the school, allowing the deaf community to utilize the school as a community learning centre, etc. Other ideas include developing programmes for retired deaf people to spend time at schools as helpers and role models.

The point of these ideas is to get deaf people more involved in the education and lives of deaf children and their hearing families (Hill, 1993). As the families, the school and the deaf community become more connected, the deaf child is not put in the position of having to reject his hearing family in order to 'become deaf'. How this is done is very important; as deaf people and sign language become more important socially and politically, hearing parents have more to cope with — learning to sign, a new language, a new culture that feels alien. It is critical that these new partnerships are created with a sense of togetherness and a recognition of the important and unique contributions that parents, school personnel (both deaf and hearing) and the deaf community all bring to the optimal development of deaf children. Although such programmes are ongoing in some schools, there has been little discussion of either best practices for success or evaluation of outcomes for children and youth.

Implication of current knowledge for educational innovation

Services for families

Based on our current knowledge of preventive mental health for deaf children and their families, the next generation of family services should consider the following components:

- Services that will teach, encourage and expand parents' knowledge and use of good problem-solving skills. For example, a problem-solving framework could be utilized as a model for parental discussion and support groups. An increase in parental success at solving problems is likely to increase their feelings of mastery and control. This, in turn, provides deaf children with influential, competent and resourceful parental role models. Just having parent groups that either teach sign language or only allow them to vent their feelings and listen to speakers will not teach them the necessary skills for effective parenting. Further, it is necessary to empower parents to create further changes in deaf education — our experiences in The Netherlands and Belgium are instructive. The PATHS Curriculum is now a central curriculum component in deaf education in these two countries — and it is totally due to the efforts of the national parents' associations, not to visionary leadership by the schools or their directors!
- Programme services should facilitate the development of strong support networks for parents, particularly for mothers because they appear to use and benefit from these networks (Meadow-Orlans, 1990,

1994; Meadow-Orlans and Steinberg, 1993; Greenberg, Lengua and Calderon, 1997). These supports might come from other parents of hearing-impaired children, friends, neighbours, extended family, professionals, community (e.g. church or other organizations), school personnel and deaf individuals.

- The development of specialized intervention programmes for fathers of deaf children, who are usually not targeted by early intervention projects.
- Parental support and guidance should continue throughout childhood. This should include advanced sign language classes (ASL), family weekend retreats, exposure to deaf adults, and problem-solving groups to address deaf adolescent issues.
- A developmental approach should be emphasized in providing services to families. Recognition of parents' different needs at different emotional and life stages, and children's varying needs at different ages, is important if families are to participate and feel that the services are meeting their needs. For example, parents of older deaf children may need not only guidance in understanding emotional reactions to their deaf child but also programmes that will facilitate peer interaction and social support for their deaf child, who may be struggling with self-identity issues.

Services in the schools

In a complementary fashion, the next generation of school-based innovations might include the following:

- The development and evaluation of preventive intervention programmes in the following areas: (a) Teaching social-cognitive abilities such as role-taking, understanding of emotions, and social problem-solving in the early school years; (b) prevention programmes for adolescents on problem-solving as it relates to interpersonal difficulties, peer pressure, drug and alcohol use, and sexuality; and (c) attributional training/problem-solving programmes to attempt to effect motivation, locus of control, and self-confidence of deaf adolescents and young adults.
- The development of curricular materials on deaf culture, deaf history, and ASL for use in school programmes for deaf children across educational settings.
- The development of programme co-ordination between vocational rehabilitation counsellors and school personnel to facilitate the transition between the worlds of school and work.

Summary

This chapter has focused on the social and emotional difficulties that are encountered by many deaf children, and on many promising ideas for educational innovation and prevention. We believe that many of the findings previously reported which show poorer social adjustment result from socialization practices at home and school that are remediable through developmentally timed preventive programming. It is clear that administrative support is critical for successful innovation. Although deaf education now occurs in a new modality (some form of manual communication), there has been very little innovation regarding the school structure and curriculum. We have discussed how educational interventions at each developmental level should be directed towards improving the risk factors and building protective factors that include child social, cognitive and communicative skills as well as enabling the family, the school and the deaf community to provide healthier ecologies for deaf children.

References

Anderson S, Messick S (1974) Social competency in young children. Developmental Psychology 10: 282–293.

Barrett M (1986) Self-image and social adjustment change in deaf adolescents participating in a social living class. Journal of Group Psychotherapy, Psychodrama and Sociometry 39: 3–11.

Benderly BL (1980) Dancing Without Music. Garden City, New York: Anchor.

Bierman KL (1989) Improving the peer relationships of rejected children. In Lahey BB, Kazdin AE (eds) Advances in Clinical Child Psychology (Vol. 12). New York: Plenum Press, pp 53–84.

Bodner-Johnson B (1986) The family environment and achievement of deaf students: a discriminant analysis. Exceptional Children 52: 443–449.

Calderon R, Greenberg MT (1993) Considerations in the adaptation of families with school-aged deaf children. In Marschark M, Clark MD (eds) Psychological Perspectives on Deafness. Hillsdale, NJ: Lawrence Erlbaum Associates, pp 27–48.

Calderon R, Greenberg MT (1997). The effectiveness of early intervention for children with hearing impairments. In Guralnick MJ (ed) The Effectiveness of Early Intervention: Second Generation Research. Baltimore, MD: Paul H. Brooks, pp 325–362.

Calderon R, Greenberg MT, Kusche C (1991) The influence of family coping on the cognitive and social skills of deaf children. In Martin D (ed) Advances in Cognition, Education and Deafness. Washington, DC: Gallaudet Press, pp 195–200.

Carnegie Task Force on Meeting the Needs of Young Children (1994) Starting Points: Meeting the Needs of Our Youngest Children. New York: Carnegie Corporation.

Cates DA, Shontz FC (1990) Role-taking ability and social behavior in deaf school children. American Annals of the Deaf 135: 217–221.

Clarke P (1993) The school/parent partnership: a role in mental health promotion. In Laurenzi C, Hindley P (eds) Keep Deaf Children in Mind: Current Issues in Mental Health. London: National Deaf Children's Society, pp 32–35.

Cole SH, Edelmann RJ (1991) Identity patterns and self- and teacher-perceptions of problems of deaf adolescents: a research note. Journal of Child Psychology and Psychiatry and Allied Disciplines 32: 1159–1165.

Committee on the Education of the Deaf (1988) Toward Equality: Education of the Deaf. Washington, DC: US Government Printing Office.

Connell JP, Aber JL, Walker G (1995) How do urban communities affect youth? Using social science research to inform the design and evaluation of comprehensive community initiatives. In Connell JP, Kubisch AC, Schorr LB, Weiss C (eds) New Approaches to Evaluating Community Initiatives. Washington, DC: Aspen Institute, pp 93–126.

Emerton G, Hurwitz TA, Bishop ME (1979) Development of social maturity in deaf adolescents and adults. In Bradford LJ, Hardy WG (eds) Hearing and Hearing Impairment. New York: Grune & Stratton, pp 221–243.

Feuerstein, R. (1980). Instrumental Enrichment. Baltimore: University Park Press, pp 314–320.

Folkman S, Schaefer C, Lazarus RS (1980) Cognitive processes as mediators of stress and coping. In Hamilton V, Warburton DM (eds) Human Stress and Cognition. London: Wiley, pp 210–248.

Freeman R, Boese R, Carbin C (1981) Can't Your Deaf Child Hear? Baltimore, MD: University Park Press.

Freeman RD, Malkin SF, Hastings JO (1975) Psycho-social problems of deaf children and their families: a comparative study. American Annals of the Deaf 120: 391–405.

Freud A (1981) The Writings of Anna Freud (Vol. 8): Psychoanalytic Psychology of Normal Development. New York: International Universities Press.

Gage S, Lou MW, Charlson E (1994) A social learning program for deaf adolescents. Perspectives in Education and Deafness 13: 2–5.

Goffman E (1963) Stigma: Notes on the Management of a Spoiled Identity. Englewood Cliffs, NJ: Prentice-Hall.

Goppold L (1988) Early intervention for preschool deaf children: the longitudinal academic effects relative to program methodology. American Annals of the Deaf 133: 285–288.

Greenberg MT (1978) Attachment behavior, communicative competence, and parental attitudes in preschool deaf children. Unpublished doctoral dissertation, University of Virginia.

Greenberg MT (1983) Family stress and child competence: the effects of early intervention for families with deaf infants. American Annals of the Deaf 128: 407–417.

Greenberg MT, Calderon R (1984) Early intervention for deaf children: outcomes and issues. Topics in Early Childhood Special Education 3: 1–9.

Greenberg MT, Calderon R (1987) Parent programs. In Van Cleve J (ed) Encyclopedia of Deaf People and Deafness. New York: Macmillan, pp 128–131.

Greenberg M, Kusche C (1989) Cognitive, personal and social development of deaf children and adolescents. In Wang MC, Reynolds MC, Walberg HJ (eds) Handbook of Special Education: Research and Practice (Vols. 1–3). Oxford: Pergamon Press, pp 95–129.

Greenberg MT, Kusche CA (1993) Promoting Social and Emotional Development in Deaf Children: The PATHS Project. Seattle, WA: University of Washington Press.

Greenberg M, Calderon R, Kusche C (1984) Early intervention using simultaneous communication with deaf infants: the effect on communication development. Child Development 55: 607–616.

Greenberg MT, Kusche CA, Speltz M (1991) Emotional regulation, self-control, and psychopathology: the role of relationships in early childhood. In Cicchetti D, Toth SL (eds) Rochester Symposium on Developmental Psychopathology, Vol. 2: Internalizing and Externalizing Expressions of Dysfunction. Hillsdale, NJ: Erlbaum, pp 21–56.

Greenberg MT, Lengua LJ, Calderon R (1997) The nexus of culture and sensory loss: Coping with deafness. In Sandler IN, Wolchik SA (eds) Handbook of Children's

Coping with Common Stressors: Linking Theory, Research and Interventions. New York: Plenum, pp 301–332.

Gregory S (1976) The Deaf Child and His Family. New York: John Wiley.

Gregory S (1993) The developing deaf child. In Laurenzi C, Hindley P (eds) Keep Deaf Children In Mind: Current Issues in Mental Health. London: National Deaf Children's Society, pp 4–15.

Gresham FM (1981) Social skills for handicapped children: a review. Review of Educational Research 51: 139–176.

Hamilton V (1982) Cognition and stress: an information processing model. In Goldberger L, Brenitz S (eds) Handbook of Stress: Theoretical and Clinical Aspects. New York: The Free Press, pp 41–71.

Hill P (1993) The need for deaf adult role models in early intervention programs for deaf children. ACEHI Journal 19: 14–20.

Hindley PA, Hill PD, McGuigan S, Kitson N (1994) Psychiatric disorder in deaf and hearing-impaired children and young people: a prevalence study. Journal of Child Psychology and Psychiatry 35: 917–934.

Hops H, Finch M, McConnell S (1985) Social skills deficits. In Bornstein PH, Kazdin AE (eds) Handbook of Clinical Behaviour Therapy with Children. Homewood IL: Dorsey, pp 543–598.

Hops H, Walker HM, Greenwood CR (1979) PEERS: a program for remediating social withdrawal in school. In Hamerlynck LA (ed) Behavior Systems for the Developmentally Disabled: 1. School and Family Environments. New York: Brunner/Mazel, pp 124–156.

Howell RF (1992) A profile of family education/early intervention services at the Maryland School for the Deaf. American Annals of the Deaf 137: 79–84.

Kusche CA, Greenberg MT (1995) The PATHS Curriculum. Seattle, WA: Developmental Research & Programs.

Lemanek KL, Williamson DA, Gresham FM, Jensen BF (1986) Social skills training with hearing-impaired children and adolescents. Behavior Modification 10: 55–71.

Loevinger J (1976) Ego Development. San Francisco: Jossey Bass.

Lou MW, Charlson ES (1991) A program to enhance the social cognition of deaf adolescents. In Martin D (ed) Advances in Cognition, Education, and Deafness. Washington, DC: Gallaudet Press, pp 329–334.

Luckner JL, McNeill JH (1994) Performance of a group of deaf and hard-of-hearing students and a comparison group of hearing students on a series of problem-solving tasks. American Annals of the Deaf 139: 371–377.

Luetke-Stahlman B (1995) Classrooms, communication, and social competence. Perspectives in Education and Deafness 13: 12–16.

Lytle RR (1987a) Effects of a cognitive social skills training procedure with deaf adolescents. Unpublished doctoral dissertation, University of Maryland. Dissertation Abstracts International 47 11-B: 4675.

Lytle RR (1987b) A social skills training program for deaf adolescents. Perspectives for Teachers of the Hearing Impaired 6: 19–22.

Marschark M (1993) Psychological Development of Deaf Children. New York: Oxford University Press.

Meadow KP (1983) Revised Manual. Meadow/Kendall Social-Emotional Assessment Inventory for Deaf and Hearing-Impaired Children. Washington, DC: Pre-College Programs, Gallaudet Research Institute.

Meadow KP, Nemon A (1976) Deafness and stigma. American Rehabilitation 2: 7–9; 19–22.

Meadow KP, Trybus RJ (1979) Behavioral and emotional problems of deaf children: an overview. In Bradford LJ, Hardy LG (eds) Hearing and Hearing Impairment. New York: Grune & Stratton, pp 414–438.

Meadow-Orlans KP (1987) An analysis of the effectiveness of early intervention programs for hearing-impaired children. In Guralnick MJ, Bennett FC (eds) The Effectiveness of Early Intervention for At-Risk Children. New York: Academic Press, pp 325–362.

Meadow-Orlans KP (1990) The impact of child hearing loss on the family. In Moores DF, Meadow-Orlans KP (eds) Educational and Developmental Aspects of Deafness. Washington, DC: Gallaudet University Press, pp 321–338.

Meadow-Orlans KP (1994) Stress, support, and deafness: perceptions of infants' mothers and fathers. Journal of Early Intervention 18: 91–102.

Meadow-Orlans KP, Steinberg AG (1993) Effects of infant hearing loss and maternal support on mother-infant interactions at 18 months. Journal of Applied Developmental Psychology 14: 407–426.

Meichenbaum D (1977) Cognitive-behavior Modification: An Integrative Approach. New York: Plenum.

Mertens DM (1989) Social experiences of hearing impaired high school youth. American Annals of the Deaf 134: 15–19.

Mischel W (1983) Delay of gratification as process and person variable in development. In Magnusson D (ed) Human Development: An Interactional Perspective. New York: Academic Press, pp 149–166.

Moores DF (1987) Educating the Deaf: Psychology, Principles, and Practices (third edition). Boston, MA: Houghton Mifflin Company.

Moores DF, Cerney B, Garcia M (1990) School placement and least restrictive environment. In Moores DF, Meadow-Orlans KP (eds) Educational and Developmental Aspects of Deafness. Washington, DC: Gallaudet University Press, pp 115–136.

Rasing EF, Duker PC (1992) Effects of a multifaceted training procedure on the acquisition and generalization of social behaviors in language-disabled deaf children. Journal of Applied Behavior Analysis 25: 723–734.

Rasing EF, Duker PC (1993) Acquisition and generalization of social behaviors in language-disabled deaf children. American Annals of the Deaf 138: 362–369.

Rasing EJ, Connix F, Duker PC, van de Hurk Ardine J (1994) Acquisition and generalization of social behaviors in language-disabled deaf children. Behavior Modification 18: 411–442.

Reagan T (1990) Cultural consideration in the education of deaf children. In Moores DF, Meadow-Orlans KP (eds) Educational and Developmental Aspects of Deafness. Washington, DC: Gallaudet University Press, pp 73–84.

Regan JJ (1981) An attempt to modify cognitive impulsivity in deaf children: self-instruction versus problem-solving strategies. Unpublished doctoral dissertation, University of Toronto.

Schlesinger HS, Acree MC (1984) The antecedents of achievement and adjustment: a longitudinal study of deaf children. In Anderson G, Watson D (eds) The Habilitation and Rehabilitation of Deaf Adolescents. Washington, DC: The National Academy of Gallaudet College, pp 48–61.

Schlesinger HS, Meadow KP (1972) Sound and Sign: Childhood Deafness and Mental Health. Berkeley, CA: University of California Press.

Schloss PJ, Smith MA (1990) Teaching Social Skills to Hearing-Impaired Students. Washington, DC: Alexander Graham Bell Association.

Schloss PJ, Smith MA, Schloss CN (1984) Empirical analysis of a card game designed to promote consumer-related competence among hearing-impaired youth. American Annals of the Deaf 129: 417–423.

Smith MA, Schloss PJ, Schloss CN (1984) An empirical analysis of a social skills training program used with hearing-impaired youths. Journal of Rehabilitation of the Deaf 18: 7–14.

Walker HM, McConnell S, Holmes D, Todis B, Walker JL, Goldenn N (1983) A Curriculum for Children's Effective Peer and Teacher Skills (ACCEPTS). Austin, TX: Pro-Ed Publishers.

Waters E, Sroufe LA (1983) Social competence as a developmental construct. Developmental Review 3: 79–97.

Watkins S (1987) Long term effects of home intervention with hearing-impaired children. American Annals of the Deaf 132: 267–271.

Watson SM, Henggeler SW, Whelan JP (1990) Family functioning and the social adaptation of hearing-impaired youths. Journal of Abnormal Child Psychology 18: 143–163.

Weisel A, Bar Lev H (1992) Role taking ability, non-verbal sensitivity, language and social adjustment of deaf adolescents. Educational Psychology 12: 3–13.

WT Grant Consortium on the School-based Promotion of Social Competence (1992) Drug and alcohol prevention curricula. In Hawkins JD, Catalano RF (eds) Communities that Care. San Francisco: Jossey-Bass, pp 129–148.

Chapter 15
Psychodynamic Therapies

Part 1 Psychotherapy

NICK KITSON, JANET FERNANDO AND JANE DOUGLAS

> 'I have learnt that the only real change that can be achieved is within ourselves, through the unconscious and the acceptance of who we are. . . . deaf consciousness, in its many different forms, is often prevented from making these discoveries and from learning to value or accept itself. (Corker, 1994)

What is psychotherapy?

Psychotherapy can occur at several levels, from supportive to exploratory, and it can take place within informal and professional relationships. At the more formal levels many different professionals may be involved. The word psychotherapy derives from ancient Greek. 'Psyche' refers to the mind or soul, i.e. the whole of that part of us which is not our bodies or their direct functions. 'Therapeia' refers to attending curatively to problems or disease. Psychotherapy has come to mean talking cures, though it can include other communication cures, such as role play, modelling behaviours and use of the arts as a medium of expression and communication (see Part 2 of the chapter). Mental health professionals' use of the term psychotherapy tends to mean 'dynamic psychotherapy', although it can refer to 'behavioural psychotherapy' (Chapter 13). Dynamic psychotherapy stems from the work of Freud and psychoanalysis. All dynamic psychotherapies explore the patient's inner worlds of thoughts, feelings and attitudes that stem from his temperament, life experiences and development, but significantly influence current feelings, thought and behaviour.

A core goal of dynamic psychotherapy is to enable the patient to gain and maintain fulfilling close relationships. There is considerable overlap between psychotherapy and counselling. The work of some counsellors with their clients is no different in depth or quality from psychotherapy. On the other hand there is 'counselling', which includes advice or which is focused on practical problems, for example, those of contraception or AIDS. The latter is clearly not psychotherapy. Psychotherapy involves exploring the unconscious mind and long-forgotten past experiences, though this can also be true of psychodynamic counselling. Psychotherapy can appear to be in the hands of practitioners who have mysterious insight into the workings of other people's minds, giving power to the therapist at the expense of the patient.

Because of the variation in psychotherapy and counselling theories and techniques and the reliance on personal experience and intuition our chapter cannot be read in context or evaluated without knowledge of the authors' own theoretical background, technique and experience.

Nick Kitson is a hearing psychiatrist for whom signing is a second language. He is also a group analytic psychotherapist, but whose main interest is in individual short-term dynamic psychotherapy (Davanloo, 1980). Although trained in behaviour therapy, he has limited experience and knowledge of cognitive therapy, but is aware there is significant overlap with short-term dynamic psychotherapy. He is more interested in technique than theory. His training and practice reflect his belief that it is incumbent on any state-funded practitioner to use the most efficient technique to assist patients to overcome their problems or, in other words, successfully gain what they need from their world. His training and personal group therapy were purely in his preferred language.

Janet Fernando is a hearing psychoanalytic psychotherapist for whom signing is a second language. Her main area of interest is working with individual patients at a frequency of at least once a week and for extended periods of time. She works with sign-language-using and oral Deaf people. She worked for many years in schools teaching deaf children. Her training and personal analysis were purely in her preferred language.

Jane Douglas is a Deaf psychodynamic counsellor for whom signing is her preferred language. She has completed a four-year advanced psychodynamic counselling training course in a hearing setting, with sign language interpretation. She has worked with signing and non-signing deaf patients as well as hearing patients, who have Deaf parents. She has experience of groups and individual work as trainee and therapist. Her training and personal therapy were mostly not in her preferred language of British Sign Language (BSL).

We are all eclectic in theoretical orientation, particularly making use of Freudian and Kleinian ideas as well as the work of Winnicott and Bowlby. We are not suggesting this theoretical background is inherently better than others. As Harvey (1993) says 'when therapists get lost in their theories, it means they've stopped listening to the client'. In fact the more we read the more we find similarities rather than differences. Unfortunately this is not always apparent. The psychotherapy world is dogged by exaggerated differences, splits with projection of the bad on to others and retention of the good. Claims to have the ultimate theory or technique are too often made. Caution is required where authors or practitioners claim to be right or reject others' approaches. Urban (1990, 1993), Farrugia (1986) and Sarlin and Altshuler (1978) provide examples of how the theories of Jung, Adler and Piaget respectively can be applied to understanding Deaf patients.

Analytic psychotherapy is, like counselling, founded on a voluntary contract between user and provider. The basic tenet is that the provider's behaviour is solely aimed at the good of the user. The core behaviour of the therapist is to provide non-possessive warmth and empathy, unconditional positive regard and genuineness (Truax and Carkhuff, 1967). Basic to analytic psychotherapy is the assumption that much of a patient's behaviour is influenced or controlled by motivations, attitudes and experiences of which the patient is unconscious. In this it is clearly different from cognitive therapy, which deals with behaviour that is conscious or readily accepted by the patient, once pointed out. As Sue O'Rourke (Chapter 17) emphasizes, cognitive behavioural therapy is scientific. It is therefore dependent on the observable and measurable. This is both its strength and its weakness. Such an approach is more efficient where the patient is largely conscious or can easily be made conscious of his problem and its ongoing causes. The cognitive behavioural approach is limited by an inability to treat deeply unconscious motivations. Earlier analytic therapists rejected behaviour therapy on the basis that it treated only the symptom, so the cause would rear its ugly head again with a substitute symptom. This has been disproved. In most cases behaviour therapy not only leads to improvement of the target symptom, but generalizes to improvements in other aspects of living. The occurrence of symptom substitution, a patient's inability to use cognitive behavioural approaches or a preference and ability for more personal exploration are indicators for a psychodynamic approach as opposed to a cognitive behavioural one.

Paradoxically, generalization as evidence in favour of the behavioural technique is also in favour of analytic theories, which view symptoms as symbolic representations of the deeper causes. Therapeutic work on the symbols of the problem will mean indirect work on the problem itself.

Classical psychoanalysis involves 50-minute relatively free floating sessions on the couch without eye contact, four or five times weekly, often over several years. Frequency and regularity contribute to the intensity and security of therapy. This in turn allows fuller expression of inner experiences associated with pain and fear. The unhurried pace allows regression to earlier more dependent relationships with associated transference of feelings and attitudes from the past on to the analyst in the present. This is referred to as the 'transference neurosis'. Forgotten experiences are then expressed in the present and available for therapeutic exploration. With some patients a 'transference psychosis' may develop. The feelings and attitudes transferred to the analyst are held as real attributes of the analyst.

Psychoanalytic psychotherapy is a modification of psychoanalysis in which the frequency of the sessions is reduced, but rarely to less than one session per week. Whereas in psychoanalysis there is time to explore all problems at all levels of personality development, in psychoanalytic psychotherapy aims are usually restricted to the resolution of key problems or conflicts. The intensity of therapy is not necessarily increased by length of therapy. Freud recognized the need to modify 'the pure gold of psychoanalysis' to 'new. . . conditions', but was referring only to the need to make it available to 'the poor man', who has 'just as much right to assistance for his mind'. Like us all, he was a man of his time. Had he seen the effectiveness of cognitive behavioural therapy and the variety of dynamic therapies, as a scientist he would have probably changed his view.

Short-term dynamic psychotherapy is an active, though non-directive form of psychoanalytic psychotherapy. Its systematic approach provides a framework to the process of therapy that is helpful in understanding the key processes of all analytic therapy. The therapist observes the patient for any behaviours that will hinder open expression of the patient's problem and accompanying feelings, attitudes and behaviours. A description in detail of an example of the problem presented is requested from the patient.

A Deaf woman, referred for depression following several overdoses with suicidal intent, describes the last time she felt really depressed. She described being at home, and her husband also Deaf being non-communicative. She is asked 'what did you do next'. 'Nothing'. 'What did you want to do?' 'There's no point' (in bitter misery). 'Did you notice you didn't answer my question.' (Sullenly) 'What question?' 'Do you remember I asked you what you wanted to do?' 'Oh. . . yes' (without enthusiasm). 'You remembered the question yet you left me to repeat it. I wonder what was happening?' 'What do you mean?' (with evident irritation). 'What were you feeling?' 'Nothing.' 'Nothing?' 'Not really.' 'You say a clear nothing then a vague not really.' 'Yes' (with a resigned expression fleetingly looking softly eye to eye). 'Were you feeling nothing?' 'You're the expert' (Irritated). 'How can I be the expert. They're your feelings.' 'You can't' (with a resigned expression fleetingly looking softly eye to eye again). 'Yet you acted as if I am the expert.' 'I know' (sadly). 'Has that happened before?' 'Yes I'm always doing it.' 'Do you want to continue' (doing it). 'No.' 'So we should look at what happened that made you do it here with me today.' The therapist then summarizes her avoiding saying what she wanted to say to her husband, leaving the therapist to do the work of remembering and asked for her feeling when she had said it was nothing. She recalled feeling anxious, then irritated, then angry as if it was only an internal state. 'With me?' (Slight wriggling, apparent discomfort and resigned nodding with a slight dismissive head shake). 'With me?' 'Yes' (calmly, but with a touch of sadness, looking me straight in the eye). 'You're looking me in the eye and telling me clearly, how do you feel now.' 'Good' (slight shake of the head indicating uncertainty). They go on in a similar way to explore how she felt towards her husband when he didn't communicate.

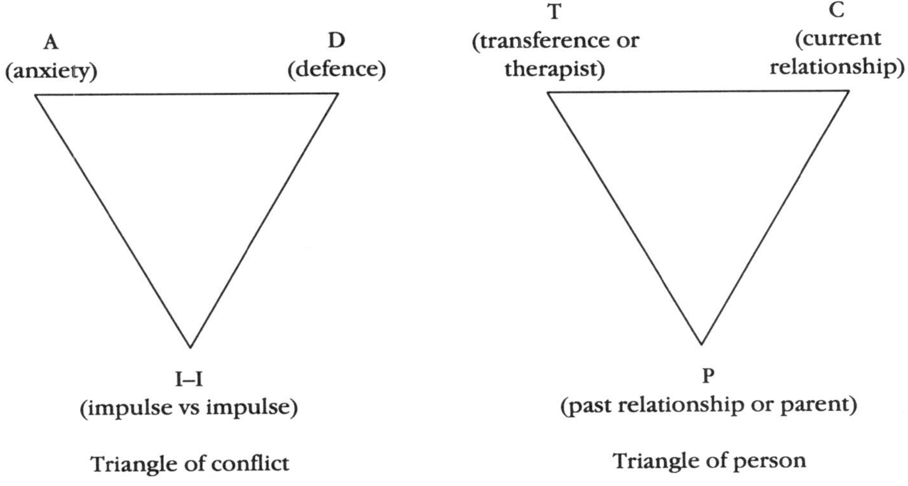

Figure 15.1 Malan's triangle. Adapted from Malan (1979) and Davanloo (1980).

What she feared if she challenged him with her anger and how she deals with her husband in the same passive aggressive way she dealt with the therapist, is explored. So what was the process of therapy?(See Figure 15.1).

Referring to the triangles, the patient very quickly assumed the need of her initial evasive, then passive aggressive defence (D) in relation to the therapist (T) for fear (A) of her conflict (I–I). She admitted she had expected the therapist (T) to be uninterested in or dismissive of her. She admitted similar behaviour with her husband (C) and that she had not really tested the hypothesis that if she showed her real feelings to him, as she had eventually to the therapist, then he might have responded more in the way she needed. She spontaneously admitted she had always been like that, which led to the therapist questioning when she first recalled feeling as she had just done in the session. She was able to recall her sullen evasive response to her father (P), who expected more of her, was wholly impatient and beat her. In simple terms, the patient's intrapsychic conflict (I–I) was 'I want to be loved and valued, but the world thinks I am no good, I am no good, therefore I fear I will be rejected'. Most common core conflicts are very similar. Of course, the therapy was not as easy as this brief account makes it appear. Her evasions and the explorations of them came up again and again in the context of different problem situations, though the therapeutic approach was essentially similar. In this example, the patient had transferred attitudes and behaviours which were relevant to her past life (P) on to present persons (C), including the therapist (T). This is the essence of the concept of 'transference', which can be explored in the here and now. The therapeutic alliance and the patient's motivation are enhanced by the positive experience or 'corrective emotional experience' (Alexander and French, 1946) and direct immediate live evidence of their own behaviour (T) that may contribute to their problems (C). Where the conflict comes from in terms of both past experiences (P) and their own conflicting impulses (I–I) are explored live in the heat of the very moment that the patient is struggling with them and their consequences in the present. Awareness of past unconscious influences on present behaviour empowers patients to change their behaviour in their own way. Inevitably with this experience and their wish for better relationships they experiment in their current relationships, spontaneously undertaking homework. Dynamic psychotherapy is by definition non-directive and is thereby more empowering. Some patients need the directive elements from cognitive behavioural therapies. The therapies can be merged in a cognitive analytic psychotherapy (Ryle, 1979).

Clearly the efficiency of classical techniques can be optimized by more active intervention, focusing on the symptoms or on a particular conflict, or by including other real relationships as in couple or family therapy, or controlled relationships as in group therapy. Setting a limited number of sessions focuses on the impending loss of support and avoids dependency which can prolong therapy. As in any sphere, a gain in one area might lead to a loss in another, though in some circumstances group, shorter-term or focused therapy would be the treatment of choice regardless of cost. Careful assessment will indicate patients who are not able to handle the emotional intensity the short-term approach demands. Patients who show a proneness to develop a 'transference psychosis', termed 'borderline patients', are examples, though this may become evident too late. An earlier indication is such intense anxiety that thought processes become disordered, or emotions are turned into action by threatened or actual harm to self, others or property, leaving therapy precipitously or manipulating appointments. Generally high impulsivity, said to be more common in deaf people (see Chapter 3), would exclude the approach.

Dynamic therapy with Deaf people

A workshop on psychodynamic counselling with Deaf and hearing professionals and interested others, including many who had experienced therapy or counselling, concluded that the psychology and therapy of Deaf and hearing people is essentially the same (Ridgeway, Kitson and Vardell, 1994). The differences noted concerned language, culture and life experience that are more or less unique to each. In this context the importance of learning from the patient was emphasized. Textbook knowledge may heighten the therapist's awareness, but should not lead treatment, particularly to those from different cultures.

Communication and culture

Psychotherapy is a talking or communication cure, so it should be done in the language of the patient, yet the majority of psychoanalytic psychotherapists working with Deaf patients are hearing, with sign as a second and only variably acquired language. Deaf therapists will usually provide the best linguistic match for patients, but on occasion it may be more appropriate for a hearing therapist to work with a deaf patient. For example, some Deaf patients may have an attitude to Deaf people that at least initially prevents work with a Deaf therapist. Others may have a need to challenge and face their assumptions about hearing or deaf people based on the past. In practice consideration can be given to the ideal deaf/hearing status of a therapist, but availability severely restricts the actual choice.

Deaf therapist (JD) finds some Deaf patients expect her to have a particularly close relationship and, for example, collude with them in a generalized paranoid attitude to hearing people. Some Deaf patients collude with their own expectations of the Deaf therapist, not wanting to show anger for fear of attacking their own culture.

There is a tendency to over-emphasize the differences and minimize the similarities between Deaf and hearing therapists. Historically, hearing people have tried to force the integration of Deaf people into a speaking world. It is not then surprising that deaf people should feel forced to emphasize the differences themselves, in order to establish an identity of their own (Fernando, 1995). We should not be too quick to say that a hearing person cannot be a good enough therapist, experience shows they can, but clearly there should be more therapists who are Deaf themselves. Deaf people should have the opportunity to choose whether they see a Deaf or a hearing therapist.

For the therapy to be as effective as possible, hearing and some deaf therapists need to consider using a transcultural model of practice. In the Deaf/hearing setting transculture can be used positively as most Deaf people have hearing parents and most of their early childhood experiences are determined by relationships with hearing people. The mere presence of a hearing facilitator in a Deaf group encouraged individual and group transferences from early childhood experiences. Defensive reactions to a life experience dominated by hearing people emerged. Some participants were in awe of the hearing facilitator, idealizing him, to avoid the pain of their experience of hearing parents, who could not meet their needs adequately. They sought 'omnipotent reassurance' to counter the 'persecutory anxiety' (Klein 1975) of the possibility that the hearing facilitator might not be good enough and their resultant destructive anger might be too much for him. Paradoxically, the hearing world's failure to provide their needs led to over-reliance on hearing people. Later the facilitator, having been put in the position of having greater expertise, was ridiculed for not living up to it. As Klein (1975) puts it, 'devaluation of the self again stirs up envy of the analyst, who is felt to be superior, particularly because the patient has strongly devalued himself'.

The therapist needs to be confident and aware enough to observe the patient's own characteristic use of sign language to express or hide information. The therapist needs to be aware that his own 'non-verbal' behaviour is likely to be more closely observed (Corker, 1994) and will influence the behaviour of the patient. Research interviews have revealed similar effects (Brauer 1989; Hindley, Hill and Bond,1993). Most Deaf people have a lifetime's experience of observing such behaviour for clues in speech and hearing environments in which they have had limited access to direct communication. They will be likely to be wiser to the unconscious motives of the therapist evident in their behaviour; on the other hand, they may be more likely to misinterpret these on the basis of their past formative experiences with hearing people. Deaf people's naturally developed observational skills of 'non-verbal' behaviour might be harnessed in their training as therapists, leading to a further advantage over hearing therapists.

It has been suggested that communication deficits, the need for immediate reinforcement, and limited awareness of social norms, militate against use of traditional insight therapies in Deaf people. This suggestion was made at a time when Deaf people and their language were more oppressed than now, though Sarlin (1984) used Deaf patients' dreams and their symbolism to clarify conflicts. The observation is true of a small minority of deaf people. Unfortunately, because of the sparsity of counselling and psychotherapy services to Deaf people, therapists have tended only to be referred the most difficult, and have extrapolated from this very biased population to the Deaf population at large. In our experience, just as with hearing patients, more sophisticated Deaf patients without cognitive disability can and do use unadapted psychotherapeutic approaches successfully. Because in the Deaf population cognitive disabilities are more common due to some of the causes of deafness, and lack of sophistication was more common due to reduced opportunities, it has, in the past, appeared to those working for the Deaf community from institutions that all Deaf people are so disadvantaged. Adaptations of the approach are necessary with some Deaf patients, just as with hearing patients, where specific disability or lack of experience requires it. Paradoxically, some Deaf patients are more likely to accept their unconscious, if it is presented as an analogy rather than a concrete link to their own behaviours. One patient, for example, whose husband was very dependent on her, told of going to the park. She saw a guide dog for the blind let off from its harness and running around and she thought 'Oh isn't it lovely, the dog running around free', but would not allow the connection with her own wishes. In the hearing world children have the opportunity of fairy tales, which help to prepare an understanding of metaphors and unconscious wishes to emotional scenarios. Most Deaf people have not had access to such stories until later life, usually with their own children.

Groups

Conducting six courses of 30 or 60 analytic group sessions for between seven and 11 Deaf trainees, each as an experiential part of the training of Deaf people in one- and two-year therapeutic counselling skills courses, has provided valuable experience of analytic psychotherapy to the able Deaf population. Initially the therapist (NK) conducted similar courses for hearing psychotherapy trainees, and lately conducted the Deaf courses with Deaf co-conductors (including JD), as well as supervising other Deaf and hearing conductors. Although not studied systematically, in essence no significant difference was observed between sophisticated Deaf and hearing groups. Both groups engaged in group and individual defences and resistances to the conductors' observations and interpretations. There was a tendency for the hearing group to intellectualize by talking about problems in a textbook fashion and for the Deaf group to use humour or long detailed story-telling in a similar fashion to avoid here and now painful emotion. These were understood by the therapist to be cultural differences (Padden, 1989) and not indicative of psychopathology. The psychopathology in both groups was fear of open confrontation or warmth, for fear of a threatening row or embarrassing or smothering warmth and intimacy.

In groups, symbolism is similar; for example, a hearing group used a slitted eye, cold monitoring robot, whereas a Deaf group used a cold ruthless roving shark to represent the paranoia induced by the facilitators' distant interpretive yet monitoring stance. At that stage both groups took the facilitators' comments as critical rather than neutral or supportive. That revealed the groups' need for approval, which they did not expect. At a later stage a Deaf group had gone on to a group cohesive metaphor of stoking or dampening the fire of the group atmosphere. They were actively exploring their individual behaviour and its meaning, as well as their relationships to each other and those significant figures outside the group or its members represented. Fears were expressed and tackled to varying degrees by different groups, Deaf or hearing. All the groups progressed at a broadly similar pace, except for those Deaf groups that had a clear mix of Deaf and partially Deaf members, including some members with limited sign language use. This probably has a similar effect to mixed Deaf and hearing groups, which places additional strains on communication (Millar and Moores, 1990). The experience of a Deaf person (JD) in an experiential group comprised of hearing trainees and two Deaf trainees adds to this picture. The facilitator was hearing with no prior knowledge of Deaf issues. An interpreter was appointed, a new experience for the hearing group members and the facilitator. The group initially perceived the interpreter as a member of the group, yet it was not always the same interpreter. Did members trust the interpreter? Both Deaf and hearing members questioned the quality of interpretation. The reality of imperfect interpretation needs to be explored, including the avoidance of that reality. Was the Deaf person's suspicion of misunderstanding of her behaviour, attitudes and talk reality or resistance? When the interpreter voiced over, the group looked in the direction of the interpreter, not at the Deaf person (the sign language interpreter usually needs to sit opposite the Deaf people to see and be seen, and adjacent to hearing people to hear and be heard). Were members failing to pick up her body language and therefore the true meaning of her contributions? Did she pick up their non-verbal communication when her eyes were concentrating on the interpreter? She became aware of having missed a member's upset, sadness and anger and then being perceived as hard-hearted. The envy towards the two Deaf members forced into a pair by 'their' interpreter and separate language and culture was an added complication. Bion (1961) states 'the group's basic assumption (unconscious) is that pairing has a sexual purpose' and 'that there would be less risk of misunderstanding in the group if the members all spoke a different language'.

On the positive side, JD's isolation within the hearing dominated group, due to the differences in language, life experience and culture, mirrored her early family experiences. The feelings of being left out, experiences of miscommunication and misunderstanding were brought forward from her unconscious. She was able clearly to recognize the statement: 'The group situation has been likened to a "hall of mirrors" where an individual is confronted with various aspects of his real identity' (Foulkes and Anthony, 1965).

Where there is no choice but to have a mixed group with an interpreter, the authors would recommend that the group facilitator/therapist is bilingual with an understanding of both cultures. Otherwise it is vital that the facilitator/therapist is open to advice from experts in Deafness and psychotherapy. The authors continue to meet too many professionals who stick dogmatically to their understanding of the rules of therapy with minds closed to the issues surrounding the interface between deaf and hearing people. On occasion this can be quite oppressive. One blatant example was a hearing counselling course organizer who insisted a deaf trainee should have a 'normal', i.e. hearing, training patient. The more subtle oppressions are more dangerous, though, as they are harder to detect or confirm.

A few members of both Deaf and hearing experiential groups made striking changes; most made significant progress and valued the experience. Some members of both groups had great difficulty. The Deaf groups revealed more traumatic past experiences and appeared to have had less opportunity to express them. The myth that Deaf people are more direct, straightforward and honest compared to hearing people's evasive talk was exposed. Fortunately for the hearing therapist, it was not necessary for him to challenge this 'foreign' cultural belief directly. Deaf trainees found they were as evasive and as careful of each other's feelings as the rest of us. This should be no surprise to many Deaf people, who complain of the Deaf community being 'back stabbing' (Redfern, 1996) and 'two faced'. These totally opposing myths existing side by side are an indication to a psychoanalytic thinker of projection and splitting, characteristic of a person or group under serious threat. In general, in the authors' experience these mechanisms are becoming less evident as Deaf people are allowed increasing opportunities, previously obstructed. The authors see this, where it exists, as a symptom of any small community and in no way directly related to Deafness.

There are minor technical differences that are none the less fundamental to group therapy with Deaf clients. In group analytic psychotherapy, whilst expression is encouraged, touching is not allowed in order to set clear boundaries on behaviour and minimize real consequences in the group. In Deaf groups it is the norm to touch in order to attract attention to oneself or others announcing entry into the conversation. Touching for this purpose clearly needs to be allowed. Chairs may need to be moved to gain adequate vision for all, including some with specific visual needs. In general, chairs will need to be a little further apart. Inevitably these behaviours, though necessary, can be used defensively to avoid group progress and may need to be explored. A Deaf group arranged the room in a semi-circle in order to see the facilitator's communication clearly. They were initially unconscious of their declaration that communication with the facilitators was more important than between themselves. In other groups, by taking up different seating arrangements they unconsciously explored separating and joining the facilitators. Many reasons were given by the participants, such as bad lighting, but inconsistencies suggested feelings of an oedipal nature were more likely behind these actions. Yalom (1985) notes 'seating patterns reveal complex and powerful feelings toward the leader'. The relevance of seating could be confirmed by the content. An unconscious attempt was made to draw the Deaf facilitator on to their side to attack the hearing person, describing the Deaf facilitator as a poodle and the hearing conductor as a rottweiler! Both were ambivalent metaphors, nice but to be petted, or dangerous but powerful.

Attempts may be made to formalize turn-taking by hand-raising on the pretext of improving communication. More often than not this has appeared to be defensive, imposing a repressive controlling structure that limits free expression. In this form it has tended to be consciously advocated by one or two members of the group. Alternatively, at times it has been necessary to avoid the chaos of many members signing over each other's communication. By and large, in the latter case it has been imposed naturally, unconsciously and spontaneously by the group for the short periods it is necessary. All these technical issues require the conductor to be aware of the communication needs of all members individually and as a group to minimize misinterpretation of behaviours necessary for communication as psychopathology and vice versa. The essence must be that the group can see clearly.

Roles, boundaries and confidentiality in groups

The small Deaf world is the most significant problem in Deaf groups in a very practical way. The world of Deaf people on higher training courses such as counselling training is even smaller. It was impossible to construct groups of trainees who did not know each other. This is not unique. All Deaf institutions such as Deaf psychiatric wards have the same problem. Confidentiality is one loser. Hearing people attending therapeutic groups are unlikely to know each other and are discouraged from having relationships outside the group with group members. This enables greater trust in the knowledge that exposing one's inner feelings to and challenging group members will not have consequences in the real world and confidentiality will not be threatened. For Deaf group members this is unlikely to be possible. Attenders from long distances have some advantage, though Deaf people are often very mobile and have roots in many areas. Worse still, members may work together or for each other, know each other's spouses, have mutual memories of school antics or even have had close personal relationships. Many will have assumptions about each other based on real past or present relationships. All these contacts add to the difficulty of working in mutual exploration of and experimentation with relationships within the group. The conductor(s) must be aware of the possibilities of real relationships, and extra emphasis often needs to be made on clarifying the fact that our assumptions about others and our resultant responses to them are often based on or biased by our own personality and experience, and reveal more about us than about the other. This can be very painful, especially in the presence of someone who has been or is the focus of one's feeling in the real world outside the group. When such real relationships become explicit in the group, the group often experiences relief, and blocks to progress, previously a mystery, become clear. For the conductors, experience in dealing with real relationships in other settings, such as family or marital work, is an advantage. Deaf conductors have a similar problem in that they will have real relationships of some depth with group members. Clear boundaries, holding clearly to the therapist role within the group, and immediately before and afterwards, and suspending the real relationship are essential to all members of the group with or without a relationship with the conductor. It is very hard for both the conductor and the group member, when strong feelings are felt towards the conductor(s) in the group, and there is inevitable confusion, whether it is a transference phenomenon generated by the group or generated by experiences of the conductor outside the group. The group needs careful exploration of the differences, but then how the reaction to the conductor in the group and to the conductor as a real person outside the group is possibly based on past experiences. The conductor in the group being (T) in Malan's triangle (see Figure 15.1) and the conductor as a real person outside the group being (C). For the conductor to manage this, minimizing his own responses to the member distorted by his own past experiences of the patient is very difficult. The support of co-conducting and supervision is necessary. Hearing conductors of Deaf groups are likely to suffer similar difficulties, though less intensely. Any hearing therapist who has sufficient sign language skill to conduct a group of deaf members with or without a deaf co-conductor is likely to have had a lot of experience in the deaf world and also have relationships of varying depth with group members. Hearing group therapists are likely to have similar though lesser problems of role, boundaries and confidentiality. They are also likely to be less fluent in communication and culture. To avoid blocks to group progress and inaccurate assumptions it is important that all these inter-relationships are in the open, as far as confidentiality and therapeutic technique will allow. Similar complications not uncommonly occur in individual therapy with Deaf people, but inevitably involve fewer people and interrelationships.

Individual therapy

Resistance

Despite the process of psychotherapy being based on a mutually agreed contract, patients inevitably become anxious and therefore defensive as conflicts are brought to the surface. They will consciously or unconsciously avoid further exploration in therapy. This is termed resistance. Rebourg (1992) reminds us that where the therapist and patient have difficulty understanding each other, resistances can always be interpreted. Either a superficial 'chat' results or the therapist (or patient) becomes an educator and treatment is effectively resisted. Hoyt and colleagues (1981) note the use of communication as resistance by looking away or signing rapidly. The latter can be pointed out, including the way the patient is defeating his own objects. Determined looking away, which cuts off any further communication, may have to be dealt with by action. Banging the table or floor may be a culturally appropriate response, opening communication through vibration. Mirroring the patient's behaviour by looking away may be effective, but this is potentially provocative. If used at all this needs to be timed sensitively and adopted in such a way as to invite communication. Such techniques are likely, in part, to be seen as persecutory, rather than supportive or exploratory, and are unnecessary in longer-term therapies. Ridgeway (1994) points out that Deaf people might need to break eye contact to enable reflective thought, and this applies as much to the deaf therapist whose action may be misunderstood. This also applies to hearing therapists with hearing patients, in face-to-face therapy. In traditional couch-based psychoanalytic techniques with the therapist out of view of the patient this, of course, is not a problem.

The lack of familiarity with the idea that feelings influence actions (Hoyt, Siegelman and Schlesinger, 1981) is common, yet, in contrast, patients also often blame their feelings for actions. In the latter case, patients are distancing themselves from their own feelings, by implication denying any possibility of having control over them. The difficulty appears to be acting on feelings in a more flexible and constructive way. Hoyt, Siegelman and Schlesinger (1981) comment positively on Deaf patients' comfort with expression of feeling, story-telling and naïve openness. The risk in this is of apparent therapeutic work, when real feelings are not expressed directly in relation *to* the therapist or others, but only in stories *about* others. This may allow some unburdening of feelings or catharsis. It does not promote exploration and modification of maladaptive behaviours. It may promote dependence on the 'understanding' therapist, rather than sorting out real relationships. Naïve openness (Hoyt, Siegelman and Schlesinger, 1981) may help the therapist to understand, but what about the patient, who may be oblivious to the consequences he needs to be aware of? All these behaviours need to be questioned as defences. Special strengths against adversity (Hoyt, Siegelman and Schlesinger, 1981) do appear to be there, but 'strengths' are resistances when they do not get the patient what they need.

Gerber (1983) observes that most Deaf people expect therapy to be 'directive, authoritative, advice-giving and brief' and are 'uncomfortable with standard approaches used in psychotherapy'. Hoyt, Siegelman and Schlesinger (1981) note the ideas that the past influences the present, that feelings can be separate from actions, regularity, commitment and responsibility are often new ideas to Deaf patients. They recommend active, directive, less abstract, educative approaches, and checking that the patient has understood. This is generally good advice, but the therapist may be adopting it as a counter-transference reaction to the transference from the patient's past. Grant and Grant (1992) state:

> 'the discussion of feelings is an abstract, complicated situation for deaf clients because it is difficult to discuss emotions without the complex English language base which many people lack.'. . . 'Psychotherapy with deaf clients proceeds slowly and has to focus on specific, concrete situations to insure that the deaf clients understand all of the factors involved in resolving their problems.'

We disagree. Ridgeway (1994) emphasizes the need for preparation as a more positive approach to the Deaf community's relative lack of awareness of therapy and the issues connected with the small Deaf world occupied by both Deaf patients/clients and therapists. She focuses on the issues of Deaf therapists with Deaf patients, but the issues are relevant to a lesser extent to hearing therapists. Deaf patients may need more education in therapy principles, most fundamentally concerning confidentiality and role boundaries. They need preparation for the almost inevitable contact between therapist and patient outside therapy. The line between inappropriate preparation that avoids necessary and constructive anxiety, and preparation which supports the therapeutic alliance, assisting the patient to use the therapy, is a fine one. There is no easy formula. Over-preparation may foster dependence, in a way that has been too prevalent in Deaf history. On the other hand, lack of preparation may leave the patient intolerably anxious and ignorant of constructive possibilities. We believe it is important to educate through the therapy, to give time to reflect and space to work through unconscious processes that reveal characteristic problems, rather than to solve them by straightforward educative means.

Some Deaf patients have never had the experience of being listened to. They expect advice. Throughout their lives it has always been a one-way process, and now it is two-way it can be difficult. Therapy can be like a mother listening to them, playing with them and using creative thought and dreams. This can really be a shock. They have a lot within them that has never been used and the therapist needs to draw this out where possible.

Virole (1992) emphasizes the need to show empathy before interpretation, and Lunden-Szczesny (1992) the need to be more emotionally present to reduce persecutory anxiety. They point out the Deaf person's common experience as a child of a mother depressed and emotionally flattened. Ridgeway, Kitson and Vardell (1994) point out the need in the small Deaf community, where the therapist may be an acquaintance of the client, to note the change of role by one's expressive style.

Apparent expression of feeling may be merely the use of formal sign language. Sign language, particularly when story-telling, includes taking the role of others or oneself in the past or predicted future. This may include expression of powerful feelings. Fluency in sign and considerable experience are needed to separate enacted emotions from real emotions in the here and now. Additionally, telling emotionally laden stories may engender feelings in the here and now. The therapist's looking for the feelings may lead to a denial by the patient accusing the therapist of not understanding that the emotional expressions of role-taking are part of sign language. It may be that the therapist is right or wrong. It takes a confident hearing therapist to challenge a Deaf person over his own language. The therapist, who is likely to need the respect of the Deaf community to be effective, may feel unable to challenge Deaf people's use of language as a defence. Some Deaf patients will use Deaf pride as a defence against, or an attack on, particularly hearing therapists in a way that hides their own anger and attributes it to the oppressed Deaf community. This is the harder to challenge as the hearing community has undoubtedly oppressed the Deaf community. A patient accused the hearing therapist of having no BSL. There was a basis of truth in the accusation. The therapist at the time had fluent Sign Supported English (SSE) and considerable BSL features to communication, though not fluent BSL. Yet what was the patient's motivation in denying the therapist possession of any BSL and in bothering to make the accusation at all? The patient could understand the therapist's communication at a linguistic level, as could the therapist the patient, though with some difficulty. The patient had revealed relatively little of himself. Later the patient was able to acknowledge the possibility that the accusation was an expression of anger with the therapist for observing the patient's difficulty in expressing past painful experiences. The anger was also related to the added difficulty imposed by a lack of linguistic matching between the therapist and patient and the emotional baggage from the patient's life-long experience of more significant difficulties with hearing people. In settings, such as groups with a Deaf and a hearing therapist, resistance by 'misunderstanding' points made by the hearing therapist can be made clearer with the aid of the Deaf therapist. Judgement of reality versus resistance is complicated in transcultural settings such as between a hearing therapist and Deaf patient.

Transference and counter-transference issues

Harris (1981) remarks 'the emotional problems of many deaf adults are rooted in the responses of their families to them as children'. Ninety per cent of Deaf children have hearing parents, yet mothers of Deaf preschool children have been found to tend to respond to them in a less permissive, more intrusive and directive manner (Schlesinger and Meadow 1972). Harvey (1984) refers to the family myth of the Deaf child as helpless, immature and not very bright. Chapter 7 records the evidence for Deaf people's experiences of abuse, including physical and sexual.

Dynamic psychotherapy explores the emotional problems through the patient's reactions to the therapist in the present. These are assumed to be based on the patient's past experience in earlier life, in other words their transference responses to the therapist. Knowledge of past experiences will help therapists to be more sensitive to a Deaf patient's responses to them, as well as to the therapists' own counter-transference reactions. Therapists should expect their patients to be likely to make them wish to behave in the ways that have been attributed to parents and other carers of Deaf children. An awareness of this will help therapists to observe their own reactions to the patient, i.e. their counter-transference, and question what behaviours from the patient lead them to feel that. Such observations can lead to helpful interpretations of the patient's behaviour and its roots. Money Kyrle (1956) stated that if the therapist is disturbed, the client has probably unconsciously contributed to it. Heimann (1950) states that 'the analyst's counter-transference is not only part of the analytic relationship but is the patient's creation and a reflection of a part of the patient's personality'. A Deaf patient, rejected by her mother in early life and brought up by multiple carers, presented with severe relationship problems. One session had to be cancelled. The following session the patient arrived very late with a melodramatic explanation that was hard to believe. There had been a disaster in which the patient was the rescuer. This was interpreted as the patient wanting to change places with the therapist (JD). The patient scoffed at the interpretations and belittled the therapist, making her feel stupid and useless. The constant dismissals of the interpretations left the therapist frustrated and angry. It seemed from the history, as well as the therapy, that the patient was expert at distressing people with fantastic stories. It is important not to deny hate that exists within the therapist. This should be sorted out within the therapist and kept in storage and available for eventual interpretation (Winnicott, 1949).

Patients can be helped to become aware of how they, by their own behaviour, now promote responses to themselves which mimic their past carers' responses to them and leave them feeling as they did in the past. This process has been referred to as the 'repetition compulsion'. It is a powerful psychodynamic, which leads to confirmation and reconfirmation of the patient's misconceptions of their present world. It is important for us all to realize the way in which we repeat behaviours that fail to get us what we want or need, and to realize why. We are then better armed to challenge them. Through interpretations, including interpretations of dreams and fantasies, the therapist can provide a corrective emotional experience transforming the patient/therapist relationship into one in which the patient feels accepted and understood.

Counter-transference can also be useful if patients' language is limited or if they are unable to express their conflict. It can be used as an aid for carers in understanding patients who disturb them. The understanding that comes from it can aid the caring of very difficult, otherwise unlovable, patients.

A criticism of counter-transference is the inherent assumption that it is generated by the patient. The patient is disempowered when the therapist's response is not a reflection of counter-transference, but of the therapist's own psychopathology. Deaf therapists will be likely to have similar life experiences to their Deaf patients and may over-identify with them, engaging in generalizations, and thereby colluding with projective defences on to Deafness or the hearing population. Equally, they are better able to be aware and empathize with patients from backgrounds similar to their own. Sorting out the confusion in the therapist's mind between counter-transference and their own psychopathology is an important reason for therapists to have personally undergone an analytic experience. Additionally, hearing therapists will need to have explored their attitudes to

Deafness and responses to Deaf people, including their own motives for working with Deaf people (Rebourg, 1992). Furnham and Lane (1984) found that deaf people had a more negative attitude to deafness than did hearing people, and expected hearing people to have a more negative attitude than they had. Corker (1994) warns that hearing therapists may be afraid of Deafness and, by projection, be afraid of Deaf people. This would affect their behaviour towards Deaf people, which in turn might be introjected by Deaf people, who see it as part of themselves, or project it on to all hearing people.

Hoyt, Siegelman and Schlesinger, (1981) refer to Deaf patients' 'heightened expectation' of therapists as 'rejecting or powerful' and a 'global sense of entitlement as compensation for handicap' compared to hearing patients. This projection on to therapists is likely to be a reflection of the Deaf patient's experience of hearing people to date, and will present differently to a Deaf therapist. Ridgeway, Kitson and Vardell (1994) argue that a Deaf patient might be more likely to confide in a Deaf therapist. In our experience, for reasons of confidentiality, some Deaf patients have felt better able to confide in a hearing therapist. Others have been comfortable with both, and others prefer a Deaf therapist. Hearing therapists are almost inevitably disadvantaged by limited fluency in sign language. On occasion incorrect use of metaphor, idiom or regional accent can be ambiguous. As with any ambiguous information, the way in which it is misunderstood by the patient will reveal something about him. Ambiguity is deliberately used in some techniques to explore patients' assumptions and responses, though clearly it is better if therapists are aware of their own interventions.

Lateness may be due to language deficits related to ordering of temporal experience (Hoyt, Siegelman and Schlesinger, 1981), but none the less needs tackling, as it is a major problem in therapeutic work. It may well be unconsciously defensive against the feared consequences of timeliness in addition to language and neuropsychological deficits. Corker (1994) also refers to its cultural origin. Unlike Corker (1994), we have not found that Deaf patients 'rarely keep to time limits', i.e. fail to arrive or arrive on time, leave early, extend sessions or have great difficulty focusing, nor have we had the significant difficulty of keeping an eye on the clock. Such problems exist, and perhaps more so with Deaf patients, yet by dealing with them in the ordered way of exploration, interpretation and clear boundaries, they can be resolved.

Conclusion

Throughout this chapter we have tried to clarify from our experience, and that of others, how psychotherapy with Deaf patients differs from that with hearing patients. We question whether Deaf-centred therapy needs to address technique in a different way to hearing-centred therapy. There are too many negative statements about therapy for Deaf people. As Sussman (1988) notes, the tendency 'to stereotype Deaf people as difficult. . . serves only to thwart their opportunity for emotional growth and psychological enhancement'.

References

Alexander F, French TM (1946). Psychoanalytic Therapy. New York: Ronald Press.

Bion WR (1961) Experiences in Groups and Other Papers. London: Tavistock Publications Ltd.

Brauer B (1989) The signer effect on MMPI performance of Deaf respondents. Unpublished paper.

Corker M (1994) Counselling The Deaf Challenge. London: Jessica Kingsley.

Davanloo, H (ed) (1980) Short Term Dynamic Psychotherapy. New York: Jason Aronson.

Farrugia DL (1986) An Adlerian perspective for understanding Deafness. Individual Psychology: Journal of Adlerian Theory, Research and Practice 42: 201–213.

Fernando J (1995) Psychoanalytic psychotherapy in a mental health setting for Deaf people. Proceedings, Third International Congress, European Society for Mental Health and Deafness.

Foulkes SH, Anthony EJ (1965) Group Psychotherapy. London: Penguin Books.

Furnham A, Lane S (1984) Actual and perceived attitudes toward Deafness. Psychological Medicine 14: 417–423.

Gerber BM (1983) A communication minority: Deaf people and mental health care. American Journal of Social Psychiatry III: 50–57.

Grant M, Grant T (1992) Psychotherapy with Deaf clients. In VandeCreek L, Knapp S, Jackson TL, Innovations in Clinical Practice: A Source Book, Vol 11, pp 99–107. Sarasota, FL: Professional Resource Exchange Inc.

Harris R, (1981) Mental health needs and priorities in Deaf children and adults: a Deaf professional's perspective for the 1980s. In Stein LK, Mindel ED, Jabaley T (eds) Deafness and Mental Health. New York: Grune & Stratton, p 220.

Harvey MA (1984) Family therapy with Deaf persons: the systematic utilisation of an interpreter. Family Process 23: 205–221.

Harvey MA (1993) Cross cultural psychotherapy with deaf persons: a hearing, white, middle class, middle aged, non-gay, Jewish, male therapist's perspective. Journal of American Deafness and Rehabilitation Association, 26(4): 34–55.

Heimann P (1950) On Counter-transference. International Journal of Psychoanalysis 31: 81–84.

Hindley P, Hill P, Bond D (1993) Interviewing Deaf children the interviewer effect: a research note. Journal of Child Psychology and Psychiatry and Allied Disciplines 34: 1461–1467.

Hoyt M, Siegelman E, Schlesinger H (1981) Special issues regarding psychotherapy with the Deaf. American Journal of Psychiatry 138: 807-811.

Klein M (1975) Envy and Gratitude and Other Works. London, The Hogarth Press and the Institute of Psycho-analysis, p 218.

Lunden-Szczesny A (1992) Issues in individual psychotherapy with with the deaf. European Society for Mental Health and Deafness, Second International Congress proceedings, p 183–186.

Malan D (1979) Individual Psychotherapy and the Science of Psychodynamics. London: Butterworths.

Millar M, Moores D (1990) Principles of group counselling and their application for Deaf clients. Journal of American Deafness and Rehabilitation Association, 23: 82–86.

Money Kyrle R (1956) Normal counter-transference and some of its deviations. Journal of Psychoanalysis, 37, 360–365.

Padden C (1989) The Deaf community and the culture of Deaf people. In Wilcox S. American Deaf Culture. Silver Spring MD: Linstock Press, pp 1–16.

Rebourg F (1992) Which way are individual therapies with Deaf people original? Proceedings, Second International Congress, European Society of Mental Health and Deafness, La Bastide, Avenue Vauban, 8,b-5000, Namur, Belgium, pp 122–137.

Redfern P (1996) Deaf professionals — a growing stream. In Laurenzi C, Ridgeway S (eds) Progress Through Equality: New Perspectives in the Field of Mental Health and Deafness. London: British Society for Mental Health and Deafness (BSMHD) Publications, p 81-84

Ridgeway S (1994) The Deaf Alliance. In Corker M (1994) Counselling The Deaf Challenge. London: Jessica Kingsley. pp 214–224.

Ridgeway S, Kitson N, Vardell T (1994) SPIG Newsletter.

Ryle A (1979) The focus in brief interpretive psychotherapy. British Journal of Psychiatry 134: 6–54.

Sarlin B (1984) The use of dreams in psychotherapy with Deaf persons. Journal of American Academy of Psychoanalysis Vol 12: 75–88.

Sarlin MB, Altshuler KZ (1978) On the interrelationship of cognition and affect: fantasies of Deaf children. Child Psychiatry and Development Vol 9 Winter: 95-103.

Schlesinger H, Meadow K (1972) Sound and Sign: Childhood Deafness and Mental Health. Berkeley, CA: University of California Press.

Sussman A (1988) Approaches to counselling and psychotherapy revisited. In Watson D, Lon G, Taff-Watson M, Harvey M (eds) Two Decades of Excellence: A Foundation for the Future. Little Rock, Arkansas: American Deafness and Rehabilitation Association.

Truax C, Carkhuff R (1967) Towards Effective Counselling and Psychotherapy: Training and Practice. Chicago, IL: Aldine.

Urban E (1990) The eye of the beholder: work with a ten-year-old Deaf girl. Journal of Child Psychotherapy 16: 63–81.

Urban E (1993) Out of the mouths of babes: an enquiry into the sources of language development. Journal of Analytical Psychology. 38: 237–256.

Virole B (1992) Indications, framework constraints and specific difficulties of deaf person's psychotherapy. European Society for Mental Health and Deafness, Second International Congress Proceedings, pp 195–197.

Winnicott D (1949) Hate in the Counter-transference. Journal of Psychoanalysis, 30: 69–74.

Yalom ID (1985) The Theory and Practice of Group Psychotherapy. New York: Basic Books, p.203.

Part 2 Arts Therapies

LAWRENCE HIGGENS AND VAL HUET

Introduction

'Arts Therapies' is a generic name used in the UK for four therapies that use the arts as part of a psychotherapeutic process. Art Therapy, Dance Movement Therapy, Dramatherapy and Music Therapy, although still relatively new professions, have been growing in many sectors and may be found in such diverse areas as psychiatry, learning difficulties, mainstream and special education, and prisons. Each of these therapies has evolved from quite separate beginnings and each has developed and incorporated therapeutic techniques relevant to their specific art form. For this reason there are similarities between them but at the same time there are notable differences. This section does not include contributions from drama therapists and music therapists and will focus primarily on Art and Dance Movement therapies. It is important to note, however, that Dramatherapy has been used very positively by deaf clients, and that many of the following remarks also apply to this type of therapy. Swink (1985) describes the successful use of the specific techniques of psychodrama with Deaf people. He notes how Deaf children's natural storytelling uses many of the concepts of psychodrama, including every sensory modality to convey the message. Music Therapy, for obvious reasons, has limited application for Deaf patients. A pilot drumming project based at the Deaf Unit at Springfield Hospital was sufficiently successful, however, to warrant further consideration of the place of music therapy with this client group. Light and vibration have been used successfully to transmit 'sound' in services for Deaf and Deaf-blind people.

The fundamentally non-verbal nature of Art and Dance Movement Therapies makes them particularly suitable for Deaf clients, providing them with an opportunity to use the arts to facilitate the expression and exploration of confusing feelings. However, it is worth noting that hearing arts therapists working with Deaf clients will need to develop signing skills. Huet (1993) points out that signing is essential when working with Deaf clients since communication cannot happen solely through the art work.

Central to all of the arts therapies is the understanding that play and exploration are fundamental to our sense of who we are. Through play, babies and young children grow to organize and make sense of their world. For this play to be possible, it is necessary for it to take place within the context of a safe environment and within a safe relationship. The infant's carer, be it mother, father or anyone else, must provide an environment in which the child feels emotionally and physically secure enough to be free to play. As we get older, our ability to play may be found in various creative and recreational endeavours. Deaf children within hearing families often lack a positive experience of play, since communication difficulties can hinder its process. Arts therapies can provide a valuable opportunity for Deaf clients to engage in a play-like activity, that is, an activity where they will not have to meet pre-set expectations, or perform to established standards. One of the therapist's initial tasks is to create a safe space within which clients can use the art form to express and explore their feelings. This means that boundaries, such as meeting regularly, on time and in the same space, are important, as is avoiding intrusion from other patients or staff during the session.

Art therapy

Art is seen by many people as being in the domain of expert artists and as requiring special skills. The art therapist attempts to overcome this potential barrier by selecting the range of art materials available to match client abilities and needs. The materials must be varied enough to be stimulating, whilst remaining easily usable by people who are unfamiliar with art making. For example, art materials such as crayons, ready-mixed paints, and felt-tip pens do not require a high degree of technical expertise to enable satisfying results to be produced.

Art is also traditionally associated with concepts of 'good' or 'bad'. The process of art making often awakens fears of being assessed on the aesthetic merits of the work and rejected if it is not up to standard. In art therapy, however, the image is seen as representing the client, and is valued as such, regardless of its aesthetic merits. This is an important issue with Deaf clients, who have often experienced processes where they have been assessed, found wanting and rejected. Consequently, the therapeutic process with Deaf clients, within the context of art therapy, usually requires a considerable period of time during which the art making process gives rise to repeated experiences of being valued and understood. The art therapist adapts to the clients' pace, allowing them time to develop trust in the therapist and confidence in using art.

> 'If the art therapist can sustain the warm holding attention described by Milner (1969), many Deaf clients will develop a sense of trust and art therapy will provide a valuable resource for people who have often been denied access to the range of services available to hearing people.' (Huet, 1993)

Dance movement therapy

Dance movement therapy taps into traditional healing rituals which have employed dance, in combination with the other art forms, for many thousands of years. On an individual level too, movement is our first 'language', facilitating our first and most important relationship, and laying the foundations for emotional, cognitive and social development. Intuitively, anyone who has ever enjoyed moving or dancing will know something of the feeling of well-being and connectedness with others that arises from it. Although dance is an inherently healing experience, dance movement therapy is much more than this. It is based on the recognition that we each have an individual movement pattern, a particular way of walking and moving, a 'movement fingerprint' as it were. Most of us become aware of this only when it is drawn to our attention by a skilful mime artist, when we experience a feeling of embarrassment when asked to move in front of others or when being described in the role shift that is part of sign language; but actors, dancers and dance movement therapists employ this knowledge of body language, and the skill of replicating it in their own bodies, as a non-verbal means of establishing communication, conducting assessments and facilitating the process of therapy. This is the ground from which dance movement therapy has developed into a profession with both artistic and scientific aspects.

When working with Deaf clients, the dance movement therapist draws on specialized movement analysis skills and research linking body movement to personality, to provide an assessment service to the mental health team which helps them to identify a patient's strengths as well as those areas of functioning in need of therapeutic intervention (Higgens, 1993). This assessment, which is not dependent on the patient's formal signing and communication skills, can be of particular value when patients have poorly developed communication skills, or are too disturbed by mental illness to communicate coherently.

Dance movement therapy has strong developmental and artistic dimensions. When working with clients individually, movement interactions are designed to help build a stronger sense of identity, and provide an opportunity to work on early developmental tasks which may have been incompletely resolved. We need only look at our language metaphors, for example: 'standing up for oneself', 'being pushed around', and 'taking a step forward', to see how movement forms the basis of tacit knowledge about ourselves and our relationships with others. Through its emphasis on spontaneous movement improvization, dance movement therapy also attempts to draw out often under-developed qualities of initiative, playfulness, and creativity which are so necessary for healthy independent living.

In group contexts, dance movement therapy is a great leveller. Regardless of a person's sign language skills and educational achievement, body movement allows a new richness of emotional expression to be discovered and shared, an experience which many Deaf clients find emotionally liberating. The dance movement therapist 'reads' subtle movement cues from the clients as indicators of the group's emotional needs from moment to moment, and uses this information to guide therapeutic movement interventions. For example, leading and following tasks may be suggested to help draw individuals out of preoccupied isolation towards an interest in other people.

Dance movement therapists combine a specialized knowledge of movement with skills drawn from dance and psychotherapy, to provide a unique service for Deaf clients.

References

Higgens LG (1993) Movement assessment in schizophrenia. In Payne H (ed). Handbook of Inquiry in the Arts Therapies: One River Many Currents. London: Jessica Kingsley. pp 138–163.

Huet V (1993) Art therapy with deaf people. Inscape Journal of Art Therapy, Summer pp 10–16.

Milner M. (1969) The Hands of the Living God. London: Hogarth Press.

Swink DF (1985) Psychodramatic treatment of Deaf people. American Annals of the Deaf, 130: 272–277.

Chapter 16
Family Therapy with Families with Deaf Members

BARBARA WARNER

Introduction

Family* systems therapy has been a developing mode of psychotherapy for the past four decades and is now an accepted form of therapy within child and adult psychiatry and psychotherapy, social work practice and the field of family and marital counselling across the world. It can briefly be described as an intervention which can be utilized with all or several family members, or indeed with individuals. When used appropriately, difficulties for families or individuals can be alleviated in more immediate and lasting ways than professional interventions aimed at an individual which define the problem as being solely within that individual.

There are many theories and ideas which have formed the basis for the development of this branch of psychotherapy and many more which are currently contributing to the continuing evolution of theory and practice. The focus of this chapter is to consider and demonstrate the value of using these ideas in the process of working with people who are Deaf and the people with whom they relate; partners, children, parents, wider family and friendship networks and social systems.

The theories which underpin the author's clinical and teaching practice are drawn from an integration of the four main branches of family systems theory:

- Structural (Minuchin and Fishman, 1981; Fishman, 1993).
- Strategic (Madanes, 1991).
- Transgenerational (Lieberman, 1980; Carter and McGoldrick, 1989).
- Milan and post-Milan systemic therapy (Jones, 1993).

---

*In this chapter all references to 'family' include those people related by birth and marriage, couple relationships of both a heterosexual and homosexual nature and other close relationships which may not necessarily be kin relationships.

Other key influences are the development of the ideas of the reflecting team (Andersen, 1990) and current developments in thinking about the issues of gender (Perelberg and Miller, 1990; Burck and Speed, 1995), culture and ethnicity (McGoldrick, Pearce and Giordano, 1982; Gorell-Barnes, 1994) which are engaging practitioners and teachers of family systems therapy.

This does not deny the roots of all these models in the nineteenth and early twentieth century development of theories of psychoanalysis and human psychology from which modern psychotherapy and clinical psychology have grown. Nor does it deny the current development in the integration of the theory and practice of both individual psychotherapy and family systems therapy by some practitioners in both fields.

There now exists a wealth of literature which gives an in-depth account of the history and current theory and practice of family systems therapy to which the reader is referred, above and in the References. Specialized training is now available at a number of levels of expertise. Those wishing to work systemically with families in any context should ensure that they have sufficient knowledge, skills, experience and supervision to undertake this work.

Emotional, psychological, developmental, physical and relationship difficulties occur in many forms within the population in general. Family systems therapy theory and techniques have been usefully applied to a wide range of families and relationships, including those which contain one or more people who are Deaf.

Deafness does not, of itself, predispose individuals and families to such problems but neither will these families be immune to difficulties that affect the general population. As the needs of people who are Deaf and their families have been recognized by psychiatric and other health and social work professionals, a limited literature relating to the use of family systems therapy with these families has developed. For some families, it has become clear, Deafness of one or more members does highlight several areas which are significant in family difficulties. Themes that have been identified and written about are:

- The cultural collision experienced by families composed of Deaf and hearing members.
- Linguistic communication.
- Triangulation and scapegoating.
- Loss and grief.

Literature

Several authors attend to the cultural collision experienced by mixed Deaf and hearing families, (Harvey, 1984; Sloman and Springer, 1987). But whilst the concept of a separate cultural identity is still waging a battle against the deviance-based model, family therapists need to attend to the concept of a 'good fit'/'bad fit' in relation to the cultural beliefs of the family as a whole, the cultural beliefs of the Deaf people in the family and the cultural beliefs of the hearing family members. The issue is wider than the acknowledgement of Deaf culture by family members, but rather how they decide to incorporate this into their own beliefs, whatever their ethnic and religious identity.

The diverse and complex issues of the transfer of information and the conceptual difficulties in interpreting across widely differing languages and cultures have been explored and documented (see McGoldrick, Pearce and Giordano, 1982; Hodes, 1989; De Zulueta, 1990), but it is the interplay between those cultures and Deaf culture that needs to be explored by family therapists working with people who are Deaf. As Scott (1984) says, 'He may belong to a subculture of the Deaf but he is not 'out' of the culture of the family' (p. 214). These cultural and language issues were explored by Hindley, Hill and Bond (1993) in relation to the effects of the interviewer's signing ability and cultural status on the outcome of psychiatric assessments of signing children and adolescents who are Deaf. Results showed that poor competence in signing skills and cultural difference in the interviewer led to the masking of a child's emotional difficulties.

A repeated theme in the early literature is the suggestion that creating clear, exact linguistic communication in therapy is the therapy itself. Shapiro and Harris (1976) focus heavily on this idea, leaving little room for the exploration of other issues.

However, it would be naïve to assume therefore that all families with members who are deaf would be problem-free because they speak the same language, in the same way that it is not expected that all hearing families are problem-free.

Although family therapists working in this area have moved on from these early views that clear communication *is* the therapy, there is not yet any documented research on the use of family therapy – either with families where all members are Deaf or where both people who are Deaf and hearing are family members.

The use of an interpreter is, however, well-documented. Harvey (1984) is clear that however well qualified in sign language, '... it is not feasible or therapeutically prudent to interpret for all of the family members while simultaneously providing treatment' (p. 207). Beyond the function of facilitating communication between Deaf and hearing family members, a further aim in using an interpreter is to draw out the more problematic elements of intrafamilial communication. Much of the work focuses on the loss, denial and guilt experienced by the family in relation to deafness, but whether this should be the sole focus for therapy is questionable, as seen in the opposing views of Harvey (1982, 1984) and Scott (1984).

Harvey (1982, 1986, 1989) has also explored in some detail the various strategies available to aid communication within the family, between therapist and family members, and the use of different forms of communication as therapeutic interventions.

He advocates a flexible stance on the direct communication between the therapist and the Deaf and hearing family members depending on the preferred communication modes of family members, the therapist's signing skills and the therapeutic aims of a particular conversation.

He has noted how the presence of an interpreter in therapy has provided a useful tool to explore the anger in some families towards Deafness.

> By arranging or requesting permission for an interpreter to be present in the session, the therapist breaks the common family rule that prohibits the use of manual communication which serves to maintain the homeostasis (or *equilibrium*). (Harvey, 1982, p. 822) (See Glossary, Appendix D.)

Harvey (1982) describes a complex series of expressed and unexpressed communications which take place between the therapist and the family in connection with the use of an interpreter. Because of the close connection between the interpreter and the child who is Deaf, the family may react towards the interpreter as if she were the Deaf child and attribute their own feelings as emanating from the interpreter, e.g. 'the interpreter is angry with me for not having learned sign language' (p. 826), when the parent is feeling angry with himself for not having done so. It is at this point, Harvey believes, the therapist can begin to utilize the interpreter's unique position by asking the family to speculate on what the interpreter's thoughts might be, as a way of understanding what the parents fear the child may be thinking. As these feelings are brought to a level of awareness they can be dealt with by the parents.

Triangulation and *scapegoating* (see Glossary pp. 445–6) are common themes in family dynamics and can also be identified in families containing people who are Deaf. One of the difficulties for the therapist is in deciding how much emphasis should be placed on Deafness and communication in the therapy. Therapists run the risk of colluding with the family if other family dynamics are not fully explored and dealt with. Robinson and Weathers (1974) found that triangulation and scapegoating also occurred towards the Deaf parents of hearing children.

A further basic theme which has been identified in families with members who are Deaf, which is also present in families with physically disabled, learning disabled and mentally ill members, is that of loss and grief associated with the lost expectations of a *normal* individual and family life. Sometimes this loss has been resolved but sometimes unresolved loss needs to be addressed in the therapy. Sloman, Springer and Vachon (1993) consider from a number of perspectives the experiences of families with members who are deaf, in particular communication, culture and loss. They bring together the grief and loss associated with the presence in the family of a child who is deaf, and the disturbances of communication which may follow, with the knowledge of the effects and treatment of unresolved grief in families.

Besides consideration of the dynamics within the family containing Deaf members, systemic theory contributes a wider view of the context within which people who are Deaf exist. Harvey (1989) suggests a six-level contextual framework which can be condensed as follows:

- **Biological**: the nature and aetiology of the hearing loss, related medical conditions, genetic factors.
- **Psychological**: consideration of the effects of deafness on the individual's cognition, behaviour and emotions. Adaptation of the individual to being deaf; responses to deafness by the family and society. Personal identity as a deaf person, i.e. as a deaf person with a strong identity within the deaf community or as a 'hearing person with a hearing problem'.
- **Family**: socialization of the deaf individual within the family. Methods of communication used by the family, patterns of interaction, family experience of and attitudes to deafness.
- **Professional network**: many professionals become involved in the life of a Deaf person; teachers, speech therapists, psychologists, audiologists, etc. These professionals will have an influence on the parents of a deaf child, and their personal and professional views of deafness may be enhancing or undermining of the deaf person and their family.
- **Informal network**: family and the individual's friends and acquaintances may influence attitudes to deafness and can reinforce both functional and dysfunctional patterns.
- **Cultural/political**: there are many different views of deafness that influence the attitudes of the culture and subculture in which the deaf person lives and which influence the political provisions made for that person. In some societies deafness is a medical problem to be alleviated by hearing aids, implants and speech therapy, a disability or a difference to live with positively. In some cultures it is seen as a curse or punishment for the family, inducing shame and guilt.

A very useful drawing together of all these themes, in relation to professionals working with families containing children who are deaf, is provided by Luterman (1987). As an audiologist he has taken account of family systems theories and applied them to the work of all professionals involved in the diagnosis, treatment and education of deaf children. He particularly emphasizes the value of building on family members' strengths, skills and attachments in the process of working with them as the children grow and develop.

Team development

The experiences of offering systemic therapy to families in which one or more persons is deaf, and upon which this chapter draws, are those of the Team for People who are Deaf and their Families at the Prudence Skynner Family Therapy Clinic (PSFTC).*

During the seven years of its existence the team has had a number of members drawn from a variety of mental health professionals working in both the adult- and child-focused teams of the South West London and St George's National Deaf Services (SWLSG NDS). The disciplines involved include clinical psychology, counselling, psychiatric nursing, occupational therapy, psychotherapy, psychiatry, family therapy and a sign language interpreter; four past or present members of the team are themselves deaf.

The team developed against the background of knowledge of family systems therapy, other people's work with people who are deaf and their families, the experience of the team, the PSFTC clinic and SWLSG NDS. There were many discussions within the team. The interaction between deaf and hearing team members, the contributions of the interpreter and family therapist and the experiences with families were always essential in coming to a resolution. This would then be worked with for a while before being revised. Throughout the life of the team, work has evolved in this way and the process of evolution continues.

Early in the process there was much to learn about how to use family therapy knowledge, skills and technical equipment in the venture of working with people who are deaf and their families. Discussion, role-play and early experiences with families led team members to the conclusion that there were three essential elements on which the team should be founded:

---

*The Prudence Skynner Family Therapy Clinic (PSFTC) is part of the SWLSG Mental Health NHS Trust. The clinic is a teaching centre with three therapy suites, each consisting of two rooms divided by a one-way mirror and equipped with video cameras and recorders. The Team for People who are Deaf and their Families is one of four specialist teams at PSFTC (the others are for people with learning difficulties, children and adolescents with eating disorders and older people and their families) and six general teams. Members of each specialist team are drawn from health and social services professionals, some of whom are also qualified family therapists, whose regular work is with the special group of clients. Liaison between team supervisors, all of whom are qualified family therapists, and the membership of more than one team by some therapists, have provided the opportunity for the transfer of knowledge between teams and aided the development of the approaches to people with special difficulties used at the PSFTC.

- At least one team member should be from among the Deaf staff members of the SWLSG NDS.
- Family therapy supervision should be provided by a qualified family therapist.
- Sign language interpretation should be provided by two interpreters, who could be long-term members of the team.

These basic elements have not changed and have proved to be as important as at first thought.

Communicating with families containing a person who is deaf

The first families seen were already known to team members or their colleagues. This made initial contacts with families less complicated, but it was necessary to find a way of explaining the reasons for seeing family members together and gaining useful information about the family members' views about themselves. The clinic already used a questionnaire and introductory letter but it was quickly realized that this and all the written contact with families would need to be revised. Deaf team members were invaluable in providing a perspective from within Deaf culture as the written material was translated into language which was compatible with British Sign Language (BSL) (see Chapter 1). Even with this revision, clients often did not complete the questionnaire and when possible a pattern was developed of both a Deaf and hearing team member visiting the family at home to introduce the clinic and questionnaire. This combination aided the *joining* (see Glossary) with families as both family members who were Deaf and hearing were made aware that they would be able to communicate directly with the team. Later in the team's development a videotape was produced using sign and voice to demonstrate the clinic facilities and explain about family therapy. This tape can be sent to families living at a distance from the clinic.

The Deaf therapists and the interpreters are also instrumental in ensuring that letters from the team are written in a style which makes them accessible to people who are Deaf. Telephone contact is facilitated by use of text telephones such as *textphone* or *Minicom* (see Glossary) and telephone relay systems such as *Relay telephone operator* (see Glossary pp. 445–6).

Communication and the clinic technology

The development of family therapy and the training of family therapists coincided with the new availablity of video technology. Training centres in the USA developed the use of cameras, video recording, the one-way screen and the observing team. The aim was to enhance the interventions of the therapist with the observations of the team members and the supervisor and to be able to review the videotape to examine in detail the therapeutic encounter between family and therapist. Supervisors were either in the observation room teaching the therapist and team or in the interview room demonstrating their own techniques. From this beginning, family therapy evolved a tradition of providing live supervision of the therapist's work together with the advantage of the team members' observations of the dynamics between the therapist and family members. As the use of this form of therapy and teaching developed, the interventions offered to families became more sophisticated and the use of the team, screen and videotape evolved within each model of family therapy. Latterly, developments in theory and practice have moved towards a more open co-operation between family, therapist and team in the therapeutic endeavour with each family (see Jones, 1993).

As the team for people who are Deaf and their families operates within a teaching centre and a national specialist service, therapy is provided in an interviewing suite consisting of a large interview room with a one-way screen, three video cameras and microphones and a viewing room with television, video recorder and mixing equipment. When developing the use of video equipment, film-makers who are Deaf were consulted and the optimum use is now made of one still and two moving cameras (see Figure 16.1). The room is as simple as possible with plain colours, no patterns, well lit, but without bright lights, and with nothing to distract the participants' attention from the signing.

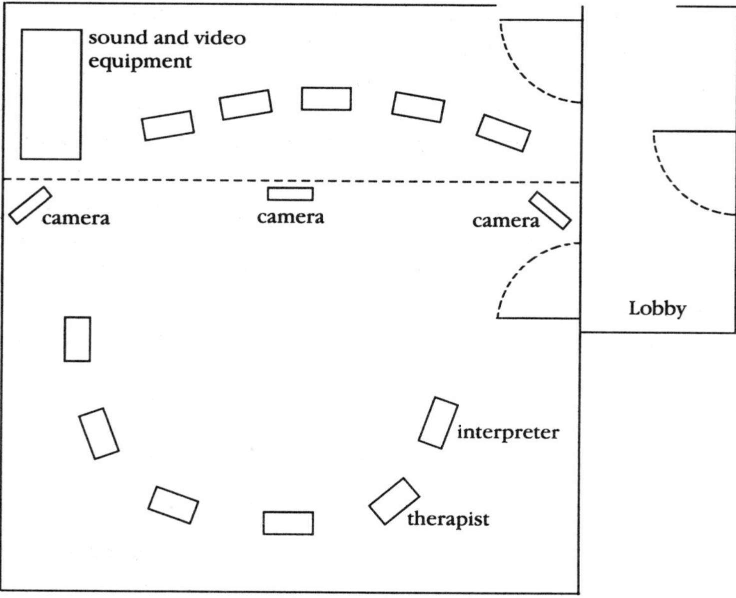

Figure 16.1

During the early life of the team, time was spent role-playing in the therapy room and following the role-play with the video cameras in order to work out the optimum positioning of the therapist, interpreter and family members. This ensured that communication within the therapy session was as clear as possible. Each person who is deaf needs to be able to see the interpreter and any other person using sign language, and to be able to see the facial expressions and lip movements of hearing family members and therapist. At first, seating positions were prescribed but as thinking and experience developed, and the style of therapy became more relaxed, family members were involved in discussions about seating. Currently, family and team are involved in ensuring appropriate seating during the session, and making changes when necessary for particular family conversations.

An example of this is a family with two adolescent children who are Deaf and their hearing parents. When a particularly emotionally laden conversation was necessary the interpreter sat between and slightly behind the parents so that parents and children could have eye contact, and facial expressions, lip patterns and sign could be read. Special care is also taken in the positioning of the interpreter if people who are deaf also have visual difficulties.

In order that deaf and hearing team members are fully able to take part in the sessions when behind the screen, people in the therapy room are positioned in a semi-circle in front of the screen. The interpreter is placed so as to be clearly visible to both those in the therapy and observation rooms. If possible, signing family members should be visible to observers without reference to the television screen. If this is not possible, the video cameras are used to facilitate the reading of sign by those in the observation room.

Communication within the team

Communication within the team, and between the therapist and team, has also been a developing process. Behind the screen it has proved essential for the second interpreter to take responsibility for interpreting within the team so that all members can express their thoughts and be available to the therapist. If the therapist is hearing then the traditional family therapy method of telephoning into the interview room or using an earpiece is employed to convey messages to the therapist. However, if the therapist is deaf then other methods are necessary. One option is for a team member to knock on the door and the interpreter to inform the therapist who then leaves the room for a signed conversation. A text telephone is now used in each room so that the therapist and team can be in direct communication in front of the family, using the telephone line. There is an argument for this to be available at all times enabling direct communication between deaf team members and a hearing therapist.

Originally the traditional model of team work was used; the therapist interviewed the family, observed by the team, with an intersession discussion between therapist and team. Therapeutic messages or tasks were then delivered to the family by the therapist.

A current development on which the team and families are working is the use of the reflecting team (see Andersen, 1990). In this model of therapy the responses and thoughts of the team are communicated directly to the family and therapist. The observing team members move into the therapy room and the family, interpreter and therapist move to the observation room. The second interpreter enters the therapy room interpreting directly towards the screen in order to be visible to the family and therapist and *voicing over* (see Glossary pp. 445–6) for signed communication by team members. It is particularly important that the use of this strategy is carefully explained to all family members and that attention is paid to ensuring the involvement and understanding of these communications by children who are Deaf.

Role and function of the interpreter

In the team

As previously stated, the interpreter is a key member of the team. Great benefit has been derived from having the same interpreter throughout the life of the team. Within the team the interpreter is necessary for communication between Deaf and hearing members. Although many hearing team members have excellent signing skills, some do not. During discussion it is not easy both to speak and sign because of the differences between spoken and signed language and the difficulty of using both simultaneously. The interpreter therefore signs for all speech and takes responsibility for voicing over for deaf team members' signed communication. Considerable attention has been paid to the process in the team between deaf and hearing people and a great deal has been learned from each other about communication within and across the Deaf and hearing cultures. Communicating ideas can sometimes be fraught with misunderstanding on both sides; this has been resolved by using each other and the interpreter as resources within each culture and then between the two cultures. Good humour and good will have often rescued situations and this learning has been taken into the work with families. The development of this level of communication and team knowledge has been a further advantage of working together over a long period of time.

Visiting interpreters have provided very useful comments on the team process and the processes between families and the team. As outsiders, they have been able to highlight some of the more political issues about how power is held and used in the team. Team members were already aware of some of these issues relating to the women and men in the team and the doctors and other professionals but it has been useful for visitors to challenge the way the hearing and Deaf team members were using their power in relation to each other. This was mainly in the form of using spoken or signed communicaton without interpretation.

In the therapy session

In the team's practice, family members' preferred communication modes are discussed and they are asked how they wish to use the interpreter for their own communications. Some hearing family members wish to sign for themselves, others prefer to use the interpreter. The team's need for the presence of the interpreter is explained. This explanation is made in terms of the communication between Deaf and hearing team members and between the therapist and the hearing family members if the therapist is using sign (usually BSL), or the therapist and family members who are Deaf if the therapist is speaking. The interpreter is used to communicate the oral communication in the room in BSL, or Sign Supported English (SSE) if more appropriate, and to voice over for signed communication.

The intrafamilial communication is then not the only focus in the team's use of an interpreter. However, once the interpreter is present and signing, many of the dynamics discussed by Harvey (1982, 1984, 1986) become apparent and family belief systems, communication patterns and dynamics associated with communication between Deaf and hearing members are challenged. The affective communication of Deaf family members may become clearer to hearing family members and vice versa.

This is illustrated by work with a mother and daughter pair. When discussing the father, who had left the family many years previously, each was able to share and appreciate for the first time the pain the other had experienced at losing a husband and a father.

Similarly, the dynamics of family communication can be revealed. The overt and covert messages contained in affective communication between family members, the playing out of family myths and the control of information passing between Deaf and hearing subsystems.

Different communication patterns emerge in families with hearing parents and Deaf children (H:D), Deaf parents and hearing children (D:H) and Deaf parents and Deaf children D:D). In the first two cases different subsystems are using different communication channels and have different access to communication with the outside world. In the final case all members use the same communication method and so effectively function in the same way as a hearing family but do not share the same communication method with all members of the team nor with the outside world.

For H:D families the parents have much greater opportunities to control their children's access to communication and information; the children have much greater difficulty in contributing to family communication and experience greater dependency on, and greater frustration with, their parents. For D:H families the hearing children have greater access to communication with the outside world, extended family, school, therapy team, etc. and find their parents depending on them to do so. Thus parental authority is undermined. As a hearing daughter of deaf parents says, 'our power is not in what we say but in what we do not say or sign'. Therefore in D:H families there is likely to be less authoritative parenting and more parentification of children, whereas in H:D families there are likely to be infantilized children and overcontrolling parents. This is not true for all families with deaf members but is certainly so in clinical populations.

It is important to realize that the addition of an interpreter does not create a situation of equal accessibility for the deaf and hearing family members any more than translation between two cultures and languages is immediate and exact. Translation is subject to temporal and content distortion. It is impossible to provide precise simultaneous interpretations of oral or signed dialogue to a third person. The person receiving the translation linguistically falls a little behind in the conversation. It is important for the therapist to be aware of this and to make sure that the family members receiving translations are given the opportunity to intervene and not to be passive observers. There may also be some content distortion in translations as it is not always possible to interpret all body language, facial expressions and gestures.

The presence of the interpreter may interfere with the intrafamilial communication patterns. Although the hearing members of the family may not sign, communication will be occuring, i.e. facial expression, gestures, idiosyncratic signing and lip-reading. As with hearing families, these communications may not always be clear to the therapist and may need to be clarified.

Experiencing fluent signing can have several effects in families. Some hearing people may react with anger, hurt or guilt at not having learned sign language, or may worry about what the team will think about their signing skills. The use of sign and the presence of an interpreter can confront the family with the reality of deafness. Hearing parents who have difficulty communicating with their child who is deaf may be surprised how well an interpreter can achieve communication and how well the child can express himself, when sign is translated into spoken language. Some parents may feel bitter about previous professional advice not to sign but to concentrate on speech and lip-reading. People who are deaf can be empowered by the experience of being able to communicate more freely and all family members can find themselves having new experiences together within the combination of the therapist's intervention and the clearer communication.

The team members are not always aware of how careful and exacting the interpreter's work is until the discussion after the session, when she will point out that language and ideas have been used which have been difficult to interpret. As with any language, individuals' understanding and use of it varies. The interpreter has the task of gauging the deaf family member's knowledge of, and facility with, sign language and adjusting her communication to fit with this. If she needs to, the interpreter will slow the session down and ensure that communication is clear. She will clarify with family members her role as interpreter if they begin to address their comments directly to her, but will answer direct questions if necessary, to ensure the family members' comfort in the session.

There may be times when it is appropriate not to have the interpreter present; for example, when wishing to join with a family containing some members who may be opposed to signing. If the therapist insists on using an interpreter the family may not engage in therapy. In this case it may be better to meet the family without the interpreter. Then when the therapist has successfully joined with the family she can demonstrate the communication difficulties they will have without the interpreter and explain the team's need of the interpreter.

Another situation in which it may be wise to omit the interpreter for part of the session may be when a hearing member of the family is struggling to communicate something important to a deaf member; for example, a parent explaining the breakdown of the marriage to a teenage child. It may be more therapeutic to encourage the parent to explain and allow parent and child to experience the direct communication together rather than have the interpreter make the explanation.

On occasion other interpreters have been involved — at holiday times or when the regular interpreter is known to the family. These occasions have demonstrated the value of the long-term involvement of interpreters but have also brought about new questions for the team as interpreters sought to understand their work in order to be effective in the session.

Like Harvey, (1982, 1984) the team has a flexible approach towards use of the interpreter when the hearing therapist has good signing skills and wishes to communicate directly with deaf family members. In these situations the interpreter will voice over for the sign and continue to sign for verbal communications for the benefit of the observing team. The therapists who are Deaf, of course, sign to signing family members and the interpreter voices over for signed communication, and signs when speech is used.

A very practical issue in signed and spoken conversations, whether as part of therapy or not, is the intense concentration needed during the session by both the people who are deaf and the interpreter. Because of this it is necessary to have a break of about 10 minutes after 45 minutes of the session; however, this is very difficult to maintain during the intensity of therapy sessions. The team interpreter and deaf team members are very tolerant of this problem but the team needs to be aware of this on behalf of the family members who are deaf.

Deaf Members of the Team

Working within a service which holds the belief that both deaf and hearing people should be part of all therapeutic work, the team began with both Deaf and hearing people as members. Currently there are two deaf team members, one woman and one man, who are vital in assessing the communication and interpersonal dynamics within the family. They are also astute in attending to the non-verbal communications used by people who are deaf and, in addition to their professional skills as mental health workers, bring with them their own experience and knowledge of living within both Deaf culture and the hearing world. Conversely, they sometimes have to be excluded from sessions because, like the interpreter, they may know members of the family. It is their intimate knowledge of Deaf culture that is so valuable, but that same intimate knowledge may preclude them from the therapy. Because the Deaf world is small and close-knit, issues of confidentiality are very important. Although clients are assured of professional confidentiality they often prefer not to be seen by team members whom they may know socially, even slightly. However, this is also the case for any therapist who knows a client socially.

At first the deaf members of the team, who had not had experience of working with families, were very uncertain about entering the therapy room. They were invaluable as team members and had very useful observations and insights to make about the therapy, the families and the context in which the team operated. Once they felt more comfortable with the setting and the techniques of systems therapy, the deaf team members were able to experiment with working in the therapy room, at first as co-therapists with a hearing colleague. This was most empowering for family members who were deaf — they felt able to communicate directly with someone from their own culture. Sometimes deaf members of the team also provided a new model of deafness for both hearing and deaf family members — someone who was functioning professionally and on equal terms within a mixed team. The same effect occurs when families experience the reflecting team, which often contains both the deaf members of the team.

Deaf members of the team now work with a variety of families. Often the team has to decide to use a hearing therapist, when a deaf therapist would be preferable.

At present the only family systems training that is provided for team members who are Deaf is that learned within the clinical setting, through reading, and some direct teaching during team discussions. This sometimes limits the scope of the direct systemic input the deaf therapists are able to make within the session. Some interventions are made during the session in *textphone* conversations between the team behind the screen and the deaf therapist in the therapy room. The reflecting team discussions also allow more systemic interventions to be made by the team. Two deaf therapists have completed the foundation training provided by PSFTC, and in the future it is planned to include deaf therapists in all the PSFTC training programmes.

It should also be stated that not all hearing team members have undertaken formal training in family systems therapy. However, written English is more readily available to them than to their deaf colleagues.

Clinical work

Engaging with families

All teams within PSFTC offer treatment to families with psychological, emotional, physical and interpersonal difficulties and this is the same for families in which one or more people are deaf. Referrals are from both child and adult departments of SWLSG NDS and from community agencies, including general psychiatric teams, GPs, Social Services departments and educational services. Criteria for treatment are broad and the most important factor is that the family members accept the value of working together in the therapy setting.

When assessing referrals, the team members consider:

- The nature of the family structure: couple relationship; parent or parents and children; extended family involvement (within the same generation or across generations); the family position in the lifecycle — a couple at the beginning of their relationship and the involvement or not of their families of origin; a family with children which is in the parenting phase; a family where children are now adults and may be moving away from the family of origin into new relationships; a family in the later stages of the lifecycle. All of these factors will have influences on the problem presented and the team members' decision about who to invite to therapy.
- The wider context of the referred family: lifecycle events within other generations and family systems; school and work settings and events such as exams; changes in school or job; unemployment or retirement; cultural issues both of race/ethnicity* and deafness/hearing and many other possible contexts which may be known at the point of referral. These issues will also influence who may be invited to therapy.

*A high proportion of clients referred to the SWLSG NDS are from minority groups, but few of those families referred to the family therapy team have accepted the offer of therapy. Engaging these families has required greater consideration. Whilst the deaf/hearing balance within the team is resolved, at present the team does not have members from any ethnic minority groups. This will be rectified as new members of staff join the SWLSG NDS and the PSFTC.

- The deafness: whether the deafness present in the family is highly significant or whether deafness is incidental to the problem; the aetiology and type of deafness (i.e. pre-lingual, acquired, specific syndrome, etc.); any other symptoms associated with the deafness; the family methods of communication and attitudes to deafness.
- The referred problem: the nature of the problem and whether it is a problem which is more significant for the referrer or whether the family members agree with the referrer's view.
- Other professionals involved with the family: who may or may not be operating as a *network* (see Glossary); mental health and health professionals, education services, Social Services, police and the courts, religious or other social organizations.

Information about these issues may be included in the referral. If this is not the case further information may be sought from the referrer. When the team members consider there is sufficient information to ensure engagement, direct contact will be made with the family.

At this stage, however, it may be decided to offer consultation to the referrer rather than becoming involved with the family direct. Experience has shown that, as a tertiary service receiving referrals from a very large catchment area (southern England), it is often wiser to consult with the referrer in detail before attempting to engage with the family. On a basic level, simply the distance between the service and the clients can prevent families who are not well prepared and supported locally, from attending on a regular basis. Often consultation is the most appropriate intervention and support from the team can ensure that current involvement by referring professionals is optimally effective.

Where direct involvement with the client family is appropriate, consultation will broaden the information available to the team and increase the possibility of the family engaging in therapy. Becoming involved too quickly and appearing to offer help can lead to failure because the family is not securely enough engaged with local professional help to take the step of making a connection with the team. There are many other levels within this triangular system which can prevent engagement from occurring. The issues of the difficulties which can arise within the triangle of tertiary treatment services, families and referrers are fully explored in family therapy literature, a seminal paper being Selvini-Palazzoli et al. (1980).

This group of Italian systemic practitioners developed a model of thinking about some of the families they had worked with, where engagement between the family and the therapy team proved particularly difficult and appeared to be hindered by the families' involvement with the original referrers. They proposed a number of models of the relationship between family, referrer and therapy team which provided a basis for the development of thinking among family therapists about the process of engagement (Roberts, 1987).

An example of consultation before engagement with the family would be the social work referral to the team of a deaf father and his two hearing sons, aged 15 and 12, because of the apparent uncontrolled behaviour of the older son: staying out late, absence from school, not responding to his father's questions and rule setting. The family lived some distance from the clinic and the team was concerned that a simple approach directly to the family would not be successful. Written communication would probably be handled by the older son, who could well view the referral to the clinic as an attempt to discipline him. The social worker was contacted and was able to clarify the situation and confirmed the team's view that the family would benefit from her presence at the initial meeting. This meeting revealed a closer and more co-operative set of relationships between father and sons than the social worker had experienced when dealing with crisis situations. Also revealed were the painful feelings each family member was experiencing following the breakdown of the parents' marriage. Further work was not undertaken by the team.

An illustration of family therapy

To illustrate some of the possibilities of family therapy with families which include deaf people, the following composite example has been devised.

> A family of hearing parents, Mr and Mrs Welch aged 50 and 47, who have separated, Mary, aged 23, who is deaf and has been experiencing psychiatric difficulties and her older hearing brother David, aged 27, who is married to Anne, with a baby, Jenny. The team has been asked by the psychiatric team treating Mary to help in re-building communication between family members who have become estranged (See Figure 16.2).
>
> On receiving the referral the team members discuss the information received and consider how best to approach the family members — who were living in separate places but communicating with and visiting the hospital where Mary was a patient. The deaf therapists in the team, in particular, considered Mary's situation as a person who is deaf: how best contact could be made with her; her point of view and possible experience within her family. The whole team thought about the relationships between the family members and the possible effects of deafness in one family member; the parents' separation; Mr Welch's relationship with his current partner, Margaret; Mary's psychiatric symptoms.
>
> It was decided to send the introductory videotape to the hospital where Mary and her family were able to view it together and see and hear the signed and spoken message about the clinic, family therapy and the questionnaire. The keyworker in the hospital helped the family to complete the form together.
>
> As Mary was still an inpatient it was decided that one deaf and one hearing team member and an interpreter would conduct an assessment session at the hospital with a member of the treatment team present.
>
> The initial session was attended by both parents, Mary, her brother, David, and the psychiatrist. Although the team interpreter was unable to attend, it was

possible to engage an interpreter with whom Mary was familiar. This meeting proved to be one of the few occasions that the whole nuclear family had been together since the parents' separation four years previously and was the first time they had experienced talking together with the aid of sign language interpretation. This was a unique experience for the doctor who had, until this point, only met with Mrs Welch and Mary and had not previously worked with a deaf patient.

The therapists decided that the hearing team member would conduct the session with the deaf member acting as the 'reflecting team' and it was explained that the interpreter would sign for her benefit. It was also explained that part way through the session the two therapists would hold a conversation together in front of the family and doctor, on which they could all comment later.

The initial part of the session revealed warmth and concern between each family member and Mary and between each parent and child, but considerable tension between Mr and Mrs Welch which David attempted to mediate.

The therapist spent the session clarifying Mary's current relationship with each family member and their concerns and questions about her treatment in the hospital.

The conversation between the therapists was used to comment on the very warm feelings apparent in the family between the two siblings and between them and each parent and to acknowledge the understandable tensions between Mr and Mrs Welch following their separation. The wish of each family member and the hospital team to help Mary recover was welcomed. The conversation then continued to explore the potential for family therapy sessions to aid this process and a number of options were considered. The possiblities of exploring: family history; the parents' decision to separate; the present and future contact between family members (which currently had become closer during Mary's admissions to the hospital); the most appropriate groupings of people with which to conduct the therapy if family members wished to take part.

This assessment session and conversation opened the way for family members and the hospital team to consider how they could work together with the family therapy team in their joint aim of aiding Mary's recovery. Mary was able to express her wish to know more of the family history, which she felt she had not fully understood due to the oral communication used within the family. The family acknowledged that they had noticed the liveliness of her signed communication with deaf friends and acknowledged that it had been difficult to explain to her some of the things that had happened in the family. David expressed his difficulty in mediating between his parents and his decision to see less of the family following his marriage three years previously. Mr and Mrs Welch agreed that it was difficult for them to be in the same room together but that they each wished to continue contact with their children.

On behalf of the psychiatric team, the doctor made a commitment that whilst Mary remained an inpatient they would provide space for sessions to take place and would maintain close liaison with the family therapy team and, with the family members' agreement, she would attend each session. Following her discharge Mary would receive community support for as long as both the family therapy and community psychiatric team thought necessary.

The subsequent ten therapy sessions, over the following year, were conducted with both Mary and David present on each occasion and with one or other parent attending. Two sessions also included David's wife, Anne.

During that time the family was able to consider the effects of the death of the second child, Janet, from multiple handicaps, and the parents' added grief when Mary was diagnosed as deaf. Mary learned for the first time the facts about her father's longstanding relationship with his current partner, Margaret and that Pauline (the daughter of Mr Welch and Margaret) was her half-sister. Although she had known that her parents were unhappy together for many years she had linked this with their disappointment with her. Both parents were able to share with their children their sense of grief and guilt over Janet's handicaps and death and Mary's deafness.

Mrs Welch's experience of post-natal depression following Mary's birth was spoken of for the first time and connected with unresolved grief over the loss of Janet. Mr Welch talked with his 80-year-old mother about his older brother who had died of multiple handicaps before he (Mr Welch) was born. Genetic counselling was sought by David and Anne.

Mr and Mrs Welch each told their children that they were not yet, and perhaps never would be, able to talk together about Mr Welch's relationship with Margaret and the breakdown of their marriage, but were able to free David and Mary from acting as mediators. David and Mary's previously warm relationship was re-established and included Anne and Jenny. Mary was able to continue her college course.

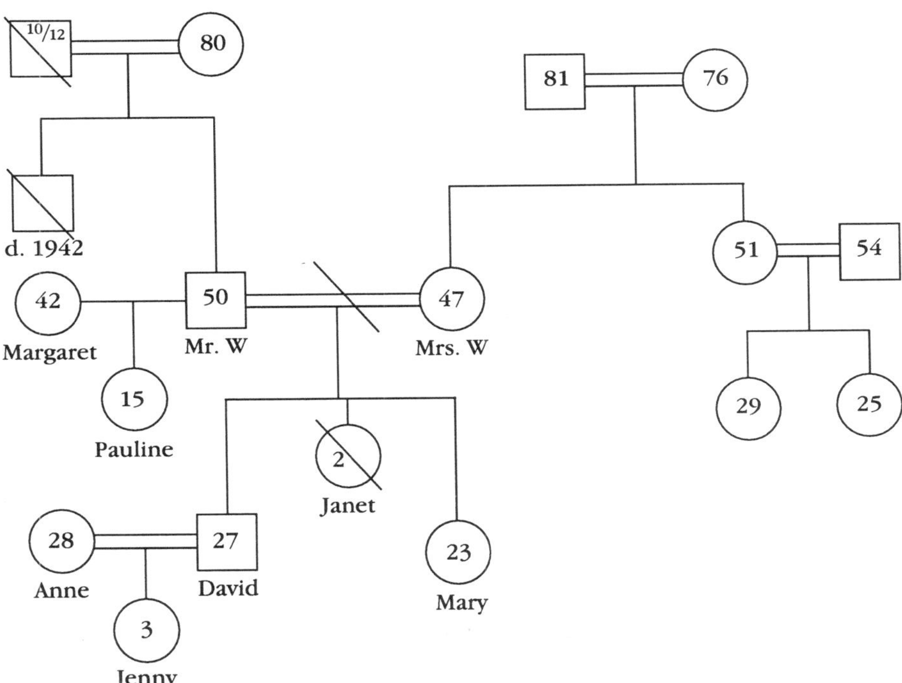

Figure 16.2.

Although this illustration is devised and not a case-study it describes issues from families seen by the team. The aim being to show the interplay between family life events and the extra dimension of deafness in one family member, which must be considered within the whole family context and not placed either in the foreground or background.

It has been the experience of the team that it is the combination of the systemic skills and techniques which are useful in all 'family' situations and the close attention to communication, not only about facts but thoughts and feelings as well, which is useful in helping families with Deaf members find new ways of being together.

References

Andersen T (1990) (ed) The Reflecting Team. Broadstairs: Borggman Publishing.

Burck C, Speed B (1995) (eds) Gender Power and Relationships. London: Routledge.

Carter B, McGoldrick M (1989) (eds) The Changing Family Life Cycle: A Framework for Family Therapy (second edition). Boston, MA: Allyn & Bacon.

De Zulueta F (1990) Bilingualism and family therapy. Journal of Family Therapy 12: 255–265.

Fishman HC (1993) Intensive Structural Therapy: Treating Families in their Social Context. New York: Basic Books.

Gorell-Barnes G (1994) (ed) Ethnicity, culture, race and family therapy. Context 20.

Harvey M (1982) The influence and utilization of an interpreter for Deaf persons in family therapy. American Annals of the Deaf 127: 821–827.

Harvey MA (1984) Family therapy with Deaf persons: the systemic utilization of an interpreter. Family Process 23: 205–221.

Harvey MA (1986) The magnifying mirror: family therapy for Deaf persons. Family Systems Medicine 4: 408–420 (expanded version of article in American Annals of the Deaf, 1985).

Harvey MA (1989) Psychotherapy with Deaf and Hard of Hearing Persons: A Systemic Model. Hove: Lawrence Erlbaum.

Hindley P, Hill P, Bond D (1993) Interviewing Deaf children, the interviewer effect: a research note. Journal of Child Psychology and Psychiatry 34: 1461–1467.

Hodes M (1989) Annotation: culture and family therapy. Journal of Family Therapy 11: 117–128.

Jones E (1993) Family Systems Therapy: Developments in the Milan-Systemic Therapy. Chichester: Wiley.

Lieberman S (1980) The extended family school of family therapy. In Walrond-Skinner S (ed) Family Therapy Collected Papers. London: Routledge and Kegan Paul, pp 339–349.

Luterman D (1987) Deafness in the Family. Boston, MA: College Hill Press.

McGoldrick M, Pearce K, Giordano J (1982) Ethnicity and Family Therapy. London: Guilford.

Madanes C (1991) Strategic Family Therapy. In Gurman AS, Kniskern DP (eds) Handbook of Family Therapy, Vol II. New York: Brunner Mazel, pp 396–416.

Meadow KP, Greenberg MG, Erting C, Carmichael H (1981) Interactions of deaf mothers and Deaf preschool children: comparisons with three other groups of deaf and hearing dyads. American Annals of the Deaf 126: 454–468.

Minuchin S, Fishman HC (1981) Family Therapy Techniques. Boston, MA: Harvard University Press.

Perelberg R, Miller A (1990) (eds) Gender and Power in Families. London: Routledge/Tavistock.

Roberts W (1987) Preparation of the referral network, the professional and the family. In Bentovim A, Gorell-Barnes G, Cooklin A (eds) Family Therapy: Complimentary Frameworks of Theory and Practice (second edition). London: Academic Press, Chapter 5.

Robinson LD, Weathers OD (1974) Family therapy of Deaf parents and hearing children: a new dimension in psychotherapeutic intervention. American Annals of the Deaf 119: 325–330.

Scott S (1984) Deafness in the family: will the therapist listen? Family Process 23: 214–216.

Selvini-Palazzoli M, Boscolo L, Cecchin G, Prata G (1980) The problem of the referring person. Journal of Marital and Family Therapy 6: 3–9.

Shapiro RJ, Harris R (1976) Family therapy in treatment of the Deaf: a case report. Family Process 15.

Simon FB, Stierlin H, Wynne LC (1985) The Language of Family Therapy: A Systemic Vocabulary and Sourcebook. New York: Family Process Press.

Sloman L, Springer S (1987) Strategic Family therapy: interventions with Deaf member families. Canadian Journal of Psychiatry 32: 558–562.

Chapter 17 Behavioural and Cognitive Approaches

SUE O'ROURKE

Introduction

Cognitive behaviour therapy (CBT) has come to mean those psychological therapies derived by the scientific process. This scientist-practitioner model has its strength in the relationship between research, in normal and abnormal psychology, and practice by the clinical psychologist. This means that the techniques used can be investigated and modified in the light of research findings. The model also lends itself to novel and peculiar cases by the use of single case-studies. CBT is used effectively to treat anxiety disorders, depression, marital and family problems, and behaviour disorders, and can be adapted to produce individualized treatment which can then be monitored and modified accordingly. Clinical psychologists working within adult mental health, with children and with people with learning disabilities, employ CBT directly and also indirectly by advising other professionals and influencing general milieu of treatment within a team approach.

Epidemiological studies of deaf populations suggest that deaf people experience the same range of psychological difficulties and disorders as hearing people (Altshuler, Rainer and Deming, 1978). Prevalence studies fail to report a greater overall psychiatric morbidity but the relative proportions of different disorders vary, with deaf people displaying greater 'problems of living' rather than overt disorder (Rainer and Altshuler, 1966). Mental health problems of deaf people fall roughly into two groups:

- Mental illness coincidental with deafness.
- Problems which are in some way related to deafness (Rainer and Altshuler, 1966; Denmark and Eldridge, 1969; Pyke and Littman, 1982; Rainer et al, 1963).

With regard to the latter, the majority present with problems of behaviour and adjustment (Denmark, 1972, 1985).

The high prevalence of behaviour disorder within the group of deaf people referred to mental health services makes behaviour therapy an attractive option for therapists. However, it should be remembered that behavioural approaches are used to treat a range of psychological disorders in the hearing population and this wide application to problems in Deaf people needs to be explored.

It has been assumed that cognitive therapies, in common with other 'talking therapies' are inaccessible to deaf people. This assumption, of course, says as much about the limitations of therapists and their communication skills as about their deaf clients. Nevertheless, when using the range of cognitive and behavioural therapies with deaf clients a number of issues need to be considered, and modifications made to therapy.

Theories and therapies

Behaviour therapy

Theories

Before the development of behaviour therapy, psychotherapeutic approaches dealt with introspection, aiming to increase the patient's insight into problems in order to alleviate suffering and facilitate change. Such therapies were eventually viewed by many as lacking in scientific rigour, being more akin to philosophical belief systems than theories open to investigation and falsification.

John B Watson (1878–1958) shifted the focus of psychology from introspection to observable behaviour. Thus, behaviour therapy, based on learning theories, was developed. Within experimental psychology, two types of learning were observed: classical conditioning and operant conditioning. These became the basis of behaviour therapy.

Classical Conditioning was originally described at the turn of the century by Pavlov in his studies of dogs. In his experiments, Pavlov presented dogs with some meat. This produced the response of salivating. He then rang a bell at the same time as presenting the meat. Soon the dogs began to salivate when they heard the bell. In other words, they had learnt that bell signalled meat and had been conditioned to respond to the bell.

Operant Conditioning involves a different type of learning concerned with the effects of consequences of behaviour rather than the stimulus–response relationship. Experiments in the 1890s by Edward Thorndike, and later by BF Skinner in the 1950s, documented operant conditioning in both animals and humans. The 'law of effect' which operates here states that a behaviour which produces a desirable, satisfying or pleasant consequence will be repeated and a behaviour which produces an unpleasant

	Pleasant Consequences	Unpleasant Consequences
Add	Positive reinforcement	Punishment or aversion therapy (behaviour)
Remove	Time out from positive reinforcement	Negative Reinforcement

Figure 17.1 Operant conditioning.

or aversive consequence, or fails to produce a satisfactory consequence, will not be repeated. Skinner coined the phrase **reinforcement** to describe this and stated that all behaviour is controlled by positive reinforcers. This radical behaviourist view denies the existence of free will and holds that the inner world of thoughts and feelings are not the proper subject matter for scientific study.

Therapies

Based on the theories outlined briefly above, and on findings from experimental psychology, behaviour therapy is used to treat a variety of psychological problems.

Anxiety disorders such as phobias or social anxiety have been treated by **counter-conditioning** and **systematic desensitization**. If anxiety is viewed as a classically conditioned response to a stimulus, counter-conditioning involves evoking an alternative response, incompatible with anxiety to that same stimulus. An example of this might be learning to use relaxation in the presence of a feared stimulus. This is incompatible with the physical changes of the anxiety response. Systematic desensitization requires the anxious person to compile a hierarchy of feared stimuli and then to imagine these stimuli while deeply relaxed until the top of the hierarchy is reached. The technique has been shown to be effective in reducing levels of anxiety. However, as a result of research it is now accepted that ***in vivo* desensitization** is even more effective in reducing fear, in other words actual **graded exposure** to the feared stimulus (Bandura, 1969).

The theory of operant conditioning has led to a number of treatments. Desired behaviour can be increased by engineering rewarding consequences (positive reinforcement) and undesired behaviour reduced or eliminated by using unpleasant consequences or withdrawing the positive reinforcement (see Figure 17.1). This has a number of applications.

Positive reinforcement can be used to teach new behaviours — giving rewards for successive approximations to a goal is called **shaping**.

Reinforcers have to be particular to an individual, and what is rewarding to one person cannot be assumed to be effective with another. Although positive reinforcement should be administered as close in time to the behaviour as possible, delays can be managed and more creative reinforcers used by the implementation of 'tokens' which can be exchanged later for rewards. A particular case of this is the '**token economy**'. Patients in a token economy are rewarded (reinforced) for appropriate behaviour by earning tokens. This idea was particularly popular in the 1960s and 1970s but has lost favour now as it is difficult to organize and requires a high level of staff expertise and a small number of patients per staff member. Also, its effectiveness over and above the additional staff input is not clear (Davison and Neale, 1982).

Aversion therapy is the introduction of negative consequences to reduce an inappropriate behaviour and is understandably controversial. This has been used to treat behaviour problems and sexual disorders such as fetishes, but the ethical problems far outweigh any possible benefits, and the idea of inflicting pain or discomfort on a patient 'for their own good' is not acceptable. Aversion techniques have long been replaced by more positive approaches, e.g. reinforcing appropriate behaviour which is incompatible with the target behaviour, known as **Differential Reinforcement of Other Behaviour** (DRO). For example, if a person tends to behave aggressively in certain situations, they may be reinforced for walking away from certain situations; or a person who habitually leaves group situations may be reinforced for staying for increasingly long periods of time. In other words, instead of punishing an undesirable behaviour, an alternative, incompatible and desirable one is reinforced by rewarding it.

The removal of positive reinforcement which is maintaining a behaviour is known as **time-out from positive reinforcement**. Frequently, the positive reinforcer at work is the attention of others. Removing this attention by turning away, or by taking the person out of the situation for a few seconds is therefore time out from positive reinforcement. This is not to be confused with the use of seclusion or removal of patients to their bed space for several minutes when they behave inappropriately. Although often called 'time out', it may either be closer to positive reinforcement due to the amount of attention received, or to punishment/aversion if the consequence is very unpleasant for the patient.

Negative reinforcement is a term often confused with 'punishment'. However, it is the withdrawal of negative consequences leading to an increase in behaviour. Observation of individuals with challenging behaviour will often reveal negative reinforcement operating to maintain the problem. For example if a person finds group work stressful and difficult, they may learn that threatening or aggressive behaviour leads to the removal of the stress as they are asked to leave the group. They therefore learn to use challenging behaviour as an effective means to avoid stressful group situations.

When tackling such situations the first step is to acknowledge when such behaviours are being negatively reinforced. The next is to alter the contingencies, i.e. the consequences of the behaviour. This might be to stop aggression allowing the individual to avoid group situations. This would be difficult to achieve in practice, and so a more effective approach might be DRO, as described above.

Cognitive Therapy

Theories

The radical behaviourists did not deny the existence of internal mental processes, but felt they were not accessible to scientific study. In addition to classical and operant conditioning a third kind of learning was acknowledged – learning through observation. The resultant treatment, known as **modelling**, allows the patient to learn through observation. It is therefore clear that in translating what is observed into action some mediating cognitive process is occurring.

Cognitive therapies, of which there are a number, have in common the basic premise that it is faulty patterns of thinking which cause psychological disturbance. Two major proponents of cognitive therapy are Albert Ellis and Aaron Beck, both of whom have done most of their research on depressed patients.

Ellis's **Rational-Emotive therapy** (RET) states that 'irrational thoughts' and illogicalities are the cause of psychological distress. People repeat internal sentences to themselves and in certain cases these can lead to emotional turmoil. Examples of irrational and unhelpful thoughts frequently encountered are 'I must be perfect in everything I do' and 'I must be liked/loved by everyone'.

Beck's cognitive therapy, relating particularly to depression, holds that it is the negative view of the world, the self and the future which is causal. The depressed person repeats to him/herself 'Negative Automatic Thoughts' (NATs) in a variety of situations and interprets events in a negative way which leads to depression. Underlying such thoughts are assumptions about the world, self and future which are rooted in the person's history and can be made explicit through therapy.

Therapy

There are a number of other cognitive therapies in addition to those of Ellis and Beck including cognitive analytic therapy or schema focussed therapy. However, all take as the focus of assessment and treatment the 'faulty' thinking of the patient. At the outset the model of cognitive therapy is explained to the patient and his/her co-operation sought to tackle his/her difficulties by looking at his/her thoughts. Once it is clear that the patient understands the therapy, the patient and therapist engage in a joint search to identify the unhelpful thoughts that are causing the distress. This is an ongoing process throughout assessment and therapy, the aim being to teach the patient to become aware of, make explicit and eventually to challenge the negative thoughts as they arise, not only in therapy, but between sessions as well.

In therapy the patient is asked to describe situations where he has felt depressed or anxious. The therapist then uses questioning to elicit the key thoughts and to challenge them.

The example which follows captures the flavour of cognitive therapy. Throughout therapy, patients keep a diary recording situations when they felt depressed or anxious, the thoughts identified and later how they challenged them. Writing thoughts down both in and between sessions helps give structure to the therapy and acts as a form of objective assessment, as well as enabling the therapist to monitor patients' progress in using the therapy.

The patient, a man in his 50s, has had a serious car accident, leaving him with some physical disability. He has been referred for depression and been seen for several sessions, and has become quite skilled at identifying Negative Automatic Thoughts.

Patient (pt): I've had a terrible week — Saturday I just broke down and cried in front of my friend. It wasn't too bad at the time — but after, well, I felt really down —

Therapist (th): let's focus on how you felt afterwards then — what was going through your mind when you were so down?

pt: nothing really — just how awful I felt

th: is that all? Anything else?

pt: only, what must John have thought — I mean a grown man crying — pathetic isn't it?

th: what do you think John did think?

pt: that I was really weak and pathetic — well I am aren't I?

th: do you think we've hit on a Negative Automatic Thought here?

pt: what do you mean 'I'm weak and pathetic?' or 'John thinks I'm weak and pathetic?'

th: maybe both? Shall we try to find challenges to both? Which one do you want to start with? Write them down

pt: OK, start with the one about John. He's a really good bloke so he might not have thought anything bad

th: so you're not entirely convinced by that thought anyway. Do you think you really know what he's thinking?

pt: well, no

th:	so you're assuming what he'll think — was there any evidence in his behaviour or what he said that he thought you were pathetic and weak?
pt:	no, actually he was very understanding
th:	I think we may have a couple of challenges then, don't you?
pt:	yes — 'I don't know what John was thinking' and 'there's no evidence that he thought I was weak'
th:	Right. I was wondering, if it was the other way around and John cried on your shoulder — would you think he's weak and pathetic
pt:	no, of course not (laughs)
th:	how are you feeling about that thought now?
pt:	well, it's daft really isn't it.

Within cognitive therapy the therapist may use direct challenges to negative thoughts, but the emphasis is on indirect or 'Socratic' questioning which engages the patient to a greater extent and leads to 'self-discovery' rather than therapist-led discovery. Examples of this type of questioning frequently involve asking if there is any evidence to support a certain thought or assumption, or merely asking the question 'Why?' or 'Why not?', when faced with assumptions such as 'I must be perfect in all I do' or 'I should not cry/get angry . . .' and so forth. This approach enables patients to explore their thoughts and be gently led down the path of challenging long-held assumptions. With practice, patients internalize such questioning and develop the skill of being their own cognitive therapist.

Cognitive behaviour therapy and Deaf people

If the strength of CBT is its scientific approach and its ability to produce individualized treatment plans then it should lend itself to adaptation to various client groups, including Deaf people. Far from applying therapy designed for hearing people in a blanket approach, this model sets itself up as one that can be tested and refined as necessary for the case in hand.

In the rest of this chapter we shall look at some of the theoretical issues when using CBT with Deaf people, and suggest how CBT might be modified when working with Deaf patients.

Setting the Scene

The Deaf population is an entity with a culture and history of its own. There is also what is known as 'culture of therapy'. Studies on the accessibility of services to minority groups have looked at this 'culture of therapy' as perhaps something alien to certain groups. This may well apply to the

Deaf community, which, with its history of oppression and paternalistic treatment by the hearing majority, may find itself at odds with the notion of 'therapy' and its aims of empowerment of the individual. Furthermore, while therapists may be equipped with the non-specific therapeutic tools of empathy and unconditional positive regard, the experience of the Deaf patient in therapy may be quite different to that intended. They are faced with a hearing person, possibly embodying a whole host of past negative experiences, who is therefore not to be trusted. The therapeutic relationship is vital regardless of the type of therapy and this issue needs to be considered and possibly made explicit at the start of therapy.

One distinct advantage of CBT, and one way in which it differs from some traditional analytic therapies, is its basic principle that the rules and agenda for therapy should be made explicit and that the goals for treatment are arrived at jointly by patient and therapist through negotiation. In other words, the therapist does not have a 'hidden agenda' of aims and is not set up as someone who knows more about the patient than he or she does. This latter position, which can exist in some other therapies, can be particularly unhelpful to Deaf patients, especially considering that the therapist is usually a hearing person.

It is good practice within CBT to explain the model of therapy at the outset, to have an agenda for the therapy, which can be flexible and changed as time goes on, and to have an agenda for each session which is written down if appropriate to the patient. The patient then knows what to expect, the therapy is 'demystified' and there is a clear focus for change. This practice can be established from the initial assessment session, and as the therapy progresses the patient may take a more active role in setting the agenda.

Assessment

As with any form of psychological therapy, the initial assessment is vitally important. However, unlike some other therapies, CBT has the advantage of being able to use a variety of media for assessment. Of course, the mainstay remains the clinical interview, but pen and paper assessments provide useful data at the start of treatment and allow the measurement of progress.

Some of these may be appropriate for use with deaf patients, others can be adapted into more easily understood English, or into 'BSL English' (i.e. English in BSL grammar). Although most questionnaires are standardized and provide norms, interpretation should be carried out with caution as they are standardized on hearing samples only. Nevertheless, the experienced clinician may find the results useful. Within the framework of CBT it is quite acceptable to devise one's own questionnaire for use with individual patients and this may be more suitable to many deaf patients who perhaps have problems very specific to their deafness. Such individualized questionnaires can then be used at intervals to provide repeated measures of a particular problem.

In addition to questionnaires, diaries are often used during both assessment and treatment and can be as simple or as complicated as the therapist and patient decide. Simple tick boxes can suffice, recording of symptoms on a scale of 1–10 may be appropriate or, alternatively, columns recording various qualitative and quantitative aspects of behaviour can be used. Diaries have the advantage of encouraging the patient to think about therapy issues between sessions and are strongly recommended for this reason, as well as for their use in ongoing assessment.

However, for some Deaf people the use of written assessments is entirely inappropriate, and for many, written English is not the medium of choice. Within Deaf culture the use of video in various settings to fulfil a range of purposes is now well established. It may be that introducing video into the assessment procedure enhances the accessibility of the therapy process to the Deaf population. This is not a new suggestion within CBT: video has been used in assessment and therapy for many years, most notably in treating problems of social interaction, i.e. social skills deficits and social anxiety. In assessment a subject may be filmed in a social setting or under certain test conditions, such as meeting a new person or having a conversation. This is then used to identify where the problems lie. A similar assessment is then carried out following treatment as a measure of improvement. Using video in this way would seem most valuable when working with deaf people whose difficulties stem from a deprivation in their learnt experiences and the object of therapy is to teach new or alternative ways of behaving. As well as being consistent with the model and goals of CBT, it has the added advantage of being in keeping with Deaf culture.

As well as the clinical interview, the use of questionnaires and video recording, many psychological difficulties lend themselves to assessment of observable behaviour: this may be carried out by the patient and therapist in an assessment session — for example asking an agoraphobic patient to travel a specified route and rate his anxiety levels, and/or be observed by the therapist. Behaviour may be observed by family and friends (with the patient's consent!) and reported back to the therapist — for example how many activities did a depressed person engage in within a 24-hour period; nursing staff/carers can record behaviour over a period of time, for example the frequency of crying episodes, the amount of time spent in bed in 24 hours, whether or not a patient was aggressive within a 24-hour period, and so on.

Assessment is not only used at the beginning of therapy, but throughout, to monitor progress and final outcome. The initial information gained from assessment, using various techniques, is used to form a treatment plan.

Ongoing assessment measures the success of that treatment and modifications can be made in the light of this new infor-mation.

Treatment

In this final section some disorders commonly treated by clinical psychologists will be considered, and modifications to treatment in the case of a deaf patient discussed. Although this is the main issue of concern to clinicians working with deaf people, little research has been carried out in this area. Indeed, much of what is written on adapting psychological interventions consists of reassurances that psychological therapies *can* be used with deaf patients if one's sign language is good enough.

Fluency in sign language may be necessary, but it is certainly not sufficient. In order to meet the needs of deaf patients the therapist has to move from the notion of 'translating' and 'adapting' therapy towards a 'Deaf-centred' approach, which might produce a very different starting point and evolve into a rather different kind of therapy.

This 'de-centring' involves two aspects: firstly, to consider that the presentation of a disorder may be different in a deaf person than a hearing person, i.e. the content of their distress may be related to their deafness; and secondly, that specific therapeutic tools may need to be modified in order for the deaf person to benefit.

Anxiety disorders, including simple phobias, agoraphobia, social anxiety and generalized anxiety states are very commonly encountered by clinicians working with hearing people — and less so by those working with deaf people. A genuine lower prevalence is unlikely; more probable is that poor access to services and a paucity of specialized mental health provision discourages presentation with such problems.

In the deaf person experiencing anxiety symptoms, the focus of their concern might be specifically related to their deafness — or rather, to their position as a deaf person in a predominately hearing environment. Their history, their beliefs and thoughts about deafness and hearing are all important here, and this is where a cognitive approach is useful. But as with hearing patients, the initial treatment of choice is usually some form of anxiety management.

Anxiety management begins with educating the patient about the nature of anxiety: its usefulness under normal circumstances, the physical changes which occur and how it can be managed. Hearing and deaf people alike often believe that the symptoms, such as sweating, palpitations, dizziness, pins and needles, etc. indicate some dreadful disease, or that they are 'going mad'. Therefore, education to the contrary is an important first step. Making this information accessible to deaf patients involves presenting it in a variety of forms as suited to the individual:

written English or written 'BSL English' is a useful adjunct to sign language, writing up key points on a flipchart, diagrams, drawings and videos may all be useful. The therapist is wise to remember that lack of access to information about 'basic' anatomy and physiology means that nothing is to be assumed. The deaf person who is intelligent and capable may need additional 'educational' input about how his or her body works, prior to education about the effects of anxiety.

Once the patient understands his anxiety the clinician may wish to use systematic desensitization, based on the classical conditioning model. Traditionally this is undertaken in the imagination, with the patient in a relaxed state. Teaching progressive muscle relaxation to the deaf patient is not a problem — using video or demonstration initially and encouraging practice at home closing their eyes and using visualization techniques. Obviously, following verbal instruction whilst lying, relaxed, with closed eyes in order to go through a hierarchy of feared stimuli, is not possible. However, since *in vivo* graded exposure has been shown to be more effective, this practical therapy can be used to great effect with deaf patients.

The cognitive element to an individual's anxiety disorder can be tackled whilst undergoing *in vivo* graded exposure, or the cognitions can be the focus of treatment. The advantage of using *in vivo* work is that the therapist can elicit 'hot cognitions' as they occur, rather than relying on the patient's reporting skills after the event. Anxiety-related cognitions frequently involve unrealistic fears about the symptoms of anxiety and are health-related, e.g. 'I'm going to die', 'I have a serious disease', etc. Others include fears of losing control, going mad, losing control of bodily functions, and thoughts of what other people might think. For deaf people, such thoughts might have an added dimension relating to deafness and how they may be seen by hearing people. This may in turn be based on difficult past experiences as a deaf person trying to cope and communicate in a hearing environment. Other thoughts might include those which 'blame' the deafness for the anxiety, and idealize hearing status as a solution to all problems: the 'if only I was hearing . . .' thought. In eliciting such cognitions one very soon comes across the individual's assumptions about deafness and hearing people and begins to look at wider issues of identity and adjustment to deafness.

Depression According to behavioural theories of depression, depressed people have little positive reinforcement in their daily lives and it is this which causes them to experience low mood and lack of motivation. This in turn leads to a further reduction of positive reinforcement, and so on. This view, whilst clearly not able to account for the full range of depressive phenomena, is useful when considering the maintenance of depression in many cases. Thus, the first stage in treating the depressed patient is often to attempt to increase their level of activity and hence rewarding experiences.

'Activity scheduling', as this is known, is a very structured and practical aspect of therapy and involves the patient and therapist timetabling activities throughout the patient's day. She is encouraged to keep a diary of activities, rating them on a scale of 1 - 10 for 'pleasure' and 'mastery', i.e. a sense of achievement. Setting practical tasks may be extremely appropriate for some deaf patients, who may have limited ability to communicate, or for whom the whole process of therapy is difficult. Creative use of drawing, cut out pictures, and simplified language may help with recording the schedule and keeping a diary. Indeed, as most depressed patients have a significantly reduced level of rewarding activity, some form of activity scheduling is often useful, even if it only involves a plan to return to a club or previously enjoyed pastime on a certain evening the following week.

Cognitive treatment of depression involves identifying the cognitions which lead to feelings of depression and challenging them in a systematic way. The aim of therapy is that the patient learns to identify and challenge these cognitions him or herself without relying on the therapist. To this end, homework tasks almost always include keeping a 'thought diary'. Events described in the diary are used as a basis for discussion and, as in the case of anxiety disorders, the therapist attempts to 'home in' on 'hot cognitions'.

When treating deaf patients, the use of the diary may be a help or a hindrance — depending on the individual's command of English. Other, more creative means of recording thoughts may occur to the therapist, but the therapy is seriously hampered without the use of a diary. One poss-ibility is to offer more frequent sessions if this is feasible, e.g. two or three times a week rather than the standard once a week. This may allow increased practice of the use of cognitive techniques in circumstances where the individual has difficulty keeping a diary, and hence is less able to generalize what is learnt in therapy. An inpatient setting may enable more frequent therapy sessions. In this instance, ward staff and other therapists can also be made aware of the specific content of therapy and assist in the cognitive therapy by dealing with the patient's distress in a previously agreed way.

Behaviour disorders CBT for behaviour disorders often consists of the clinical psychologist working indirectly, by advising nursing staff or carers how to manage challenging behaviours or increase desirable and adaptive behaviours. Using techniques based on operant conditioning, described earlier, an individual's behaviour can be observed, recorded and a programme of behaviour modification set up.

Theoretically, behaviour modification does not require the understanding of the patient in order to be successful. Indeed, having identified the reinforcers operating to maintain inappropriate behaviours in a ward environment, staff can frequently make changes in *their* behaviour to the benefit of a number of patients, without involving those patients specifically.

For example, it is frequently the case that severe shortages of staff lead to a 'crisis management' approach in a residential setting. Patients are attended to when they present a problem, and left when they are behaving appropriately. However understandable this may be, it is reinforcing challenging behaviour, and omitting to reinforce acceptable behaviour. When staff begin to recognize this and make the necessary changes, there can be a dramatic improvement, to everybody's benefit.

Programmes to modify an individual's behaviour can be implemented as easily with a deaf person as with a hearing person. Many of the techniques used were described earlier, and since behaviour modification largely involves changes in staff or others' behaviour in order to manipulate reinforcers, it has as much potential with deaf as with hearing patients.

Frequently, in deaf and hearing patients alike, the origins of maladaptive behaviour lie in damaging experiences or lack of opportunity to learn appropriate behaviour. In such cases the person not only has a problem behaviour, but also has a skills deficit. While using a behaviour modification approach to reduce inappropriate and increase appropriate behaviour on a day-to-day, moment-to-moment basis, the patient may well benefit from individual therapy to address skills deficits.

Skills deficits The behavioural approach comes into its own when dealing with patients whose difficulties stem from a skills deficit. Many deaf adults were brought up in an impoverished environment by virtue of being deprived of an effective means of communication. In an oral/aural education system the child is unable to communicate effectively through speech and may never learn sign language. Without communication, the child is deprived of basic information and lacks knowledge which is acquired informally through incidental learning, as well as being at a disadvantage educationally. Lack of communication can also deprive the child of meaningful reciprocal relationships in which to develop social and other skills. As a result there is a risk that he or she reaches adulthood with deficits in social and personal skills. Deaf people with such problems are in need of habilitation rather than rehabilitation (see Chapter 19).

The teaching of new skills by behavioural means is often carried out in conjunction with behaviour modification to reduce challenging or inappropriate behaviours. Reinforcement of other behaviours is all very well, but first the patient may need to be explicitly taught alternatives to challenging behaviour.

Social skills training may be carried out in a group or with individuals. Assessment involves discussion and possibly observation/video recording of patients to identify skills deficits. New ways of behaving are taught through modelling, role play and feedback, again preferably using video. Groupwork can be particularly fruitful in such cases as feedback is provided by other patients as well as the therapist. Also having a therapist who is deaf or a deaf co-therapist is invaluable as a means of ensuring that skills taught are appropriate to Deaf culture. Examples of areas covered by such groups might be: anger control, sex education, assertiveness training. More specific examples of what might be covered are how to ask someone out; how to ask for help when you are upset/angry; recognizing emotions in others; 'listening' skills; taking turns in a conversation; being served in a shop; and so forth.

To illustrate how this structured approach might be undertaken, an outline for anger control is given below:

- **Week 1 — Assessment**
  What makes you angry? — list what you do when you are angry
  Homework: diary of aggressive behaviour

- **Week 2 — Consequence/risks**
  Recap on week 1
  Discussion of angry feelings as 'normal'
  Discussion of risks of behaving aggressively, i.e. consequences
  Homework: diary

- **Week 3 — Recognizing anger**
  Recap on previous weeks

  (a) discussion of bodily symptoms of arousal — learn relaxation
  (b) triggers: identify individual 'trigger' situations to increase awareness of risky situations (e.g. alcohol, certain people, anxiety-provoking situations)

  Homework:
  (i) diary of aggressive behaviour and angry feelings
  (ii) practise relaxation

- **Weeks 4–6 — Alternatives to aggressive behaviour**
  Recap on previous weeks

  (a) video teaching: video of Deaf people arguing and behaving in different ways. Patients comment on likely consequences of each/what happens next and decide which is preferable and why.
  (b) Role play: enacting situations from patients' diaries and practising new skills, e.g. walking away, talking it through, punching a cushion!

  Homework:
  (i) diary
  (ii) relaxation
  (iii) using new techniques as discussed during sessions

- **Week 7 — Review**
  Recap on all sessions
  Discuss particular concerns and worries for the future
  Plan follow-up

The experiences of deaf people growing up in an environment where communication is limited and access to information is generally poor makes them vulnerable to problems in relationships with others. Possible over-protection by parents and therefore limited experiences in adolescence constitute a risk that relationships in adulthood are fraught with difficulties.

This particular area of skills deficit may require marital and sexual therapy or family therapy. Within the framework of CBT, relationships and sexual difficulties lend themselves to a structured, educational approach along the lines discussed for social skills training. Contractual marital therapy involves the identification of difficulties in the therapy sessions by encouraging direct and frank communication and the negotiating of agreements and compromises (contracts) to overcome these difficulties.

Conclusions

The strength of CBT lies in the scientist/practitioner approach. The basis of this model is that therapy is a scientific process in which hypotheses are formed, tested and revised. That CBT is based on empirical research, and is adapted and modified to meet the needs of the individual makes it extremely suitable for use in new areas. Rather than practising therapy under the assumption that what is applicable to hearing people is also suited to deaf people, CBT allows for the possibility of testing that assumption and developing treatment accordingly.

Within the framework of CBT lie a number of therapeutic techniques, many of which are practical in nature. This variety allows therapists to be creative and adapt their techniques according to the needs of the patient. As a result, CBT has a particularly wide application with patients from different cultures or who have difficulty communicating. Indeed, some of the techniques used, such as video teaching/assessment and the use of other visual aids, are particularly culturally appropriate for use with the deaf population.

Any therapy which claims to be useful to deaf people must not only be applicable to the variety of psychological difficulties found in hearing people but must also address issues peculiar to the deaf population. Techniques devised under the umbrella term 'behaviour therapy' are particularly valuable when treating skills deficits discussed earlier. Cognitive therapy can be a useful adjunct to these techniques addressing some of the beliefs and assumptions underlying anxieties about engaging in new ways of behaving. Some of these cognitions may reflect the position of the deaf person in a hearing society, beliefs about hearing people, or what hearing people think about deaf people. With regard to the latter, a commonly held belief is that 'hearing people think Deaf people are stupid'. Of course, there is evidence in history and probably in the deaf person's experience to support this belief. However, to say that all hearing people believe this is clearly not the case, and more importantly the holding of this belief can affect the deaf person's ability to function from day to day. In challenging such thoughts and beliefs, it is a matter of weakening the strength of the thought by questioning it gently, rather than denying the person's experience of ignorance and prejudice on the part of hearing people.

Using cognitive therapy to address thoughts and beliefs about deafness and hearing is important when working with deaf people with low self-esteem. Most patients referred to mental health services fall into this category, and feelings of worthlessness often relate to difficulties in accepting deafness or resolving issues of identity in relation to deafness. Some patients are desperately trying to be 'as hearing as possible'; others are comfortable only with deaf people and antagonistic to the hearing world. Most, of course, are in between. Research has shown that the most psychologically healthy position is to be able to relate to both deaf and hearing people and to have a 'dual identity' (Weinberg and Sterritt, 1986; Cole and Edelmann, 1991). Underlying difficulties are often thoughts, beliefs and assumptions that are open to discussion and modification. Many of these relate to the relative positions of deaf and hearing people: 'hearing people are more intelligent/attractive/likeable/confident . . . than deaf people', 'hearing people don't have problems/communication problems/mental health problems . . ., don't feel shy/anxious/stupid . . . .' and so forth. Thoughts and assumptions about communication are particularly interesting. All through a deaf person's life the issues of speech, language and communication are at the forefront of people's concern. It is hardly surprising then, that many people develop the belief that all their problems would be solved if they could hear and talk. It often comes as a great surprise to learn that hearing people have difficulty communicating clearly, have frequent misunderstandings and may need professional help to aid communication in relationships. This relates to a further group of cognitions which blame deafness for all one's problems: 'if only I was hearing . . . my marriage would be OK/my parents wouldn't have split up/I wouldn't get in trouble with the police', etc. In research carried out by the author, Deaf adolescents at residential schools were asked to identify whether they experienced common adolescent problems. They were also asked if they thought that hearing adolescents experienced each of the problems as a measure of the extent to which problems were attributed to deafness. In this study 28.5% of problems were attributed to deafness on average, and many inaccurate and negative ideas about deafness were expressed. For example, it was frequently held that while deaf schools were boring, hearing schools were not, and that in hearing schools children worked harder and there was no trouble. In other words, perfectly ordinary complaints about school life were erroneously attributed to deafness (Cole, 1989).

If everyday concerns and complaints are blamed on being Deaf, it is likely that more serious problems are also seen in this light. As well as being at least partially inaccurate and detrimental to self-esteem, inherent in blaming deafness is the notion of being unable to change, or helplessness. One 'solution' to this problem is depression. Another is to try to get rid of the deafness, for example by having a cochlear implant operation. Cochlear implants are very high-cost, high-profile 'miracle' operations. Increasingly, psychologists are being asked to be involved in cochlear implant programmes to assess suitability for treatment. The operation is controversial and viewed with suspicion by many within the Deaf community and by some professionals working with deaf people. A major concern is that deaf people who have difficulty accepting their deafness and who have psychological problems as a result of or in addition to this, may present as candidates for the implant rather than seeking appropriate counselling and therapy. The way in which cochlear implants have been portrayed by the media makes it all the more likely that people coming forward have unrealistic beliefs and expectations concerning the operation and its likely effect on their lives. Assessment of candidates using a cognitive approach can make explicit their thoughts, beliefs and expectations about the implant. This information can then be used to provide a psychological element in preparation for the operation and rehabilitation afterwards. Alternatively, following psychological assessment, other needs may be addressed as an alternative to pursuing cochlear implant.

The use of CBT in working with candidates for cochlear implants is just one example of how this approach is flexible and can be tailored to meet individual needs. When considering different psychological problems and a variety of techniques, three requirements emerge, common to all eventualities. The first is the need to be 'deaf-centred' — this means perhaps abandoning traditional notions of how therapy should be carried out and looking towards the Deaf community and Deaf culture to find what is acceptable and appropriate. It also means considering how Deafness may impinge on a particular psychological problem giving rise to new aspects of a particular disorder.

The second requirement is to be creative. CBT is a broad-based approach and can encompass new and evolving therapeutic techniques, with the proviso that they can be researched within a scientific framework. Again, looking towards a Deaf community for inspiration the therapist can use video, drama, written material, cartoons, drawing, etc. to meet the needs of the patient. Therapies should continue to develop, ideally within the Deaf community, to ensure real access by deaf patients.

Finally, it almost goes without saying that the therapist should be able to communicate fluently in sign language. It has been said that since many patients have poor communication skills in sign language, staff do not have to be highly trained. Far from it — it is precisely these patients that particularly need a therapist with good signing skills in order that they can be creative with language.

All this points to one glaringly obvious conclusion — the need for deaf therapists. At present there are hearing professionals with sign language and a few deaf mental health workers, mostly without professional qualification. The two can work well together, but there is a desperate need for equal access to professional training for deaf people in order that deaf patients receive mental health care on equal terms with their hearing counterparts.

References

Altshuler KZ, Rainer JD, Deming WE (1978) Mental health and the Deaf: a first step toward epidemiology. Mental Health and Deafness 2: 14–24.

Bandura A (1969) Principles of Behaviour Modification. New York: Holt, Rinehart & Winston.

Cole SH (1989) Cultural Identity and Coping in Deafness: A study of Deaf Adolescents' Problems & Self-Perceptions, Unpublished Thesis. University of Guildford.

Cole SH, Edelmann RJ (1991) Identity patterns & self- and teacher-perceptions of problems for deaf adolescents: a research note. Journal of Child Psychology and Psychiatry 32(7), 1159–1169.

Davison GC, Neale SK (eds) (1982) Abnormal Psychology (third edition). New York: John Wiley.

Denmark JC (1972) A psychiatric unit for the Deaf. British Journal of Psychiatry 120: 423–428.

Denmark JC (1985) A study of 250 patients referred to a department of psychiatry for the Deaf. British Journal of Psychiatry 146: 282–286.

Denmark JC, Eldridge RW (1969) Psychiatric services for the Deaf. Lancet 2: 259–262.

Pyke JM, Littman SK (1982) A psychiatric clinic for the Deaf. Canadian Journal of Psychiatry 27: 384–389.

Rainer JD, Altshuler KZ (1966) Comprehensive Mental Health Services for the Deaf. New York: Department of Medical Genetics, New York Stage Psychiatric Institute, Columbia University.

Rainer JD, Altshuler KZ, Kallman FJ (eds) (1963) Family and Mental Health Problems in a Deaf Population. Springfield, IL: Charles C Thomas.

Weinberg N & Sterritt M (1986) Disability and identity: a study of identity patterns in adolescents with hearing impairments. Rehabilitation Psychology 31(2) 95–102.

Chapter 18
Drug Treatments

JEREMY BIRD AND NICK KITSON

Introduction

The treatments in psychiatry with medications known as 'psychotropic' drugs are aimed at changing (tropic) the function of the brain and thereby the mind (psych). Gerber (1983) noted there is 'no evidence that the use of psychotropic medication, ECT, or other somatic therapies differs in indications or method of use between deaf and hearing persons'. We would not quite agree. Generally the indications in Deaf people are the same as for hearing people, but the side effect profile necessitates special care in prescribing for Deaf people. We shall refer exclusively to drug treatments, but it is important these should be kept to a reasonable minimum necessary by other treatment approaches, such as the psychotherapies. This is especially necessary in Deaf patients, many of whom will both be more prone to develop side effects, and also more disturbed by those side effects that affect vision or movement, as these interfere with sign language communication and general awareness. It is unfortunate that both Deaf and hearing programme staff were found to ascribe Deaf patients, versus identically described hearing patients, as more in need of supervision and medication (Dickert, 1988). It is to be hoped this attitude test is not mimicked by practice with deaf patients.

Psychotropic medication may be divided according to several classifications, for example chemical structure, pharmacology, mode of action within the body once a drug has been ingested. For the purpose of this book, it is convenient to classify medication according to its clinical uses, and then consider subgroups of each category (Table 18.1). It is important to realize that treatment of any one clinical disorder may not dovetail neatly with the use of a single category of medication by this classification. Combinations of treatment may be useful, and drugs conventionally within one group may have clinical uses outside it; for example carbamazepine, an anticonvulsant, also has mood-stabilizing and antidepressive properties.

Table 18.1 Classification of psychotropic drugs

Antidepressants
- Monoamine oxidase inhibitors (MAOIs)
- Non-MAOIs: tricyclic, non-tricyclic

Antipsychotics
- Dopamine blockers: phenothiazines, butyrophenones, thioxanthenes
- Atypical antipsychotics

Minor tranquillizers

Mood-stabilizing drugs
- Lithium
- Anticonvulsants: carbamazepine, sodium valproate

Others
- Beta blockers
- Stimulants

The functioning of the brain is understood through its anatomy, physiology and chemistry. Psychotropic drugs act by promoting or inhibiting natural chemistry and physiology throughout the brain or in specific parts of it. Messages in the brain are transmitted by chemicals, known as neurotransmitters, crossing between the end of one nerve and the start of another, a junction called a *synapse*. A nerve's receiving junction is not unlike staff letterboxes or 'pigeon holes'. What is put in may inhibit or encourage staff action. The outcome will depend on the type of message, from where and to whom. Drugs act to reduce or increase the general flow, to enable or disable the messages (neurotransmitters) at specific or groups of sites or to increase the sensitivity or reduce the sensitivity of the receiver or receivers. The brain thus consists of a very complicated and sophisticated network system. As a result even those drugs with relatively specific actions at specific sites may have complicated ramifications which lead to wanted or unwanted side effects. Unfortunately these can be common effects of psychotropic medication.

Antidepressant medication

The most well-established antidepressant medications are amitriptyline and imipramine. First used in 1951, they are still used widely in clinical practice today. They are members of the tricyclic group of antidepressants whose name derives from a triple ring in their molecular structure. As a general rule antidepressants act mainly upon two neurotransmitter systems within the brain, noradrenaline and serotonin. The tricyclic group of drugs acts upon a variety of other neurotransmitter systems, leading to side effects which can be convenient (e.g. sedation in agitation) or unwanted. Tricyclic antidepressant medication increases neurotransmitter availability in the brain by inhibiting re-uptake. Similarly, monoamine oxidase inhibitors (MAOIs) increase availability by inhibiting the enzyme systems which break down neurotransmitters.

Antidepressant drugs which act in a more specific way, either with respect to a very specific neurotransmitter, or to a particular site within the brain, have been developed more recently. Specific serotonin re-uptake inhibitors (SSRIs) which are now a widely used class of antidepressant, have fewer and more predictable side effects.

At the time of writing there is an intense debate over the overall effectiveness of prescribing any particular type of medication in terms of cost, dropout rate (the number of people who abandon treatment because of side effects) and prophylaxis against relapse of the original depression. These are important discussions as depression is a common clinical condition, with a high morbidity, whose treatment and prevention requires use of medication over extended periods to be properly effective.

An established episode of clinical depression needs to be treated with an appropriate dose of antidepressant medication for an adequate length of time. Although there are clear differences in chemical structure, pharmacology, precise mode of action, and side effect profiles, and individual patient responses to one drug or another, as a general rule each episode of depression will need sustained treatment for between three and six months, and no one medication has been shown to be clearly superior to the original tricyclic group of compounds.

A wide range of antidepressant drugs is now available. In deciding which to use to treat an episode of clinical depression, the psychiatrist will consider, firstly, the patient's pattern of clinical symptoms; whether sleeplessness is a major problem; the level of agitation and anxiety symptoms; whether suicidal ideas are expressed. Secondly, there may be medical problems which make the use of certain medications less desirable, for example whether there are cardiac, renal or urinary problems (more common in those deafened by maternal rubella); whether the patient has epilepsy (more common in all those deafened by traumatic causes); whether they are taking any other medication which might interact with the drugs selected. If they have previously been treated effectively for the same disorder it may make sense to use the same drug. A history of any close relative who has suffered depression of similar pattern may also give helpful information.

Traditional tricyclic antidepressant drugs act variably to influence the effects of the neurotransmitters, noradrenaline and serotonin. Some, for example desipramine, are selective for noradrenaline, others such as clomipramine affect mainly serotonin. Altshuler (1986) reported that psychomotor retardation was rare in Deaf patients, which he attributed to psychological immaturity. He notes depressed children similarly rarely show psychomotor retardation and are more responsive to amitriptyline, which acts more to enhance serotonin. He questioned whether Deaf depressive patients were also differentially responsive to serotonin-enhancing medications. This is worthy of further research, though experience to date with Deaf depressive subjects does not indicate a differential response to the serotonin agonists. Maybe Deaf depressive patients, like other Deaf people, now have the advantage of better upbringing, making them more similar to hearing patients.

It is important to note that although a particular compound may be selective for one or other neurotransmitter, once the drug is metabolized within the body, active metabolites may have a different pattern of activity.

The traditional group of tricyclic antidepressants also influence the neurotransmitters, acetylcholine and histamine, blocking their natural receptors, and causing side effects. Side effects may include sedation, dry mouth, palpitations, difficulty reading small print, gastrointestinal disturbance, sweating, giddiness upon standing, difficulty urinating, and interference with sexual function. Most of these are not specifically difficult for Deaf people, but the blurred vision associated with the anticholinergic side effects of tricyclic antidepressants can very significantly affect communication in more drug-sensitive patients.

The antihistamine side effects may be useful in sedating agitated patients, but sedation might be undesirable in a taxi driver or one who operates complex machinery, and can be particularly troublesome for Deaf patients in a hearing setting where communication requires concentration. People may not spontaneously volunteer all side effects, especially changes in sexual function, which may need specific enquiry.

In a depressed person, unexplained physical changes may increase already high levels of anxiety or despondency and careful explanation may be necessary beforehand and at each clinical evaluation. It is particularly important to provide Deaf patients with clear explanations of possible side effects and opportunities to report them, as they will have had fewer opportunities to learn about the problems and more difficulty communicating in predominantly hearing health settings.

In view of the delayed positive effect and high incidence of negative side effects it is important to make it clear to the patient at the outset that the onset of action of an antidepressant drug may be delayed, and that relatives or carers may notice improvements before the sufferer does. It may be between three and six weeks from beginning the course of medication that its full effectiveness begins to be seen, and treatment may need to be continued for 6–12 months before an episode of depression is fully treated.

The side effect profile of these drugs is clearly important as it influences people's initial willingness to persist with the treatment, and in some individuals, who may need prophylactic treatment for repeated episodes of depression, it is important that the medication is tolerable in the long term. To this end, some effort has been made to develop antidepressants with fewer side effects, which usually implies less activity on such a wide range of neurotransmitters and more specificity, for example serotonin alone. These drugs are often considerably more expensive but may be much more effective overall if people are willing to continue taking them over long periods. These are less sedative than the standard tricyclics and safer in overdose. As this group also have fewer anticholinergic effects they are safer in those with existing cardiac problems and generally better tolerated by deaf people. Nearly all antidepressants lower the seizure threshold in people with epilepsy, with the possible exception of viloxazine. Again, deaf people are at greater risk.

Monoamine oxidase inhibitors

This group of drugs inhibits the enzyme, monoamine oxidase, to increase available noradrenaline and serotonin at brain synapses, but they also inhibit the same process in the gut and blood. As a result of this action, naturally occurring amines present in food, which would normally be destroyed in the gut and liver, may enter the bloodstream and cause symptoms such as flushing, headache and a potentially dangerous rise in blood pressure. To avoid this hazard, patients are carefully advised to avoid a list of foodstuffs containing monoamines, such as mature cheese, game, pickled herrings, yeast extracts, beer, Chianti wine and broad bean pods, any of which may trigger this so-called 'cheese' reaction. In addition, over-the-counter (OTC) cold remedies and other medicines may contain hazardous ingredients. Deaf people with poor reading skills will have difficulty reading the detail of the food labels or seeking the pharmacist's advice on medicines, so extra caution is indicated.

MAOI side effects include low blood pressure, difficulty passing urine, interference with sexual function and sometimes insomnia, though blurred vision and aggravation of glaucoma are less common. In theory the MAOIs might be less of a nuisance to Deaf people than the tricyclics, as clear vision is so valuable. In practice this is outweighed by the risks of the cheese reaction and the differing indications.

Although this group of drugs may be used in the treatment of major depression, they are usually identified as being more useful in depression where strong features of anxiety, hypochondriasis or phobic anxiety are predominant. They may also be useful in major depression where other groups of antidepressants have proved disappointing. Finally, they may be used in combination with tricyclic antidepressants in treatment-resistant depression.

A more recent reversible MAOI, moclobemide, is indicated for major depression. It does not seem so prone to cause troublesome interactions with diet and may prove to be particularly useful in those with a risk of glaucoma.

Antipsychotic medication

Antipsychotic medication consists of several related groups of compounds also known as neuroleptic or major tranquillizing medication. The usual clinical indications for their use are major psychiatric illness, especially the psychoses such as the florid delusions and hallucinations of schizophrenia or calming the agitated phases of bipolar affective disorder. They may also be used for treating behavioural disturbance or aggression, especially in those with organic brain damage, though the risk of lowering the seizure threshold needs to be taken into account. In lower doses they may be anxiolytic or antidepressive.

There may be a very wide dose range which is potentially useful, haloperidol being useful in doses ranging from 1.5 mg daily to up to 80 mg daily in different disorders. Often, low-dose antipsychotic medication may be useful in conditions where higher doses would be sedative or side effects outweigh any clinical benefit. It is important, therefore, to be clear about the intended purpose of antipsychotic prescription, to assess clinical effects, and use incremental regimes to minimize side effects whenever possible.

In the same way as antidepressants, classical antipsychotic medication may be subdivided according to chemical structure, or clinical usage. Original antipsychotic medications such as chlorpromazine (commonly known as Largactil) also act upon a variety of neurotransmitter systems, including dopamine, serotonin, adrenergic receptors, histamine and acetylcholine. The common property of the original antipsychotic agents was their blockade of dopamine receptors, which broadly correlated with their clinical potency.

Blockade of dopamine receptors may lead to the emergence of a number of movement disorders, both short and long term. In order to achieve maximum efficacy whilst minimizing unpleasant or persistent movement disorders, more recent antipsychotic drugs have been derived which are highly selective for particular dopamine receptor subtypes or, in the case of newer drugs such as the 'atypical antipsychotics' (or substituted benzamides), appear to achieve antipsychotic potency by affecting a number of neurotransmitters without high potency dopamine blockade.

Classical antipsychotic drugs fall broadly into three groups:

- **Phenothiazines**, such as chlorpromazine, as a group affect many of the neurotransmitters described above. The main complaints from Deaf users are poor concentration, sedation and blurred vision. It is important to note that visual impairment due to pigmental retinopathy is a rare side effect of the phenothiazines, especially thioridazine, when prescribed at high doses for a prolonged period.
- **Butyrophenones**, such as haloperidol, have more specific and potent dopamine blockade, but result in more movement disorder, which can affect signing fluency.

- **Thioxanthenes**, such as flupenthixol, have moderate levels of dopamine blockade.

Selection of antipsychotic agents takes into account the same broad general principles described under antidepressant therapy above. It may be necessary to continue antipsychotic medication for many years to prevent relapse of schizophrenic illness or to stabilize mood in treatment-resistant affective psychoses. It is important to choose medication with a tolerable side effect profile which also relieves illness symptoms. To ensure compliance in people who are chaotic or have little insight into their disorder, depot preparations of several antipsychotics are available in injectable form which ensures a reservoir of drug is always available in the body from a once-weekly or less frequent injection.

Motor side effects

It is important that motor syndromes are recognized and treated appropriately, as they are unpleasant, interfere with the fine movements and subtleties of sign language and may be mistaken for further symptoms of the psychotic illness. They broadly fall into early syndromes of acute onset and late or chronic side effects.

The early movement disorders include Parkinsonism, acute dyskinesias or dystonias and akathisia. The first line treatment of early movement disorders is to reduce the antipsychotic dose or potency to the minimum possible. They all respond to the administration of anticholinergic medication, though it is less effective in akathisia.

Akathisia is an acute motor restlessness, which is distressing and may be identified by an inability to sit and repeated tramping movements of the feet or limb crossing. It may be mistaken for agitation. It also responds to benzodiazepine or beta-blocking drugs.

Acute dystonias or dyskinesias are abnormalities in muscle tone or pattern of movements of a wide variety of muscle groups, particularly in the face and limbs. These disorders are more likely in patients with organic brain damage (including those 30% or so Deaf people with a traumatic cause of deafness), more severe forms of schizophrenia or those already disposed to similar movement disorders (for example hereditary dystonias) which may be released or triggered by first administration of these agents. They also respond to benzodiazepine medication.

Parkinsonism arising from antipsychotic medication is characterized by similar symptoms to those seen in Parkinson's disease: altered gait, reduced facial mobility, increased muscle tone, characteristic tremor, decreased arm swing and altered posture. The facial immobility and slow movement may be mistaken for the unusual emotional responses or psychomotor retardation which can also be characteristics of the disorders treated by the drug. This is particularly so in Deaf people for whom facial expression is an important grammatical part of sign language.

Long-term movement disorders include the tardive syndromes: tardive dyskinesia, tardive dystonia and tardive akathisia. These consist of characteristic patterns of muscle tone or movements affecting predominantly the face, limbs or trunk. A wide variety of dyskinetic patterns occur, the signs of which may vary from subtle to gross. It is important to balance the long-term risk of chronic movement disorders against the suppression of disabling symptoms of mental illness. Again, these long-term movement disorders appear more likely in individuals with pre-existing organic brain damage or the more severe forms of schizophrenia. A good deal of research interest is presently focused on evolving novel antipsychotic agents that will not trigger or exacerbate these symptoms.

It is therefore important to monitor carefully those taking long-term antipsychotic medication, and to use minimum doses consistent with good control of clinical symptoms of the illness itself. Breakthrough of the original clinical symptoms may come in the form of non-specific symptoms of anxiety or mood disorder rather than psychotic experiences in the first instance. In those subjects on depot medication, minimum doses can often be used if a supply of 'rescue medication' in oral form is given to settle such breakthroughs, enabling lower doses of depot medication to be used in compliant patients.

The use of low-dose antipsychotic medication in the treatment of behavioural disturbances, anxiety, tic disorders or autism carries a lower risk of motor side effects. There is also a lesser likelihood of longstanding tardive dyskinesia at these doses.

Other side effects which occur may include photosensitive dermatitis and effects upon the bone marrow, which produces red and white blood cells. The latter is particularly important with the drug clozapine. Clozapine is a very useful antipsychotic, which does not appear to act by potent dopamine blockade and avoids movement disorders described above. It is also effective in treating the negative symptoms of schizophrenia, such as apathy, amotivation and inertia, in addition to the positive symptoms of delusions, hallucinations and abnormal perceptual experiences. Unfortunately, if not monitored regularly it may allow potentially serious irreversible bone marrow depression to evolve, so at present is available in the UK on condition that regular blood counts are monitored. Other novel antipsychotics such as risperidone show similar promise to clozapine in otherwise treatment-resistant patients, without such undesirable effects.

The neuroleptic malignant syndrome is a medical emergency with a significant death rate. It is characterized by overheating, muscular rigidity, disorders of the autonomic nervous system and changes in mental state. There is a 1% life-time prevalence in those treated with neuroleptics, but it is more frequent and a greater risk in those with pre-existing brain damage. Lazarus (1992) describes the syndrome in a congenitally brain damaged deaf sign language user.

Kitson and Fry (1990) note that schizophrenia is generally less responsive to antipsychotics in deaf patients, often requiring higher doses, or combinations with mood-stabilizing drugs such as carbamazepine. It may be due to coexisting behaviour disorder which they noted often emerged once treatment was successful. Checinski (1991) also noted behaviour disorder as a secondary diagnosis to schizophrenia in Deaf patients.

Mood-stabilizing medication

Mood-stabilizing medication can be very effective in the treatment and prevention of recurrent affective disorders with both depressive and manic phases. Lithium carbonate has been shown substantially to reduce the long-term morbidity of recurrent affective disorders. More recently it has been established that anti-epileptic medications, sodium valproate and carbamazepine, may be used alone or in combination with each other or lithium in certain types of cycling affective disorder.

Lithium carbonate

Lithium is used for the acute treatment of mania and for the prophylaxis of bipolar disorder (manic depression) (Guscott and Taylor, 1994). It may be used to treat recurrent aggressive disorder, especially associated with organic brain damage. Altshuler, Abdullah and Rainer (1977) reported on the successful treatment of a few Deaf patients with impulsive, aggressive behaviour, including those with concurrent schizophrenia. To be effective in manic depressive psychosis the drug must be taken regularly on a long-term basis, including regular blood tests to avoid toxic levels. Unfortunately the difference between a therapeutic blood level and a toxic one is relatively small. Changes in blood levels may be caused by different brands of lithium at the same dose and variations in renal function due to drugs or illness. Caution is particularly necessary in rubella-deafened patients whose renal, cardiac and thyroid function may be affected. Lithium suppresses thyroid function and may contribute to permanent damage. Autoimmune damage to the thyroid is a recognized sequela of both lithium treatment and maternal rubella and it may be that there is even greater risk when both are present.

The mode of action of lithium is thought to be upon central serotonin manufacture. Although it may be effective alone to prevent a cycling mood, it may be more effective in conjunction with a variety of other agents which may help prevent the breakthrough of mania or depression: these may include antiepileptic medication, antipsychotics, antidepressants and thyroxine.

Minor side effects include skin rashes, polyuria, polydipsia, weight gain, gastrointestinal disturbances, unsteadiness, tremor and weakness. The rate of occurrence of these side effects is often related to blood lithium concentrations. More severe central effects, such as drowsiness, confusion and ultimately stupor and seizures, are the result of toxic blood levels and represent an urgent medical emergency in order to effect a reduction in blood lithium level. The patient should be warned about side effects and maintained on the minimal effective levels with an easy dose regime.

Interactions with some other psychotropic medications may increase the likelihood of neurotoxicity, particularly with haloperidol. Such interactions again are more likely to occur in those with pre-existing organic brain damage. It is important to be aware that side effects may occur at lower dosages in patients taking more than one drug.

Benzodiazepines

Benzodiazepine drugs are a group of compounds which would be subsumed within the group of minor tranquillizers. They are used for a variety of purposes:

- Anxiety reduction.
- Anticonvulsants.
- Hypnotics.
- Adjunctive sedation during treatment of major mental illness to avoid excess antipsychotic medication.

There is a wide variety of these compounds, which vary according to their half-life (the time it takes in hours for the body to eliminate enough drug for its concentration to be halved).

Clearly, short-acting compounds with a half-life of four to eight hours are of value as hypnotics to avoid a hangover effect, but they appear to be more addictive. Longer-acting compounds are of value as anticonvulsants or anxiolytics.

These drugs were once widely prescribed as a panacea for stress and anxiety, and were claimed to be much safer than the barbiturate group of compounds they replaced, which had significant addiction potential and were dangerous in overdose. In recent years it has become clear that benzodiazepine dependence can be a major problem in some individuals, beginning to occur relatively early in treatment. It may be difficult to distinguish the symptoms of the benzodiazepine withdrawal syndrome from the symptoms of the original anxiety disorder that the drug was used to treat. Physical symptoms accompanying agitation and even frank psychotic episodes may occur if the dose is withdrawn too quickly. For this reason it is now recommended that the use of this group of drugs should be sparing and on a short-term basis, with the exception of some compounds used as adjunctive third line anticonvulsants.

In elderly, frail or brain-damaged individuals, problems may occur with over-sedation, memory and concentration difficulties and occasionally paradoxical effects such as over-stimulation and increased aggression. The risk of disinhibition and increased impulsivity may be a particular risk to those Deaf patients who historically have been described as impulsive.

More recently, hypnotics and anxiolytics such as zopiclone and buspirone have been available which appear not to have such a high potential for dependence, but are not sufficiently tested in Deaf patients, particularly those with brain damage.

Before treatment, a thorough analysis of the pattern of anxiety symptoms should be undertaken, as they may accompany clinical depression, obsessive compulsive disorder or a major mental illness, in which case the appropriate antidepressant, SSRI or antipsychotic medication would be a more suitable. In the case of individuals unable to tolerate moderate or large doses of antipsychotic medication this group of drugs may be a useful adjunct for sedation and control of aggression. Withdrawal should always be done with caution.

Beta blockers

The beta blockers are drugs which block a specific (beta) subtype of adrenergic receptor. They are a useful group of drugs in the treatment of anxiety, particularly where the physical symptoms of anxiety predominate, such as rapid heart rate, over-breathing, sweating, tremor and flushing. The blockade of these symptoms in the body may reduce subjective anxiety. They are particularly useful against performance anxiety in exams or major presentations.

In addition to this central use they may be valuable in treating the movement disorders of antipsychotic medication, particularly akathisia or lithium-induced tremor. They are also useful in individuals with brain damage or autism who seem to be in a state of over-arousal with liability to explosive, intense and sudden outbursts of rage.

Larger doses have been suggested as valuable in the treatment of schizophrenia, but it is unclear whether this potentiates antipsychotic medication or is of direct value in its own right. If added to phenothiazine antipsychotics there can be a marked increase in blood levels of the former.

Before commencing therapy it is important to rule out conditions such as asthma, which would be worsened by the onset of beta blockade. Side effects may include dizziness, depression and sedation, low heart rate and decreased blood pressure, indigestion, constipation and abdominal discomfort and occasional difficulty urinating, and interference with sexual function. It is therefore important to obtain an appropriate medical history before commencing this form of treatment.

Aggression

People with aggressive behaviour may be excluded from opportunities which may lead to an enhancement in the quality of their lives. Medical treatment of aggression can be criticized as a means of control or solely for the ease or protection of staff or others, but aggressive behaviours in patients may put at risk their own safety, safety of others and, more broadly, influence how the wider public respond to them, individually or as a group.

It is tempting to look for a simple explanation for aggressive behaviour, but problems are usually multiply determined. Sovner and Hurley (1991) list ten hypothetical causes of aggression. They were described for a developmentally or learning disabled population and are directly useful for that significant part of the Deaf population with such disorders. Though useful for any population, they are also particularly helpful in those Deaf people with impulsivity. Chapter 3 reviews the relationship between immaturity, traumatic cause of deafness and impulsive behaviour in deaf people. Such impulsive deaf people can be considered to be suffering a developmental delay, and similar considerations may apply to those with permanent developmental disorders.

Sovner and Hurley's (1991) hypotheses are, firstly, that aggression may reflect a physical illness (a 'dangerous' deaf patient transferred from a locked disturbed ward to a signing environment was able to report severe pain from a large peri-anal abscess requiring immediate operation); a medication side effect; or be a seizure-related mood change. Each of these hypotheses requires a medical team reasonably fluent in sign language to consider them and instigate appropriate alternative remedies, medication or anti-epileptic drugs respectively.

Hypotheses linked to psychiatric rather than physical disorders are that aggression reflects irritability secondary to mania, depression or acute or established organic brain damage. Specific paranoid ideas may arise in major mental disorders such as mania, schizophrenia or, in severe personality disorder, leading to opportunistic or planned assaults. Lastly, aggression may be due to rage attacks.

Recognition of the psychiatric, physical, emotional and environmental factors are of great importance before treatment can begin with an appropriate drug, such as lithium or an appropriate antipsychotic drug for mania or schizophrenia, antidepressant medication, or anti-epileptic medication for an organic mental syndrome.

The final group of causes of aggression include an inability to express needs in those with severe communication difficulty, as a result of task-related anxiety, as an escape or avoidance behaviour in the presence of an aversive situation or as a means of obtaining positive reinforcement, such as subjugation of another or the close attention of staff.

It is important that due weight is given to both personal and environmental factors. The former include abilities and disabilities, ability to interpret events around the person, past and recent experiences, personality, psychiatric disorder, physical and emotional state and beliefs. Environmental factors include physical environment (e.g. noise, heat, crowding), social environment and occupation at the time of event.

It is important to consider this diversity of causes of aggression in order to determine accurate and appropriate management. In any group of individuals with frustrated communication and other developmental disabilities, such as autism or organic brain dysfunction, the clear distinctions between classes of medication traditionally used to treat depression, cycling mood disorder and psychosis may need to be revised. A further caution is that psychotropic medication may cause more side effects and sometimes paradoxical aggressive reactions.

States of excitement arising from organic mood disorder may be treated with lithium, sodium valproate or carbamazepine, as may states of persistent irritability which are not themselves part of a major mood disorder. In addition, low-dose antipsychotic medication and SSRI antidepressants may prove useful in irritability. Rage outbursts, which may occur without other major psychopathology, may respond to propranolol.

Conclusion

It is important to realize that physical, psychological and emotional factors may be more difficult to detect in people with developmental difficulties, including autism. If there is any doubt about these diagnoses, referral to a specialist service which can carry out an appropriate multidisciplinary assessment is advisable. Such a service will be familiar with the impact of focal and global cognitive impairments, and how these may influence personal and environmental factors.

We have emphasized the side effects of the commonly used drugs in psychiatry as these lead to the principal differences in prescribing for deaf patients. We want to emphasize that these drugs, despite their side effects can be very effective in reducing the severe distress of the major mental illnesses and disorders, as well as being life-saving for some.

References

Altshuler KZ (1986) Perceptual handicap and mental illness, with special reference to early profound Deafness. American Journal of Social Psychiatry 6: 125–128.

Altshuler KZ, Abdullah S, Rainer JD (1977) Lithium and aggressive behaviour in patients with early total Deafness. Diseases of the Nervous System 38: 521–524.

Checinski K (1991) Preliminary findings of the study of the prevalence of psychiatric disorder in prelingually Deaf adults living in the community. Proceedings, Mental Health and Deafness Conference. London: St George's Hospital Medical School.

Dickert J (1988) Examination of bias in mental health evaluation of deaf patients. National Association of Social Workers, pp 273–274.

Gerber BM (1983) A communication minority: Deaf people and mental health care. American Journal of Social Psychiatry 3: 50–57.

Guscott R, Taylor L (1994) Lithium prophylaxis in recurrent affective illness: efficacy, effectiveness and efficiency. British Journal of Psychiatry 164: 741–746.
Kitson N, Fry R (1990) Prelingual deafness and psychiatry. British Journal of Hospital Medicine 244: 353–356.
Lazarus A (1992) Neuroleptic malignant syndrome and pre-existing brain damage. Journal of Neuropsychiatry l4: 185–187.
Sovner R, Hurley AD (1991) The functional significance of problem behaviour: a key to effective treatment. Habilitative Mental Healthcare Newsletter 10: 10.

Suggested further reading

Cookson J, Cranmer J, Heine B (1993) The Use of Drugs in Psychiatry (fourth edition). London: Gaskell.
Kendall RE, Zealley AK (eds) (1993) Companion to Psychiatric Studies (fifth edition). Edinburgh: Churchill Livingstone.
Trimble MR (1988) Biological Psychiatry. Chichester: John Wiley, pp. 350–400.

Chapter 19 Rehabilitation

NICK KITSON AND SARAH WILSON

> Recovery from mental illness means becoming able to fulfil tasks which contribute towards your own well-being or the well-being of others. It means being able to manage your own life and have some practicable vision of your future towards which you can plan and take action. It means sufficient supports, rewards and consolations in your everyday life to endure commonplace adversity or misfortune. It means assuming social roles and a way of life which define you in your own eyes and those of others as a 'well' person. (Patmore, 1987)

What is rehabilitation?

The word 'rehabilitation' means to reskill. The word as used in the mental health setting refers to all the skills of daily living required to function successfully in human society. A number of Deaf people who present to mental health services have never attained sufficient living skills and the slogan 'habilitation not rehabilitation' has been used. Their lack of living skills can be due to impoverished life experience, which is a failing of society, or learning disabilities, which are secondary to the cause of deafness. Throughout this chapter we use the term rehabilitation as inclusive of habilitation.

The World Health Organization describes rehabilitation as 'all means aimed at reducing the impact of disabling and handicapping conditions in individuals and enabling them to achieve maximum integration into the community'. It categorizes impairment, disability and handicap (WHO, 1980). *Impairment* is defined as the physical problem of function or structure. *Disability* is that daily living function that cannot be performed (unaided) as a result of impairment. *Handicap* is the problem caused by the person's or society's response to the impairment and/or disability. The British Royal College of Psychiatrists (RCPsych, 1980) states that rehabilitation services need to concentrate on psychiatric impairment and dysfunction, social disadvantages and personal reactions to impairment and/or disadvantage. Wing and Morris (1981) describe how these three can be causes of 'social disablement' and define this as 'the state of an individual who is unable to perform socially up to the standards expected by himself, by people important to him or her or by society in general'. They define rehabilitation as:

> the process of identifying and preventing or minimising these causes (of social disablement) while at the same time helping the individual to develop and use his or her talents and thus to acquire confidence and self esteem through success in social roles.

Although detailed labelling is important for clear thinking and communication about problems in daily human functions, the labels themselves can add to the 'handicap' (as defined by WHO, 1980). Our aim should be to enable patients to successfully gain what they need and to express themselves in their world as fully as possible, becoming independent and responsible, but able to be appropriately dependent on others for help and love (Kitson, 1992). Rather than focus on symptoms, deficits and deviances, we should build on strengths, talents and skills (Cook, Graham and Razzano, 1993).

Needs

Rehabilitation is artificially separated from the specific treatments, such as psychotherapy for neuroses or drugs for schizophrenia, as it is severely restricted without them. Similarly, specific treatment of the disorder is of little point in most patients without rehabilitation. If mental health problems are not affecting the living functions then it is dubious whether to treat, particularly as most treatments have negative side effects.

Mental illness

Mental illnesses commonly cause a deterioration from previous function. Schizophrenia is particularly associated with withdrawal from human society and loss of intrinsic motivation. Some patients present with this change in personality as the first indication of illness, though more commonly it is a slow relentless decline following episodes of more florid illness. It seems that the decline is a primary function of the illness and is associated with changes in brain structure. Kraepelin's early name for schizophrenia, dementia praecox, is particularly apt for such patients. The decline is difficult to predict, but occurs in about one-third of patients. Another third will have significant impairments in function following schizophrenia. Generally a slow insidious onset with predominantly negative symptoms has a poorer prognosis for daily living functions. Acute onset of florid symptoms, such as delusions and hallucinations, that readily respond to medication have the best prognosis. Cook, Graham and

Razzano (1993) found, contrary to expectation, that the diagnosis of schizophrenia in Deaf patients treated in a model Deaf-centred psychosocial rehabilitation programme, did not correlate with a poor rehabilitation outcome. Unfortunately, whether the schizophrenic illness was florid or of a slow insidious onset was not clear.

Medication

Most medications for mental illnesses have a sedative effect. The treatment of acute mania is essentially the same as that of schizophrenia, the drugs being classed as major tranquillizers. In addition to sedation these drugs can cause visually obvious movement disorders and an inner restlessness, akathisia. Specific drugs for manic depression aimed at stabilizing mood swings can cause an emotional flatness. These drug side effects will have a significant effect on rehabilitation prospects and will tend to be more pronounced in those whose deafness is not hereditary (see Chapter 18).

Dependence

In any mental illness or disorder that has required a period of increased dependence on others, there is a risk of the attractions of dependence and riddance of the stress of personal responsibility. Mania, for example, may give the patient experience of outrageous irresponsibility, that may provide the patient with immediate personal gains in the mental hospital or care culture, but to the detriment of the person in the outside world. Effective taboos may be broken and be difficult to re-establish. The effects of mental illnesses or the drugs to counteract them can lead to behaviours that, while necessary for recovery, become habits. Institutionalization, a product of the old asylum approach to mental illness, is hopefully being prevented by the community approach to psychiatry.

Rehabilitation in practice

The planned 'teaching' or practice sessions of a rehabilitation programme, whilst important, play a relatively small role in the success or otherwise of an individual's progress. More importantly, the attitudes of those around the patient, those of the peer group and staff, the day-to-day interactions that reinforce a move towards responsibility and independence, will be crucial. For this reason there can be no individual profession or group solely responsible for rehabilitation. Rather, the whole team needs to be involved in regular planning and liaison. Traditionally in the UK, nurses, occupational therapists and social workers have been those most involved with patients on a day-to-day basis.

A few examples of the type of issues involved in rehabilitation are:

- Self-care — personal hygiene.
- Domestic — from snack and beverage preparation to weekly menu

planning and cooking skills, safety in the home, simple house maintenance (changing light bulbs, etc.), laundry and cleaning, budgeting.
- Community — use of public transport, banks, post offices, road safety, use of public amenities such as libraries and sports facilities.
- Social skills — assertiveness skills, making friends, dealing with conflict, relationships and sex education.
- Task and work performance skills — concentration, motivation, decision-making, sequencing activity, planning, specific employment training.
- Environment — adaptations in the home, adaptions at work, involvement of benefits and work support agencies.

Specific adaptation to the environment will be needed for Deaf people. Many will also need Deaf awareness training, introductions to the Deaf community and intensive teaching of skills that were not learned prior to an episode of illness. Otherwise the mental health rehabilitation programme for a Deaf person is essentially similar to that for hearing people.

Group work is traditionally used particularly by mental health rehabilitation workers — in the UK 'occupational therapists'. Groups are essential for some aspects of a programme, e.g. social and recreational skills. However, for practical issues such as domestic and community skills it is generally necessary to work individually with a Deaf client. Mental health services for Deaf people cater for a particularly wide range of needs. This is accompanied by a variety of communication skills and cognitive or developmental levels. Forming groups that share similar goals and communication modes can be extremely difficult.

Apart from the obvious need for fluent signing staff, the use of visually presented material is often vital. Breaking material into simple steps, the use of diagrams, 'stick people', role-play demonstration, mime and video can all be useful, particularly for those patients with delayed language skills.

Careful grading of programmes is always important but for many Deaf patients with fragile self-esteem this is essential to enable success experiences and encourage motivation.

During the initial stages it frequently becomes necessary for negotiation between staff and clients to agree the immediate goals of treatment.

In order for patients to move out of hospital into a more independent setting there are some issues that must be covered, such as safety in the home and on the roads, basic self-maintenance and self-care skills.

Time often has to be spent working with clients in order to agree these goals. Many have unrealistic initial aims either as a result of mental illness (delusions, for example, that distort their understanding of the world) or due to a naïvety about the world leading to expectations of a high status job purely on the basis of fairness, despite experiences that the world is not a fair place. Negotiation is often necessary to try to assist patients to become involved with those goals considered immediately necessary by professionals and others, whilst enabling individuals to have control over their own lives and take responsibility for themselves. We have referred to *needs* not *wants* throughout this chapter quite deliberately. Unfortunately, what some patients want in immediate terms has, when pursued directly, led repeatedly to consequences not wanted by them. Reminding patients of past experiences or allowing them to repeat their behaviours whilst subject to staff observation and clarification can be effective.

Those involved in this negotiation need to consider some basic theories of motivation. Maslow (1968, in Creek, 1990) reminds us that it is pointless to address issues of esteem or of relationships if basic physiological and safety needs are not met:

- Self-actualization and realizing one's full potential.
- Cognitive and aesthetic needs.
- Exploring and appreciating the physical and social environment.
- Need for esteem.
- Love and belonging.
- Safety.
- Physiological.

Maslow's model allows for a hierarchy of needs which can be considered in order starting with basic physiological ones. An example that includes the full hierarchy is sexual needs — an area neglected in the past. The relatively high incidence of sex offenders amongst Deaf mental health service users (Hamblin and Kitson 1992), the inappropriate sexual experience (see Chapter 7) and the lack of sexual education (Tripp and Kahn 1986) amongst Deaf people indicate an increased need for social and sexual education and skills training.

Dependence and Deafness

The history of the Deaf adult with mental health problems has to be considered when planning a rehabilitation programme. The experience of being a Deaf child, adolescent and adult can have a profound effect on any mental health rehabilitation aims. There are three main reasons for this:

- Education.
- Risk-taking and dependency issues.
- Motivation.

Education

Many Deaf people have experienced difficulties during their school years. Most (but not all) Deaf people who are denied access to fluent signed communication during school years will be delayed in social, emotional, linguistic, educational, domestic and occupational skills development despite their innate ability. If prior to an episode of mental illness there is already an issue of delay in acquiring social, domestic or occupational skills, these obviously have to be addressed during rehabilitation.

Risk-taking and dependency issues

Opportunities for risk-taking and experiment can be limited if figures of authority are concerned about lack of skills or have lowered expectations of a Deaf person. Many Deaf psychiatric patients have experienced long histories of institutionalization in residential care or schools, or of over-protection by carers or families. These can seriously affect the level of skills in independent living an adult may have prior to an episode of illness.

Motivation

The co-operation and motivation of the patient to progress to a more independent situation is always crucial to the success or otherwise of a rehabilitation programme. Intrinsic motivation is the urge to use one's capacity to have an effect on the environment independently of any external reward. Everyone is born with this urge, but experiences throughout life affect how it develops and is used. The pleasure in being able to act competently can be strong enough to motivate activity even when the action itself causes pain, e.g. a marathon runner. Intrinsic motivation prompts people to try out and master new skills throughout their lives.

When a child tries out an activity and receives positive feedback, self-respect is enhanced and a self-image as a competent performer begins to build up. The child will try again. Frequent experience of failure, unsatisfactory outcomes or prevention of risk-taking will reduce the urge to try out activity, along with a reduced self-image and learned helplessness.

The communication barriers with the hearing world can be perceived as difficulties negatively affecting success in establishing social contacts; asking for needs to be met and joining social activities can be challenges to be mastered. Many Deaf psychiatric patients have a low sense of self-esteem and efficacy and hence a hesitancy to involve themselves in activity or risk-taking.

Deafness and mental health rehabilitation

We are not considering Deafness as an impairment, disability or handicap. It could be argued that those who see it as such, including some Deaf people themselves, are promoting mental health problems, the opposite of the aim of rehabilitation. The story of Martha's Vineyard (Groce, 1985), where at one time a significant proportion of the population was Deaf, demonstrates that Deafness need not lead to any dysfunction, just differences. If everyone was Deaf would the world be disadvantaged or merely different? Clearly, in purely statistical terms Deafness is abnormal, but so are many things that in common parlance are considered normal. The 'medical model' often referred to, but which many medics would not own, considers Deafness an impairment (nerve or ear damage), which causes disability (inability to hear) and may lead to handicap (social disadvantage). Chapter 1 gives an account of how Deaf people view themselves, and are increasingly viewed by others, as an ethnic cultural group.

There is significant evidence that deafness leads to handicaps, but this is by definition a product of society or an individual's response. Deaf people in a Deaf environment can perform all functions of daily living, from the most simple to the most sophisticated. In such environments it is hearing people who are almost universally handicapped. Mental health rehabilitation in a Deaf context has nothing to do with 'treatment' of Deafness, though it may have a lot to do with 'treatment' of attitudes to Deafness. Dickert (1988) examined bias in the mental health evaluation of Deaf patients and found that while Deaf programme staff had a better attitude, both Deaf and hearing programme staff gave Deaf patient case descriptions more need for supervision and medication versus identical hearing descriptions.

Mental health skills need to reflect the patient's problems. The increased prevalence of behaviour and communication disorders (Denmark, 1985) suggests the services of a professional language therapist (unfortunately, in a Deaf context, titled 'speech therapists' in UK) as vital for the detection and remediation of specific language disorders associated with minimal brain damage and language delay. The characteristic psychiatric descriptions of Deaf patients as concrete-thinking, rigid, showing decreased empathy, projecting of responsibility, lacking insight or self-reproach, having unrealistic views of abilities, increased demands, impulsivity and poor control of rage (Altshuler, 1971) need to be taken into account. These descriptions, though an exaggerated caricature of the Deaf mental health rehabilitation patient, are a useful summary of the challenges presented to Deaf psychiatric rehabilitation services. It is common for such behaviours to co-exist with mental illness and emerge once treatment of the mental illness is effective (Kitson and Fry, 1990).

A variety of psychotherapies need to be integrated into rehabilitation work to modify behaviours, reduce fears, question assumptions, challenge defences, encourage expression of emotions and reveal unconscious motives, so the patient can successfully get their needs from society (Kitson, 1992). The recommendations of Hoyd, Siegelman and Schlesinger (1981) for psychotherapy for Deaf people of active, directive, less abstract, educative approaches are refuted in Chapter 15, but are applicable to many Deaf mental health rehabilitation patients, many of whom need basic education. The negative assumptions made by psychiatrists who are not specialists with Deaf patients (Altshuler and Rainer, 1970) need to be guarded against, and the daily living problems of Deaf patients, which are secondary to Deafness rather than mental illness, will have a better prognosis, as will behaviour and personality disorders (Basilier, 1964; Kitson and Fry, 1990).

The most noted difference in Deaf patients has been impulsivity (Altshuler, 1986), yet rehabilitation is disturbing (RCPsych, 1980). Quadenfeld and Farrelly (1983), for provocative therapy, note that interventions are designed initially to provoke the client's maladaptive behaviours, assumptions, and feelings and how important this is for successful work. Kitson (1992) notes that behaviours must be overt for rehabilitation to start. In rehabilitation, maladaptive responses are not directly deliberately provoked, but patients need to be progressively faced with the demands of life outside the protection of hospital or residential care. Any maladaptive responses then need to be worked with. A peaceful mental health rehabilitation setting is likely to be one that is not working. It is not the aim of rehabilitation to protect people from disability or handicap; rather it is to enable them to face their challenge and 'have the experience of success and thus the motivation to aim towards greater things' (Clark, 1984).

The rehabilitation environment for impulsive Deaf people will need to be well contained and able to manage impulsive acts effectively in a way that does not reward and encourage them, nor further lower the patient's self-esteem. Although such behaviour may have to be controlled physically it is important to acknowledge the patient's feelings, affirm him as a valuable person, and work towards more effective ways of expressing his feelings. This is a fundamental role of Deaf ward nurses and community housing staff.

Self-esteem

Self-esteem has been found to appear high in Deaf students (Garrison and Tesch, 1978), but is often fragile except for those integrated into the Deaf world (Meadow, 1975). It seems likely that self-esteem has been held up by low expectation, which will encourage dependency. Rehabilitation sets higher aims and reduces self-esteem. A common hospital story is of young Deaf adult patients avoiding group activities where there might be an element of competition or need to perform. Once encouraged to attend they often explode in rage on some minimal pretext and dramatically distract from their own performance anxiety. It takes a brave patient (and therapist!) to face the real causes of the explosion and work through the problem, but such work with patients in live situations is crucial to them ultimately being able to cope with their impulsivity out of a protected environment.

Disability

The Deaf rehabilitation literature is full of examples of papers on rehabilitation of multiply handicapped or deprived Deaf people. Though not the focus of this chapter, clearly Deaf psychiatric patients also suffer at least the same surfeit of disadvantage as the non-psychiatric Deaf population. Mental health rehabilitation is primarily aimed at the deficits induced by mental illness. In the interests of 'normalization' and 'integration' the disadvantages not part of or secondary to mental illness should ideally be referred to outside Deaf agencies. Unfortunately, some patients are too disturbed to use them and some services are not sufficiently available, so mental health rehabilitation may also have to include the rehabilitation of co-existing problems, for example Deaf blindness or cerebral palsy. To give an indication of the size of the challenge, approximately 25% of the Deaf population has physical disabilities. Hamblin and Kitson (1992) found a 30% prevalence in Deaf patients referred to SWLSG National Deaf Mental Health Service based in London. Ten per cent had significant visual impairment and 10% had more than one additional disability. Many Deaf patients have suffered brain damage and have a range of subtle intellectual disorders in addition to the 10% with clear neurological impairments. Expert neuropsychological assessment may be required to indicate appropriate coping strategies or therapies.

Prevention

Rehabilitation starts with prevention. From first contact with a potential patient, thought must be given to the preservation of skills, effective attitudes, thoughts and emotional responses as an inherent part of treatment for the particular mental health problem. The aim of treatment is not simply to cure or ameliorate the presenting mental disorder. It is for the patient to leave the service as able as possible to gain successfully what they need from their world for as long as possible. Modern nursing, residential care or the work of other carers should address rehabilitation from the start of care.

Service models

Models of service are as important to rehabilitation as the actual direct work with patients. In general this means services as near to home as possible and which promote the continuation of patients' usual domestic social and work life.

For Deaf people this is not so true. Proportionately more Deaf people have missed opportunities to develop their lives and have been overprotected in their families or other carer worlds. As 90% have hearing parents, most of whom do not use sign language, they are cut off from meaningful communication. This may be the cause, an aggravator or independent of their mental health problem. It is not surprising that many

Deaf patients do not see their parents as a major source of support (Pyke and Littman, 1982). Most patients will require at least a period in a Deaf world for their mental health interests.

Some patients will be unable to communicate fluently in any language. Most will have had ample opportunity to learn spoken language, but limited or no opportunity to learn sign language. Sign language needs to be provided in units large enough to allow a signing therapeutic community of patients and staff. Markowitz and Nininger (1984), on the basis of one patient, claim the provision of interpreters limits regression in the inpatient setting, allowing Deaf patients, for whom dependency is a key issue, to make their fullest contact to date with the hearing world. They claim confinement on an inpatient unit for the Deaf would have returned their patient to a potentially regressive environment, and stress the positive outcome achieved by mainstreaming. Gerstein (1988) comments that 'grouping Deaf patients to simplify interpreting needs' is 'an all-too-frequent practice'. His service uses interpreters extensively for a maximum of six Deaf patients at one time and 'hearing patients learned the rudiments of fingerspelling'. It is inconceivable to the authors that this approach is the right one for Deaf people. How do they manage peer group effects? How do those with limited language learn to sign as a natural day-to-day language? How do the Deaf patients accommodate for the lack of interpreters in the external world? It should be noted that the supply of sign language interpreters does not meet the demand, let alone the need, nor is it ever likely to. Many Deaf people enjoy experiencing the hearing world, but this is not their usual choice. At a time when Deaf patients are already suffering and in need of significant help, it seems totally inappropriate for them to have the extra strain of difficult communication and lack of adequate peer support and interaction. On the other hand, the authors are not aware of any mental health treatment setting internationally, where the hearing world is anywhere nearly totally excluded. Deaf people's skills in managing the interface with the hearing wider world are unlikely to be lost. To allow for the variety of patients' communication needs and to maximize their communication potential, it is important that the staff mix allows for fluency in sign language, spoken language and pidgin varieties, although Deaf staff generally provide the best access to communication in an appropriate culture and environment. Staff and patients also need to be aware of communication in different settings and have available expertise in sign and spoken language development and pathology (Thacker, 1990).

Brant (in Gore and Critchfield, 1992), referring to South Carolina, recommends: a statewide continuum of services; that outpatient services be established on a regional basis; that an inpatient unit be established for Deaf persons who use sign language; and that deaf people in need of housing be placed in appropriate supported living situations where sign language is used. For Deaf mentally ill people to live successfully in the community a comprehensive array of services is necessary, not a 'patchwork quilt' (Cook, Graham and Razzano, 1993).

Over ten years ago the two National Health Service (NHS) as well as the principal non-NHS Deaf mental health services in the UK were largely institutional. They focused on hospital admission or a few years' residential 'rehabilitation' in large 30-bedded institutions. Although a few other countries had effective outpatient services, most similarly concentrated on inpatient or residential work. Services and attitudes have changed very significantly over the last ten years, during which the countries with the most developed mental health services for Deaf people, including the UK, are now providing non-institutionalized approaches for the significant majority of patients, including those with serious mental illness.

The ideal model of service will depend on the locality to be served. It will be a compromise between local availability and service size necessary for viability or quality. The forum of psychiatrists for Deaf people in the UK agreed a minimal critical mass of 10 (acute illness or active rehabilitation) beds with 20 community places, and an ideal of about 20 beds with 40 community places, based on services in the large densely populated cities such as London, Birmingham and Manchester. There will be many variables affecting the minimal critical mass required to achieve and maintain a good enough service. In small countries with their own unique sign language, or geographically isolated populations, inevitably qualities such as range and depth of professional expertise will have to be sacrificed. Gerstein's (1988) model may be an appropriate compromise in such circumstances.

The level of need of services will be a crucial factor in deciding the quantity and quality of services needed by a particular region. It seems the statistic of one per 1000 of the general population being born Deaf or Deafened in early childhood holds true internationally, at least in the developed nations. Though less well demonstrated, it seems there is no greater prevalence of the most significant mental illness, schizophrenia, in the Deaf population. The lifetime prevalence of schizophrenia is generally reckoned to be just under 1 per cent. Of the 55 million UK population, a maximum of 300 000 (0.54%) have been diagnosed in their lifetime and around 150 000 (0.27%) remain significantly affected (Office of Health Economics, 1989). Services being equivalent to those of the hearing population, a maximum of 300 (0.54%) of the UK Deaf population would have been diagnosed in their lifetime and 150 (0.27%) remaining significantly affected and in need of ongoing care. The Deaf schizophrenia caseload figure will be nearer 150 than 300. Fifty per cent of SWLSG's National Deaf Mental Health caseload suffers from schizophrenia. When doubled to account for other diagnoses, the national Deaf mental health caseload figure will be between 300 and 600, i.e. between five and ten per million of the general population.

Look at it another way; using the SWLSG National Deaf Service in London as an example, it has well-developed, wide-ranging modern community psychiatric services. It is as accessible as any regional service is likely to be to the population of the two Thames regions (focused on London), as it has taken full advantage of its chance geography. The two Thames regions' population has about 13 000 Deaf people (total population 13 220 000 at one Deaf person in 1000). The two regions accounted for about 75% of the caseload in 1992. The Annual Report 1991/1992 shows a caseload for the adult service of 164, to which the then 17 hospital residents must be added. Extrapolating to a national figure, the national caseload would be 500, or approximately one per 100 000 general population. In the USA it is estimated that there are approximately 3500 Deaf chronically mentally ill persons, i.e. 1.4 per 100 000 (Nickless, 1994).

Returning to the London figures, by similar extrapolation the number of Deaf mental hospital residential places should be about 50 or one per 1 000 000 general population. The number in supported mental health community housing should be about four per 1 000 000 general population. These figures are, of course, extremely crude approximations, based on the operation of one service situated and operating fairly ideally. It appears they hold fairly well internationally, which is not so surprising as both mental health and Deaf statistics also do so. Clearly, less advantaged services, through geography or finances, would have to make modifications. For example, in services providing for less densely populated areas, more residential hospital and community places are likely to be needed due to difficult access. Hopefully these figures will provide a guide to service development elsewhere, once local factors are taken into account.

For hearing patients, rehabilitation started in the 1950s, for Deaf patients it has been much more recent. Studies have shown that there were too many Deaf people in mental hospitals (Denmark, 1966; Cornforth, 1972) and they stayed far too long (Denmark, 1966; Timmermans, 1989). Timmermans (1989) showed, for example, that the Deaf people admitted to mental hospitals up to 1985 stayed an average of 21 years compared to a 1982 figure from the same country's hearing population of only 148 days. The studies have shown that up to ten times as many Deaf people were in mental hospitals than there should have been if they are assumed to have had the same need as hearing people. Deaf people have been in mental handicap services despite normal intelligence (Cornforth and Woods, 1972) and other institutions have an excess of Deaf people (Sainsbury, 1986). The authors are not aware of clear evidence that these figures have been improved upon, as there have been no more recent studies. Anecdotally, the experience of specialist Deaf mental health services is that fewer long-term hospital patients are being referred and it seems that with the greater awareness and better specialist services for Deaf people these figures will have decreased considerably. We do, of course, still receive some patients who have been institutionalized long term. More worryingly, as all large mental hospitals are shrinking or closing, with patients transferred to community housing, we are aware of some deaf patients being more isolated in small houses of hearing patients. Those we see are likely to be only the tip of the iceberg.

We believe the majority of Deaf patients need specialist deaf community housing. Deaf culture is needed for adequate rehabilitation. Kitson (1992) states that for mental health most deaf patients either are, or would be, better off in Deaf communities, primarily as communication fluency in group situations is possible only through sign language. Initially, overt disturbance is to be expected in a communicating environment (Denmark and Warren, 1972) but this should not be a reason to avoid communication for Deaf people. The ideals of most disability politicians — 'normalization' and 'integration' — must usually be within the Deaf community. Normal Deaf people marry Deaf partners (Rainer and Deming, 1963), seek company in Deaf clubs and centres (Phoenix, 1988) and more recently Deaf culture has been widely celebrated (Padden and Humphries, 1988). Staff need knowledge of, and links with, Deaf culture to see behaviour in perspective and to introduce or re-introduce patients to the Deaf community. Deaf mental health rehabilitation workers form the natural bridge.

The South West London and St George's National Deaf Mental Health Services, London: A Model?

Most models of need and care suggest a pyramid (Figure 19.1). The apex represents the most intensive treatment in hospital for the smallest minority with the most disorder — usually schizophrenia — and the base, the majority in the community with minor disorders. The services available to hearing people roughly match the pyramid of need found in community surveys forming an appropriate pyramid of care. Checinski postulated the familiar pyramid of need, but observed psychiatric services for Deaf patients to have a funnel of care (Kitson and Checinski, 1992) (Figure 19.2). The pyramid is distorted with blunting of the apex by all those Deaf people in hospitals and institutions, and the base is narrowed by a lack of services to the less disturbed. To enable Deaf people with mental health problems to live optimally we need to convert the funnel of care for Deaf people to the usual pyramid of mental health care. An upward force needs to help the inpatient — usually with schizophrenia and/or challenging behaviour — out of more restrictive services. A downward force needs to help the silent sufferers with depression and anxiety into services.

Our upward force is provided by a wide range of domestic and occupational services for Deaf people in ten different signing environments for about 70 patients (Figure 19.3). Rehabilitation is an ongoing process that

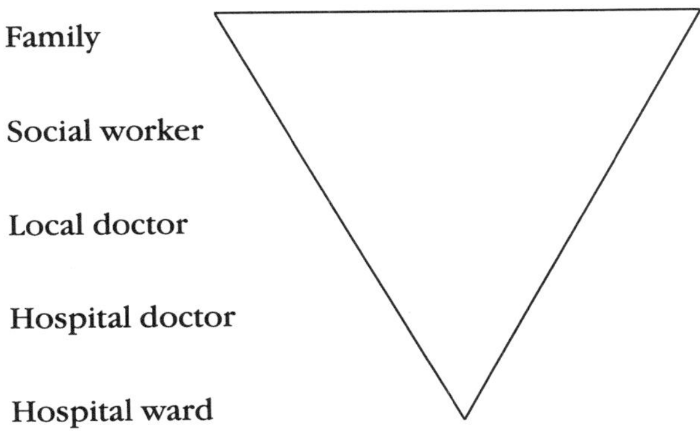

Figure 19.1 The pyramid model of need and care.

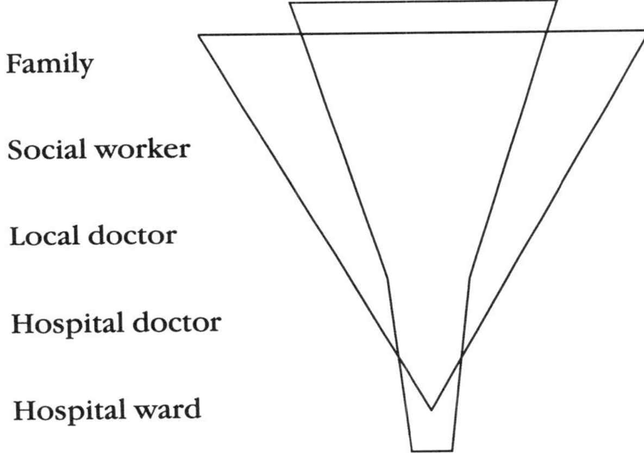

Figure 19.2 The funnel of care.

should continue after discharge from hospital in a series of steps towards independence. SWLSG's National Deaf Services provide a framework in which this can be ensured.

SWLSG's Deaf Services are provided from a converted building in an ordinary south London inner-city residential street. The service offers:

- Eighteen assessment, treatment or rehabilitation 'hospital' beds.
- One bed for emergency admission from linked homes.
- Eighteen 'day hospital' places on the ward.
- Twenty 'Clubhouse' places at a different site.
- Visiting community staff.

Other closely associated agencies provide 45 beds in the community in:

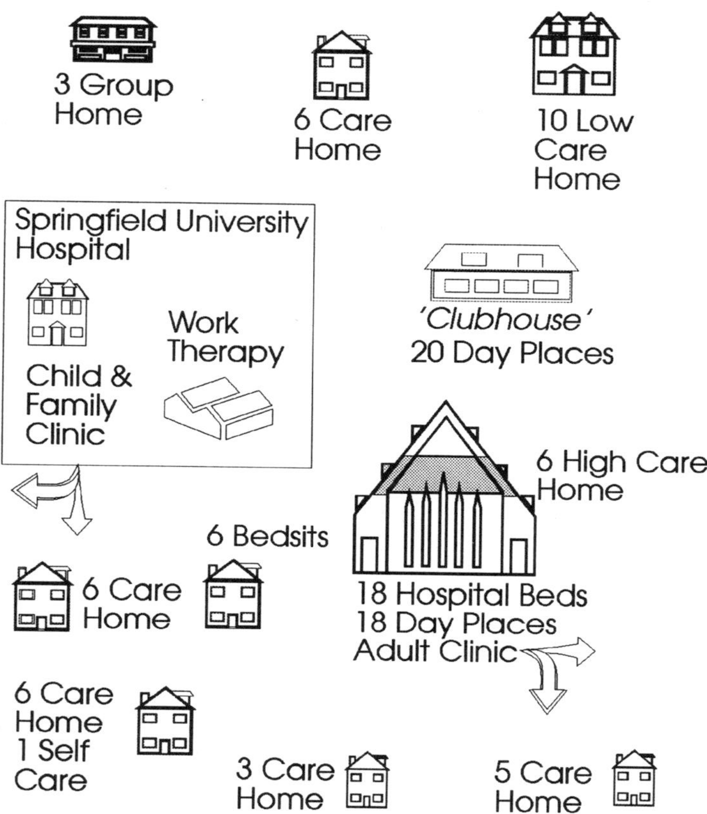

Figure 19.3 The South West London and St George's (formerly Pathfinder) National Deaf Services framework.

- A staffed rehabilitation home.
- Two staffed living skills assessment single bedsits.
- Four staffed long-term homes.
- Two shared houses of long-term bedsits.
- A group home.
- Ordinary flats and bedsits.
- Various supported work schemes.
- Open employment.

Springfield University Hospital, from which the service moved in 1996, continues to provide work schemes on the hospital site and in the community, including a sheltered workshop, work experience and a 'social firm' run as a small business. Further work and rehabilitation to work is being developed through the 'Work Ordered Day' and 'Transitional Employment Programme' of 'Falcon House', the 'Clubhouse' purchased by SWLSG from Sign. The Clubhouse Model (Beard, Propst and Malsmud, 1982) 'is a social invention in community rehabilitation of the severely disabled psychiatric patient'. The model attempts to convey the 'profoundly important' message to members that it is a club belonging to them and that their attendance is expected (anticipated and needed). The programmes are set so the members feel wanted as contributors. There are four fundamental beliefs:

- The potential productivity of the most disabled.
- Work is a deeply generative and integrative force for all human beings (every opportunity is taken to convert every activity into a productive activity for members enabling a 'Work Ordered Day').
- That all human beings require social interchange.
- Human beings require pleasant, affordable residential accommodation which provides supportive companionship.

The programmes include pre-vocational, transitional employment, evening and weekend activities, residences, outreach, thrift shop, house name and newspapers, psychiatric and other medical consultation and evaluation and accountability. The Transitional Employment Programme (TEP) provides a guaranteed opportunity for members to maintain temporary entry-level employment through a series of placements. The TEP placements are in ordinary commercial businesses at ordinary pay and performance expectations, but staff members will have performed the job as an assessment of suitability; individual jobs may be shared by any number of Clubhouse members; and the Clubhouse staff will stand in temporarily where no member can work. The opportunity to fail is also valued as both a normal and learning experience. Social activities are not carried out during working hours, both to promote the 'Work Ordered Day' and to enable members in open employment to benefit from the support of the Clubhouse's social activities. Fountain House, the founding Clubhouse in New York, opened in the mid-1950s. From the start it accepted Deaf patients, but in a predominantly hearing environment, and Deaf people have inevitably not had full access to all programmes all of the time. Falcon House, which opened in London in late 1995, is the first Clubhouse specifically for Deaf people.

In addition to specific treatments, SWLSG National Deaf Mental Health Services tries to modify maladaptive behaviours through a separation anxiety model.

> The base from which an adult operates is likely to be either his family of origin or else a new base which he has created from himself. Anyone who has no such base is rootless and intensely lonely. (Bowlby, 1975)

Through signing clinical staff — approximately 30% of whom are Deaf themselves — we hope the hospital base provides sensitive 'good enough mothering'. Community patients are encouraged to return to the ward to throw a tantrum, seek help or chat. They do all three. The emergency bed is kept for similar reasons. It provides for very short stays, usually a day or two, with rapid return to the greater independence in the community. Deaf mental health patients have been noted to be impulsive, and can be very temporarily beyond their community carers. Paradoxically, as with mothers, providing a readily accessible secure base leads to a reduced need for it.

The London experience clarifies the importance that mental health services for Deaf people are as far as possible placed in large densely populated metropolitan areas (Kitson, 1992). They provide a wide network for healthy Deaf people such as Deaf clubs, centres, college facilities, theatre and meetings. Deaf patients under rehabilitation are able to get out and avoid their staff. There is flexibility with independence, but staff and resources to fall back on. The large Deaf population, and Deaf people's migration towards it, provide a source of Deaf staff. A sufficient range of rehabilitation and resettlement facilities can be absorbed without saturating the normal Deaf or hearing communities. There are ample opportunities for Deaf patients to be trained in the use of public transport, providing progressive access to the service. There is a very wide range of general hearing services. Specifically, metropolitan mental health services tend to be speciality centres for whole regions, allowing availability of specialist resources too rare to be provided viably within Deaf services, yet close enough to be easily supported. Similarly, specialist medical services needed by Deaf patients with associated illnesses or disabilities are more easily available. There are also some disadvantages. Some antisocial and dangerous patients can be given more freedom in isolated institutions away from the public, and a minority of Deaf patients with schizophrenia can do better in a less stimulating environment.

In the community, like the therapeutic community of the hospital ward, the normalizing effect of peer pressure is monitored and at times managed by the staff of the inpatient ward in team work with the staff of the residences. Patients pop into each other's residences for social recreation and help. They are brought closer together by a language not shared by the wider community, and by similar experiences and culture. In spite of greater adversity, our Deaf patients with schizophrenia tend to be more lively and sociable. We are able to function as a therapeutic community in the community, with patients venturing out from the secure ward base, then the care home, then their own homes. For our patients, with all the disabilities and handicaps secondary to mental illness, avoiding further obstacles to communication and a good enough emotional life is all the more important. We do try to enable patients to be involved, as far as they can cope, with the range of Deaf clubs and Deaf activities that London offers.

Some need continuing asylum at some level. Resettlement, the adaptation of the environment to the patient, is a necessary part of rehabilitation, as well as its result or alternative. As far as possible it is provided by resettlement in our or other Deaf communities. Some return to their local region.

Our services provide an example of how the attributes required by Gore and Critchfield (1992) are practically feasible. Although our qualified mental health professionals with fluent sign language are not yet sufficiently available at strategic locations throughout the state and we do not have crisis telephone lines sufficiently accessible, these are a matter of funding. Gore and Critchfield (1992) found regional community mental health counsellors for the Deaf at one per 800 000 of general population in their State inadequate. The UK equivalent would probably be social workers with Deaf people, though they are not specifically providing for mental health. They also estimated the length of time necessary to develop an appropriately trained mental health professional in Deafness as between three and five years. Our experience would support this. Their professional communication and collegiate support systems are necessary for a rural state, where professionals are working at significant distances from one another. If possible, we would recommend such support is based from a central well-established service to promote the highest possible Deaf mental health standards. Even in such established services, the additional areas of expertise required by most members of staff most of the time, together with the problem of relationships between Deaf and hearing staff and the stress of training in Deafness and communication (Denmark and Warren, 1972) and inadequate resources to meet a huge need, require very good staff support systems. Hartman and Kitson (1995) describe a study of staff members' (n = 30) attitude to a staff support group in a Deaf mental health setting. The importance of such support is emphasized by the fact that 81% of staff wanted the group to continue, though most concerns expressed were not Deaf-specific.

Physical environment

The architecture in which Deaf services are provided should clearly optimize the preservation or acquisition of independence. Patients with explosive tendencies, and trapped by limited communication, need airiness, space, freedom to avoid frustration. Medication or tolerance of violence will encourage dependence or encourage learned maladaptive habits. Building and furnishings should be designed to take considerable wear without deterioration. It is important that those with destructive tendencies are not rewarded by visual damage to the property or staff's attention to it. Effective techniques to gain long-term satisfying attention is the aim for patients. Interview rooms need to be sound and vibration proofed. Deaf people are noisier. Some staff and patients have to concentrate on distorted speech. Hearing aids pick up extraneous sounds excessively. In public rooms vibration is an important orientating sense and essential for dancing to music. The environment needs to be light for visual manual communication and easily observable for monitoring, yet this conflicts with confidentiality in sign.

Conclusion

Gerber (1983) summarizes the key issue: many Deaf rehabilitees will have had significant discrimination in the home, education and employment bringing more problems of living to the clinical situation. We hope we have gone some way to answering Gerber's three significant issues to consider in rehabilitation — rehabilitation from what, to what and how. As Gerber (1983) states, all these have differences in Deaf people with mental health needs, the last being dictated largely by the first two.

References

Altshuler K (1971) Studies of the Deaf: relevance to psychiatry theory. American Journal of Psychiatry, 127(11), 1521–1526.

Altshuler KZ (1986) Perceptual handicap and mental illness, with special reference to early profound Deafness. American Journal of Social Psychiatry 6: 125–128.

Altshuler K, Rainer J (1970) Observations on psychiatric services for the Deaf. Mental Hygiene 54: 538.

Basilier T (1964) Surdophrenia: the psychic consequences of congenital or early acquired Deafness. Acta Psychiatrica Scandinavica 40: 362–372.

Beard JH, Propst RN, Malsmud TJ (1982) The Fountain House model. Psychiatric Rehabilitation 5: 1.

Bowlby J (1975) The Making and Breaking of Affectional Bonds. London: Tavistock Publications.

Checinski K (1991) Preliminary findings of the study of the prevalence of psychiatric disorder in prelingually Deaf adults living in the community. Proceedings, Mental Health and Deafness Conference. London: St George's Hospital Medical School.

Clark PH (1984) The development of a psychiatric rehabilitation service. Lancet 2: 625–627.

Cook JA, Graham KK, Razzano L (1993) Psychosocial rehabilitation of Deaf persons with severe mental illness: a multivariate model of residential outcomes. Rehabilitative Psychology 38: 261–274.

Cornforth A (1972) Disturbed and Deaf. Nursing Times 68: 139–141.

Cornforth A, Woods M (1972) Subnormal and deaf. Nursing Times, 68: 177.

Creek J (ed) (1990) Occupational Therapy and Mental Health: Principles and Practice. Edinburgh: Churchill Livingstone.

Denmark J (1966) Mental illness and early profound Deafness. British Journal of Medical Psychology 39: 117–124.

Denmark J (1985) A study of 250 patients referred to a department of psychiatry for the Deaf. British Journal of Psychiatry 146: 282–286.

Denmark J, Warren F (1972) A psychiatric unit for the Deaf. British Journal of Psychiatry 120: 423–428.

Dickert J (1988) Examination of bias in mental health evaluation of Deaf patients. Social Work 33: 273–274.

Garrison W, Tesch S (1978) Self concept and Deafness: a review of research literature. Volta Review 80: 457–466.

Gerber BM (1983) A communication minority: Deaf people and mental health care. American Journal of Social Psychiatry 3: 50–57.

Gerstein AI (1988) A psychiatric program for Deaf patients. The Psychiatric Hospital 19: 125–128.

Gore TA, Critchfield AB (1992) The development of a state-wide mental health system for Deaf and hard of hearing persons. Journal of the American Deafness and Rehabilitation Association 26: 1–8.

Groce NE (1985) Everyone Here Spoke Sign Language — Hereditary Deafness in Martha's Vineyard. Boston, MA: Harvard University Press.

Hamblin L, Kitson N (1992) Springfield supra-regional Deaf unit: a retrospective case note survey. Abstracts, Royal College of Psychiatrists Annual Meeting, p 73.

Hartman D, Kitson N (1995) An examination of a staff group at a supra regional Deaf unit. Psychiatric Bulletin 19: 82–83.

Hoyt M, Siegelman E, Schlesinger H (1981) Special issues regarding psychotherapy with the Deaf. American Journal of Psychiatry 138: 807–811.

Kitson N (1992) Mental health rehabilitation for Deaf people. Proceedings, Second International Congress, European Society of Mental Health and Deafness. La Bastide, Avenue Vauban, 8, b-5000, Namur, Belgium, pp 243–249.

Kitson N, Checinski K (1992) Community care needs of Deaf people. Abstracts, Royal College of Psychiatrist's AGM.

Kitson N, Fry R (1990) Prelingual Deafness and psychiatry. British Journal of Hospital Medicine 44: 353–356.

Markowitz J, Nininger J (1984) A case report of mania and congenital Deafness. American Journal of Psychiatry 141: 894–895.

Meadow K (1975) The development of Deaf children. In: Review of Child Development Research (Volume 5). Chicago and London: University of Chicago Press, pp 441–508.

Nickless C (1994) Program outcome research in residential programs for Deaf mentally ill adults. Journal of the American Deafness and Rehabilitation Association 27: 42–48.

Office of Health Economics (1989) Mental Health in the 1990s: From Custody to Care? Office of Health Economics, 12 Whitehall, London SW1A 2DY.

Padden C, Humphries T (1988) Deaf in America: Voices from culture. Cambridge, MA: Harvard University Press.

Patmore C (1987) Living after Mental Illness — Innovations in Service. Beckenham: Croom Helm.

Phoenix S (1988) An interim report on a pilot survey of Deaf adults in Northern Ireland. The Northern Ireland Workshop with the Deaf.

Pyke JM, Littman SK (1982) A psychiatric clinic for the Deaf. Canadian Journal of Psychiatry 127: 103–108.

Quadenfeld C, Farrelly F (1983) Provocative therapy with the hearing impaired client. Journal of Rehabilitation of the Deaf. 17(2), 1–12.

Rainer J, Deming W (1963) Demographic aspects: number, distribution, marriage and fertility statistics. In Rainer J, Altshuler M, Kallmann F, Deming E (eds) Family and Mental Health Problems in a Deaf Population. Department of Medical Genetics, New York State Psychiatric Institute, Columbia University, pp 13–27.

Royal College of Psychiatrists (1980) Psychiatric Rehabilitation in the 1980s. Report of the working party on rehabilitation of the social and community psychiatry section.

Sainsbury S (1986) Deaf Worlds: A Study of Integration, Segregation and Disability. London: Hutchinson.

Thacker A (1990) Giving Deaf clients more than lip service. Speech Therapy in Practice (Special Supplement) December: x–xii.

Timmerman S (1989) Research Project European Society for Mental Health and Deafness. European Congress on Mental Health and Deafness Proceedings, Utrecht, 87–91.

Tripp AW, Kahn JV (1986) Comparison of the sexual knowledge of hearing impaired and hearing adults. Journal of the Rehabilitation of the Deaf 19: 15–18.

WHO (1980) International Classification of Impairments, Disabilities and Handicaps. A Manual of Classification Relating to the Consequence of Disease. Geneva: World Health Organization.

Wing JK, Morris B (1981) Handbook of Psychiatric Rehabilitation Practice. Oxford: Oxford Medical Publications.

Appendices

Appendix A

Protocol for interviewing Deaf and hard-of-hearing children and adults about abuse (see Chapter 7)

Center for Abused Children with Disabilities, Boys Town National Research Hospital

I. Statement of Purpose

1. Inform the person being interviewed about the investigation process.
2. The deaf or hard-of-hearing person must understand that he or she is not in any trouble. This is a frequent misconception of deaf or hard-of-hearing persons who are interviewed.
3. Explain the purpose of the interview and clarify your role as an impartial investigator whose function is to gather information.
4. To the best of your knowledge, give the person being interviewed honest answers about what is likely to happen as a result of the investigation.
5. Respect the person's privacy in conducting the interview, and arrange for a setting that allows privacy.
6. Inform the person that you will maintain confidentiality and that information given to you will be released only to those persons with the authority to receive it, i.e. law enforcement agencies, prosecutors, etc.
7. Ask the person to maintain confidentiality by not discussing the case with anyone other than the investigators. Emphasize particularly that other members of the Deaf or hard-of-hearing community should not be given information about the contents of the interview.
8. Watch your vocabulary and avoid technical terms the Deaf person may not understand, i.e. alleged, perpetrator, etc.

9. Use simple subject/verb/object sentence construction, rather than complex questions with complex grammatical structures. With deaf and hard-of-hearing persons, Yes-No questions cannot be avoided. Use them after the person has indicated an abusive event to clarify what specifically occurred.
10. Look for consistency in the story and congruence between language statements and non-verbal communication.

II. Establish Communication

1. Ask the individual if they know the interpreter and whether or not they feel comfortable in discussing private information about themselves in the presence of that particular interpreter. Do the same for all interpreters who may become involved in the communicative interaction with the deaf person.
2. Arrange the room to be conducive to the use of an interpreter. Sit directly across from the individual being interviewed. Have the interpreter sit at either your left or right side, whichever is more comfortable for you and the deaf or hard-of-hearing person. Maintain eye contact with the deaf or hard-of-hearing person and attend to the deaf or hard-of-hearing person rather than to the interpreter. Make sure there are no bright lights shining directly in the deaf or hard-of-hearing person's eyes, i.e. have them sit with their back to the window rather than facing it. This will ensure optimal use of the interpreter.
3. Speak in a normal tone. It will not help to make exaggerated lip movements or to talk loudly. The most common mistake hearing people make in interviewing deaf or hard-of-hearing people is that they sometimes talk loudly, and this is no help at all.
4. Indicate a willingness to listen through maintaining eye contact with the person being interviewed, nodding your head, displaying interested facial expressions, and having a normal tone of voice. Avoid interruptions and expect to take a long period of time in interviewing persons with hearing impairments. Repeat key words as necessary and paraphrase what the person has told you in making notes. You can check for your own comprehension of what the person is saying by repeating back your understanding of the person's statement. *Caution: in repeating the statement, be sure that an expanded answer is not suggested.*
5. Use the person's name, and be non-judgmental in your approach.

III. General Questions

1. As a warm-up period to allow the interviewee to become accustomed to using an interpreter, it is good to ask some general questions. This has the added benefit of allowing the interpreter some time to get used to the interviewee's type of sign language and become comfortable in reading their sign language. Ask general questions about the individual's name sign, how he or she got the name sign, their family, and their job, their likes and dislikes.
2. Some general questions about the school with the yearbook can be asked here, 'Where was the dorm, gym, school, etc.', 'Where are the pictures of you in the yearbook?'
3. Some general questions may also be asked about the home situation, including the physical placement of rooms in the home, sleeping, eating and bathing arrangements, and pictures of family members within the home.

IV. Sexual Abuse Interview

1. Begin the interview by telling the individual that you want to gather information about different people (adults and children) in his or her life at home and at the school. Go through each item and ask the individual to provide names for you. Use family pictures or albums to identify family members, including extended family members and live-in companions of either parent. It is also helpful to identify friends who visit the home often and to include the friends of siblings and siblings of peers as well. Use the school yearbook for the person to identify the specific individual named. The name sign for George, Gerry and Gregory will all be the letter 'G'. It will be most important for you and the interviewee to become comfortable in identifying the exact names of individuals mentioned. In many cases, the hearing-impaired person from a residential school only knows the first initial name sign of the individual rather than their full name.
2. Show the individual the 'Who, What, When and Where' paper which identifies both adults and children, witnessing sexual abuse or being the victim of it, and various sites in school and home where it may have occurred:

   'Adults–Kids'
   'Saw–Happened to me'
   'School–Dorm–Bathroom–Shower–Bus'
   'Home–Bedroom–Bathroom–Shower–Basement'

Tell him or her that you are going to ask a series of questions and you want to have them assist you in filling in those columns. It is important to also communicate the following to the child or adult being interviewed to avoid suggestibility issues in questioning (Saywitz, Geiselman and Bornstein, 1992):

A. There may be some questions you do not know the answer to and that is all right. If you do not know the answer, simply tell me that you do not know. Do not guess or make anything up. It is very important that you tell me only what you really remember. Only what really happened.
B. If you do not want to answer a question you don't have to answer it. Tell me you don't want to answer it.
C. If you don't know what something I ask you means, tell me you don't understand. Or tell me 'I don't know what you mean'. Tell me to say or sign it in new words.
D. I may ask you some questions more than one time. Sometimes I forget that I already asked you a question. You do not have to change your answer. Tell me what you remember the best you can.

3. Ask the individual the following list of questions:
A. Was there punishment in your home? What type of punishment? Who administered the punishment? Was there punishment in your school? What type and who administered the punishment?
B. Have you ever been hit, kicked or slapped? By your parents? By fellow student(s)? By a staff member(s) at school? Others?
C. Have you ever been forced to do anything which you felt was not proper or what you wanted? By parents? By fellow student(s)? By staff member(s)? Others?
D. Has a staff member ever touched a private part of your body? (You may need to show the individual the body parts for the male and female and ask them to give you their specific signs for those private parts.) Ask if he/she knows what private parts are and their location. Has any fellow student touched them? Any staff member? Have your parents or siblings touched you?
E. Have you ever been threatened? Form of threat? By whom? Fellow student(s)? Staff member(s)? Parents? Siblings? Others?
F. Have you ever talked to anyone about this problem? If, yes, who? If not, what was the reason for not telling anyone about it?
G. Have you ever seen anyone hit any other child or individual; kick; or touch their private parts? Who? Where? When?
H. If the individual indicates sexual behaviour, have them show you specifically what occurred by using anatomically correct dolls. This is imperative, because Deaf or hard of hearing individuals frequently over- or under-generalize the meaning of a sexual term. For example, rape can mean kiss and touch can mean rape.

4. Ask the following questions:
A. What is your favourite memory of your home, school, or current living situation?
B. What is your worst memory of your home, school, or current living situation?
C. What is your happiest memory of your home, school, or current living situation?
D. What is your saddest memory of your home, school, or current living situation?
E. What is your most fearful memory of your home, school, or current living situation?
F. What is your funniest memory of your home, school, or current living situation?

V. Summary/Confirmation

1. Use this time to summarize what you have understood from what the interviewee has reported to you.
2. It is most helpful to have paper with the following on them:
   A. Adults, Kids
   B. Saw–Happened to me
   C. Home, School, Dorm, Bathroom, Shower, Bus
3. Establish some type of closure with the person interviewed. Thank them for sharing the information with you. Reassure them that it will be shared only with those persons with the authority to receive it. Inform the interviewee that they are in no way to blame for what happened to them. Some persons are not aware that some experiences are abusive. Inform the person that the information given in the interview will help make deaf or hard-of-hearing children safer. If needed, consider making a referral to a mental health agency where the person can receive counselling, if they desire it.

General points about interviewing Deaf or hard-of-hearing children and adults about abuse

1. Your own comfort level in talking with deaf or hard-of-hearing children or adults is critical. If you are uncomfortable with deaf or hard-of-hearing people, you should find someone else to conduct the interview.
2. If the person is hearing-impaired, **ALWAYS** use an interpreter. **NEVER** write notes to communicate or assume the individual can lip-read you adequately to conduct the interview. Hire only certified interpreters. Do not use volunteers or relatives of the person to interpret the interview. Ideally, the person should be allowed to choose interpreter(s) for the interview.

3. Use open-ended questions as much as possible. With the hearing-impaired, it is not always possible to avoid Yes-No questions entirely. Remember, it is important to keep your grammatical structure as simple as possible. This will ensure adequate comprehension on the part of the individual being interviewed. For example, do not ask a question such as 'Now isn't it true that on several occasions you went to the gym and had a good time with Mr Smith?' Several questions are embedded in this. It is better for you to ask several small questions, i.e. 'Did you go to the gym?', 'How often?', 'With Mr Smith?', 'Did you have fun?', 'How?'.
4. It is imperative that you keep your vocabulary as simple as possible. Use simple terms and do not assume the individual understands everything you are asking. Re-ask or rephrase questions as necessary. Ask the question in several different forms, if you feel it is not being understood. **Remember, never suggest the answer.**
5. Don't assume the individual is not comprehending because they do not answer the question the first time it is asked. Wait for the person to complete the answer and then re-ask the question if you do not comprehend the answer. Care must be taken here not to suggest answers and not to give the person the impression that they are giving an incorrect answer. There are no incorrect answers in interviews of this nature.
6. Avoid contaminating questions by implying a desired response, or associating the question with individuals or groups who might have an intimidating effect on the child, i.e. 'Didn't Joe Jones have sex with many of the high school boys?'
7. The pace of the interview will be very different with a hearing-impaired individual. Be comfortable in silence. Learn to be patient and give the individual time to arrive at a response. Be sensitive to the individual's needs for a break due to powerful emotions, exhaustion, limit of attention span, etc. Advise the interviewee at the onset of the interview to take their time in answering questions, because you want them to be sure of their answers. Remove the feeling that if they have to think about the answer, then it must not be true.
8. Questions that probe the memories of feelings and sensations provide important information and may help the individual recall significant details. For example, 'How did that feel?' 'What did you see?' 'What did it look like?' 'What kind of smells do you remember?' 'Did you taste anything?'
9. Give the individual the choice of using tools of symbolic representation to assist in telling their story; for example, anatomically correct dolls or drawings.
10. Questions about sexual abuse may be avoided because of embarrassment. When the individual seems embarrassed or expresses embarrassment, let the person know that you understand that it is

embarrassing to talk about sex because it is a very private subject. Let the individual know that it is part of your job to talk to individuals about problems with touch and sex. Reassure them that you will not get angry or blame them for anything that might have happened. If you yourself are embarrassed talking about sex, get someone else to do the interview.

11. Avoid any comments that would seem to blame or be critical of the individual, either for their behaviour in this situation under investigation or in the interview situation. For example, if you cannot understand what the individual is trying to communicate, avoid implying that the individual is to blame for the lack of understanding. Accept the responsibility for the communication failure and come back to the area of confusion at a later time.
12. Repetitive questioning by the same or different interviewers or investigators may lead to accusations of coaching or rehearsal of the story. However, it may be necessary to conduct several interviews to elicit all the details and to evaluate consistency in the story. The first interview closest in time to whatever incident or incidents that occurred will be given the greatest weight, so concentrate on who, what, where, when, during this interview. Subsequent interviews are for clarification of specific areas only.
13. Don't take statements or comments at face value. Your meaning and the individual's meaning may be very different. It is imperative that you understand specifically what the individual means by terms such as rape, touch, kiss, etc.
14. Look for consistency and congruence between the individual's sign language statements and displays of emotion. Does the individual appear anxious, fearful, ashamed or angry when talking about the abuse?
15. Interview the individual in a neutral setting, away from the site of the alleged abuse. It is imperative that the interviews do not take place at the site where the abuse is suspected of occurring.
16. When investigating sexual abuse, find out what terms the individual uses for body parts and sexual functions, and use those terms. Don't assume that the hearing-impaired individual knows the meaning of sexual terms. If they use the term 'intercourse', ask them to show what that means with the anatomically correct dolls.
17. Make sure the interpreter used feels comfortable in communicating about sexuality and knows the specific signs for sexual behaviour used by the Deaf community. Inform the interpreter not to show disgust or to display emotion when interpreting sexual events. Ask the interpreter to use the same signs that the individual uses. Do not rely on fingerspelling to communicate signs for specific sexual activities. Make sure the interpreter has contacted members of the Deaf community to learn the idiosyncratic school signs for sexual behaviour. If possible learn these signs yourself.

18. If you do not understand the information that is being conveyed to you, be honest and let the Deaf person and the interpreter know. Tell them you do not understand and ask them to show you through either a drawing or with the use of the anatomical dolls what is being communicated.
19. Hearing-impaired people may have difficulties remembering past events and may have confused time concepts. Questions about time can be linked to concrete milestones or events during the years, such as birthdays, Christmas, who was your teacher that year; Whose dorm group were you in, etc.
20. The individual will most likely have both positive and negative feelings about the same perpetrator. It is important to ask them to give you information about both positive and negative experiences with the person.
21. Hearing-impaired adults may feel uncomfortable about revealing abuse by peers with disabilities to others. They may feel they will be labelled by this contact. In some cases, hearing-impaired individuals have been mislabelled regarding their sexual preference by the Deaf community. If the person is obviously uncomfortable, ask if they would prefer to discuss these events with a person of the opposite sex to the perpetrator(s).
22. One study has been conducted on interviewing deaf and hard-of-hearing children (Porter, Yuille and Bent, 1995). This study involved using the Step-Wise Interview (Yuille, 1988) with a small sample (15) of deaf school-aged children attending a mainstreamed programme in British Columbia and included a hearing comparison group. The authors found that the deaf children were not as accurate when provided with very directive questions and concluded that deaf children were more suggestible than hearing children. They recommend a free-recall method of questioning deaf children. However, a relay interpreter was utilized with the deaf children wherein a deaf person 'relayed' the communication from a hearing interpreter to the deaf child. In effect, a relay interpreter is an interpreter for the interpreter. This communicative interaction involves three individuals: the hearing speaker, the hearing interpreter, and the deaf relay interpreter before the communication reaches the child. The potential for error and/or embellishment of the original utterance is obvious. The researchers did not establish the accuracy of conveying information through a relay interpreter. Thus a significant confound compromises the interpretability of these data. A comparison using interviewers who sign for themselves is needed before it can be concluded that deaf children are more suggestible than hearing children. More importantly, a similar relay system for the hearing comparison group was needed to determine if the accuracy of hearing children is affected by relaying the communication between three adults before it reaches the child.

23. It has been our clinical experience that Deaf and hard-of-hearing children respond best to direct questions rather than to free-recall questions. Deaf and hard-of-hearing children frequently need to have the topic identified for them. This is consistent with the work of Saywitz (1992) and her colleagues who have found that young children are most accurate when asked direct questions than in free-recall situations.

Appendix B

List of psychological tests and test publishers (see Chapter 8)

AAMD Adaptive Behavior Scale. Washington, DC: American Association on Mental Deficiency.

Bender Gestalt Test for Young Children. New York: Grune & Stratton.

Brigance Diagnostic Inventory of Basic Skills. North Billerica, MA: Curriculum Associates.

Bronfenbrenner Hearing Attitude Scale. In Levine, ES (1981). The Psychology of Early Deafness (pp 366–370). New York: Colombia University Press.

California Achievement Tests. Monterey Park, CA: CTB/McGraw-Hill.

Central Institute for the Deaf (CID) Preschool Performance Scale. Wood Date, Illinois: Stoelting Co.

Children's Apperception Test. Larchmont, NY: CPS Inc.

Columbia Mental Maturity Scale. New York: The Psychological Corporation.

Hiskey–Nebraska Test of Learning Aptitude. Lincoln, Nebraska: Marshall Hiskey.

Impact of Childhood Hearing Loss on the Family Questionnaire. In Moore DF, Meadow-Orlans KP (eds) Educational and developmental aspects of Deafness, pp 321–338.

Kaufman Assessment Battery for Children. Circle Pines, MN: American Guidance Service.

Keymath. Circle Pines, Minnesota: American Guidance Service.

Leiter International Performance Scale. Wood Dale, Illinois: Stoelting Co.

Meadow-Kendall Social-Emotional Inventory for Deaf and Hard of Hearing Students. Washington, DC: Gallaudet University Press.

Metropolitan Achievement Tests. New York: The Psychological Corporation.

Minnesota Multiphasic Personality Inventory. Minneapolis: University of Minnesota Press.

Peabody Individual Achievement Test. Circle Pines, Minnesota: American Guidance Service.

Piers–Harris Children's Self-concept Scale. Los Angeles, CA: Western Psychological Services.

Raven's Progressive Matrices and Vocabulary Scales. New York: The Psychological Corporation.

Rorschach. New York: Grune & Stratton.

Scales of Independent Behavior. Allen, TX: DLM Teaching Resources.

School Behavior Checklist. Los Angeles: Western Psychological Services.

Sequential Assessment of Mathematics Inventories. Columbus, OH: Charles E. Merrill.

Sixteen Personality Factor Questionnaire. Champaign, Illinois: Institute for Personality & Ability Testing.

Smith–Johnson Non-verbal performance Scale. Los Angeles, CA: Western Psychological Services.

Snijders–Oomen Non-verbal Intelligence Scale, SON. 2-1/2-7. Netherlands: Swets Test Services.

Snijders–Oomen Non-verbal Intelligence Scale – Revised, SON-R. Netherlands: Swets Test Services.

Stanford Achievement Test Series, Eighth Edition. San Antonio, Texas: Harcourt Brace Jovanovich.

Tennessee Self-concept Scale. Los Angeles: Western Psychological Services.

Test of Early Reading Ability – Deaf or Hard of Hearing. Austin, Texas: Pro-Ed.

Appendix C

The policy of the European Society for Mental Health and Deafness (Kitson and Monteiro, 1991) includes that members of the society are expected to:

- Encourage the employment of Deaf* people fluent in sign language and part of Deaf culture in mental health services for Deaf people.

*(Deaf with a capital 'D' is used in this document to refer to deaf people who are part of Deaf culture or would function better in that culture.)

- Enable Deaf people to gain recognized qualifications and full status in such services.
- Recognize that Deaf people should lead and provide the services for Deaf people, but not as a right. This should be achieved by proper training, qualifications and experience.

Appendix D

Glossary of terms used in family therapy (see Chapter 16)

Definitions below are highly simplified to provide information for readers new to these ideas. For in-depth definitions of systemic family therapy terms see Simon, Stierlin and Wynne (1985).

Equilibrium (homeostasis) — these terms, taken from cybernetic and biological theory, are used to describe the relative stability and balance maintained within family systems. Early therapists used these ideas in a simplified manner and construed dynamics in some family interactions as 'homeostatic' and 'stuck'. Current thinking and practice understands that families, and the individuals within them, are constantly changing and developing new interactional and internal mechanisms which can be highlighted and enhanced in the therapeutic encounter.

Joining — a term, originating in structural family therapy, describing the need for the therapist to join with the family system in order to observe and understand family rules and interactions. Joining with the family system, and individuals within the family, produces a new system — the therapist/family system — within which change can be explored and developed.

Network — used in family therapy thinking to describe the social, and sometimes the ecological, environment of the family. As used in this chapter 'operating as a network' means communication between the members of the professional network around the family.

Relay telephone operator — relays messages between a Deaf person using a textphone and a hearing person using a voice phone. He/she types spoken messages from the hearing person and voices typed messages from the Deaf person to the hearing person.

Scapegoating — this biblical metaphor has been used in family therapy theory to describe situations in which one family member (often a child or the symptomatic person) has become the focus of family difficulties, masking conflicts between other family members.

Textphone/Minicom — brands of type telephone which can be used by each partner to a telephone conversation. The normal telephone receiver is rested on the transmitter which has a keyboard. The typed messages are displayed both on the transmitter and receiver. A simple communication code is used to signal when each person has completed their side of the conversation.

Triangulation — describes the process whereby the parties in a dyadic relationship draw in a third party in order to defuse intense emotions. There are a number of models of this process within family therapy theory.

Voicing over — the interpreter reads the sign language of the Deaf person and speaks the interpretation for the hearing people present.

Appendix E

Further information on services in the UK

National Health Service's Specialist Mental Health Services' Headquarters: (providing hospital, day and out patient care in addition to community mental health teams, each covering approximately one third of Great Britain. Services include diagnosis and treatment of mental illness, access to community housing, as well as a range of psychotherapeutic and counselling approaches):

Adult Team
National Deaf Services
South West London and St George's Mental Health NHS Trust
Old Church
146a Bedford Hill
London SW11 9HW

Telephone:	Voice:	020 8675 2100
	Minicom:	020 8675 2200
	Fax:	020 8675 2266
	Video:	020 8675 9707
Email:	deafunit@btinternet.com	

Deaf Child & Family Service
National Deaf Services
South West London and St George's Mental Health NHS Trust
Hightrees
Springfield University Hospital
61 Glenburnie Road
London SW17 7DJ

Telephone:	Voice:	020 8682 6925
	Minicom:	020 8682 6950
	Fax:	020 8682 6461
	Video:	-

National Centre for Mental Health and Deafness
John Denmark Unit
Bury New Road
Prestwich
Manchester M25 3BL

Telephone:	Voice:	0161 7723400
	Minicom:	0161 7723407
	Fax:	0161 7985853
	Video:	0161 7737011

Mental Health Service for Deaf People
Queen Elizabeth Psychiatric Hospital
Mindelsohn Way
Edgbaston
Birmingham B15 2QZ

Telephone:	Voice:	0121 6272930
	Minicom:	0121 6978284
		0121 6272871
	Fax:	0121 6272934

Providers of Community Housing:
Sign (Nationwide provision of mental health care community housing for the Deaf community, including Deaf people with disabilities)
Headquarters:
13 Station Road
Beaconsfield
Bucks HP9 1YP

Telephone:	Voice/Minicom:	01494 816777
	Fax:	01494 812555
	Video:	-

Harding Housing Association (South London, but to a nationwide catchment, provision of mental health care community housing for the Deaf community)
Headquarters:
48 Wandsworth Common Northside
London SW18 2SL

Telephone:	Voice:	020 8870 7577
	Minicom:	020 8877 1866
	Fax:	020 8874 6270
	Video:	-

Royal National Institute for Deaf People (Nationwide provision of community housing for Deaf people, including those with disabilities or in need of mental health care. Also provides interpreting.)
Headquarters:
19–23 Featherstone Street
London EC1Y 8SL

Telephone:	Voice:	020 7296 8000
	Minicom:	020 7296 8001
	Fax:	020 7296 8199
	Video:	-

SENSE (Nationwide provision of community housing for Deaf people with disabilities, including those in need of mental health care.)
11–13 Clifton Terrace
London N4 3SR

Telephone:	Voice:	020 7272 7774
	Minicom:	020 7272 9648
	Fax:	020 7272 6012
	Video:	-
Email:	inquiries@sense.org.uk	

Other Providers

Royal Association in Aid of Deaf People (Provision of community support to the Deaf community, including Deaf people with disabilities or mental health problems, including interpreting, pastoral care, chaplaincy, advice and counselling.)
Walsingham Road
Colchester CO2 7BP

Telephone:	Voice:	01206 509 509
	Minicom:	01206 577 090
	Fax:	01206 769 755
	Video:	-
Email:	info@royaldeaf.org.uk	

Email: info@royaldeaf.org.uk

Relevant Associations

British Society for Mental Health and Deafness
Care of, Hon. Secretary: Peter Hindley
Deaf Child and Family Service
Hightrees
Springfield University Hospital
61 Glenburnie Road
London SW17 7DJ

Telephone:	Voice:	020 8682 6925
	Minicom:	020 8682 6950
	Fax:	020 8682 6461
	Video:	-

European Society for Mental Health and Deafness
Director: Bob Clowes
'Daylesford'
Stokeinteignhead
Newton Abbot
Devon TQ12 4QD

Telephone:	Voice:	0162 6873332
	Fax:	0162 6872745
	Video:	-
Email:	esmhd@dial.pipex.com	

British Deaf Association
1–3 Worship Street
London EC2 2AB

Telephone:	Voice:	020 7588 3520
	Minicom:	020 7588 3529
	Fax:	020 7588 3527
	Video:	-

Council for the Advancement of Communication with Deaf People (A national organization setting standards of communication training and examination as well as keeping the register of interpreters.)
Pelaw House
School of Education
University of Durham
Durham DH1 1TA

Telephone:	Voice/Minicom:	0191 3743607
	Fax:	0191 3743605
	Video:	-
Email:	durham@cacdp.demon.co.uk	

National Deaf Children's Society
15 Dufferin Street
London EC1Y 8PD

Telephone:	Voice/Minicom:	020 7490 8656
	Fax:	020 7250 5020
	Video:	-
Email:	ndcs@ndcs.org.uk.	

Index

A letter n following a page number refers to the footnote on that page